RENEWALS 458-4574

DATE DUE			
GAYLORD			PRINTED IN U.S.A.

Interdisciplinary Statistics Series

STATISTICAL CONCEPTS
and
APPLICATIONS in
CLINICAL MEDICINE

CHAPMAN & HALL/CRC
Interdisciplinary Statistics Series

Series editors: N. Keiding, B. Morgan, T. Speed, P. van der Heijden

Interdisciplinary Statistics Series

STATISTICAL CONCEPTS
and
APPLICATIONS in
CLINICAL MEDICINE

John Aitchison
Jim W. Kay
Ian J. Lauder

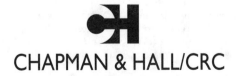

CHAPMAN & HALL/CRC

A CRC Press Company
Boca Raton London New York Washington, D.C.

Library of Congress Cataloging-in-Publication Data

Aitchison, J. (John), 1926–
  Statistical concepts and applications in clinical medicine / John Aitchison, Jim W. Kay,
Ian J. Lauder
    p. ; cm. -- (Interdisciplinary statistics ; 14)
  Includes bibliographical references and index.
  ISBN 1-58488-208-5
  1. Medical statistics. 2. Clinical medicine--Research--Methodology.
  [DNLM: 1. Biometry--methods. 2. Clinical Medicine--methods. 3. Data Interpretation,
  Statistical. 4. Models, Statistical. WA 950 A311s 2004] I. Kay, J. W. (Jim W.) II.
  Lauder, Ian J. III. Title. IV. Series.
RA407.A38 2004
610'.072'—dc22   2004058293

Visit the CRC Press Web site at www.crcpress.com

© 2005 by Chapman & Hall/CRC

No claim to original U.S. Government works
International Standard Book Number 1-58488-208-5
Library of Congress Card Number 2004058293
Printed in the United States of America 1 2 3 4 5 6 7 8 9 0
Printed on acid-free paper

Contents

Preface

The role of the statistician in society is to undertake the quantitative study of uncertainty and variability whatever the source of these disturbing yet fascinating features of our daily experience. Of all the subjects studied by the human mind the greatest uncertainty and variability are undoubtedly to be found in the human body itself, not least in those aspects of its existence which concern the function and malfunction of the body. The medical statistician, who concentrates statistical argument and techniques on the problems of uncertainty and variability in clinical practice and medical research, may thus have an important contribution to make both to the well-being of the individual and to the progress of clinical science.

To be effective the medical statistician, like any consulting statistician, has to adopt a truly applied mathematical approach. He or she must recognize that the aim is to analyse and answer the medical problems presented and not, as can so easily happen in branches of applied mathematics, to invent and develop statistical theory which may be applicable in medicine if the kind of problem imagined in the theory chances to come along. The emphasis in such work must be in tackling real problems with the aim of providing customer satisfaction. It may be thought that this requirement of practicality must inevitably lead to dull application of standard statistical techniques and to limited intellectual satisfaction. The contrary is the case. Some of the most challenging of theoretical statistical questions arise from such practical problems and the requirements of practice provide a sense of direction to the theory. Nowhere is greater satisfaction to be found than in the happy combination of stimulating theory and useful application.

It will be clear from these introductory remarks that medical statisticians are faced early and repeatedly in their careers with new and non-standard statistical problems. Any book which claims to expound the principles and practice of medical statistics must therefore instil in its readers a confidence and capability to approach new problems with an open mind, must demonstrate the arts of problem formulation and statistical modelling and must provide techniques for developing statistical models towards solutions which are relevant to the practical problems posed. In attempting to fulfil these injunctions in this book we have, for illustrative purposes, drawn mainly on those practical medical problems in which we have ourselves been substantially involved over more than fifty man-years. One difficulty facing us has been how to retain this open view of the subject as one of consultative statistics through the challenge of actual problems and yet provide a connected and developing account of the subject. The expository technique by which we have attempted to resolve this issue has been to introduce the practical problems in such an order that they provide a natural development of the relevant statistical concepts and techniques as they relate to medical applications. How far this has been successful must be left to the reader to judge. What cannot fail to be appreciated is that medical statistics is a challenging and stimulating field in which to enjoy the use of statistical abilities.

The participation of the statistician in a particular problem of medicine may be an ephemeral one. For example, when called in to assist in devising a system of differential diagnosis, based on a combination of tests possessing only incomplete powers of discrimination, the statistician should realise that the purpose of medical research may be to discover new and better diagnostic tests to replace the existing ones and so indeed to make the statistician redundant. Consultant statisticians must accept, and indeed welcome, such advances. They may be assured that other urgent and equally intriguing problems will soon arise to test their skills. These advances do, however, create a substantial and insuperable problem for the authors of a medical statistical textbook. The period between the conception of a book and its publication may be many years, in the present case over twenty years, so that events may overtake the relevance of the medical aspects reported. All that authors can do in such unavoidable circumstances is to report the problem as it was presented and analysed at the time of their involvement. Since this book is concerned with approach and analysis, and not with the current state of medical knowledge, we hope that the reader will be generous enough to accept this limitation and will not fall into the trap of quoting any conclusions as the last word on present medical knowledge or practice.

Special features of this book which are worth noting in this preface are as follows.

1. Most books on applied statistics develop their subject by way of statistical topics, such as estimation, significance tests, analysis of variance, contingency tables, illustrating each statistical technique by an appropriate application. In the true spirit of applied mathematics this book takes as its starting point the particular field of application, with the consequence that the natural development of the subject proceeds by medical subdivisions. Thus we have chapter titles such as observation, diagnosis and prognosis and treatment. This approach has the advantage of providing a unified development through the stages of the complicated clinical process which attempts to transform a patient from a state of disease to one of health.

2. Most books on medical statistics confine attention to the types of statistical problem arising in medical research. A much more extensive view of medicine is taken here, including the actual practice of medicine as well as medical research. We shall even investigate statistical problems of assessing the performance of clinicians in their decision making. Moreover, in problems of medical statistics, no less than in the actual practice of medicine, the individual patient is of paramount importance and so in all our formu-

lation of statistical models and development of statistical methodology we shall focus attention on how best to serve the interests of the individual patient.

3. The approach is problem-oriented. As has already been explained we typically present each consultative problem in its original form as a challenge to the reader and follow this successively by the process of problem formulation, the construction of a suitable statistical model, the motivated development of the model on statistical principles and finally the interpretation of the statistical analysis in the context of the real problem. The reader wishing to select examples of specific statistical techniques can do so in two ways. First, the subject index provides for each statistical technique references not only to locations of theoretical consideration but also to locations of applications. Secondly, within the chapters reviewing statistical methodology, Chapters 3 and 4, the locations of further developments and applications are provided.

4. There is no prealignment with any particular ideology of statistical inference such as Bayesian, so-called classical or frequentist, fiducial, neo-Bayesian or structuralist. The reasons for this are obvious. Each practical problem is examined on its own merits. Thus for one problem there may be features which suggest that a classical frequentist approach is more suitable; for another problem the natural way of proceeding may be Bayesian. Often more than one approach will be used, for example classical hypothesis-testing techniques forming the basis of the first stage of arriving at a suitable statistical working model, and Bayesian techniques subsequently supplying an appropriate development of the analysis within the framework of the selected statistical model. Bayesian methods have often been dismissed as theoretically elegant and philosophically satisfying but of little practical value. In so far as the book demonstrates that, for an appreciable proportion of the problems investigated, the Bayesian approach has a decided practical edge over a classical approach at the analytical stage, and so speaks against this too glib dismissal of Bayesian methods, it may appear to have some pro-Bayesian message. We re-emphasize, however, that a satisfactory resolution of the medical problem presented to the consulting statistician must be the primary concern.

5. In any textbook which is aimed at a level of readership ranging from advanced undergraduate, through postgraduate to consultant statistician and research worker, some basic knowledge of statistical concepts and techniques must be assumed. The extent of this prerequisite knowledge is approximately the content of such textbooks as Hoel (1971), Silvey (1975), Cox and Hinkley (1974) and the comparative review of Barnett (1982). In our experience statistical consultative work in medicine, and indeed in other disciplines, is considerably eased through familiarity with aspects of statistical methodology mostly scattered throughout research journals and seldom touched upon in textbooks. A connected account of the principles

and technicalities of these statistical methods, with special attention to their role in serving the individual patient, is presented in Chapters 2–4. They have a generality and wide applicability which can stand the consulting statistician in good stead and make less daunting the approach of any consultee with a new and probably non-standard problem. Some recent and newly developed techniques are applied for the first time in this book.

6. To help in the provision of such training we have supplied at the end of each chapter a further collection of problems in clinical medicine, against which the reader may develop formulatory, analytic and interpretative skills. Although the situations described in these problems are not real they are, we believe, realistic and the reader should find them a significant challenge to statistical modelling skills.

7. Although our concern is with the application of statistics to a particular field the book is in its outlook a suitable basis for a course of data analysis either at advanced undergraduate or at postgraduate level. Indeed the problems have been successfully used in data analysis classes in three universities, providing in the appreciation of the reality of the data and in the urgency of the questions posed a strong stimulus to the student's search for satisfactory answers. There is, of course, no substitute for real consultation, but any training in consultation must inevitably be preceded by analyses of as many real problems as possible.

8. Finally we express our grateful thanks to the many anonymous clinicians and patients depicted within this book. In all our consultative work there has been an agreement between consulting statistician and clinical consultee that the statistician may use the data for the purposes of illustrating statistical concepts and methodology. This is what we have tried to achieve in this book and we hope that we may thereby have advanced the state of clinical medicine by demonstrating ways in which the data of experience may be brought to bear on the needs of the present patient. We also thank our colleagues at the universities of Glasgow, Hong Kong and Virginia, the anonymous reviewers for helpful comments on earlier drafts of the book and also the staff at Chapman and Hall/CRC for their helpfulness.

CHAPTER 1

The Field of Application

1.1 The role of the consulting statistician

The aim of every medical worker – general practitioner, consultant clinician, radiologist, surgeon, psychiatrist, research biochemist, pharmacologist, physiologist – is to provide through knowledge, experience and technical skill the best possible medical care for each individual patient. Such is the commitment of the Hippocratic oath, and for many of the day-to-day problems of clinical practice and medical research the achievement of such an aim has fortunately been reduced to effective routines; in such problems the statistician has no significant role to play.

Human beings, however, often show great variability in the ways their bodies function and malfunction and in their responses to treatment. There is thus a large number of medical problems where uncertainty plays a dominant part, and much of this chapter will be devoted to giving challenging examples of this variability and uncertainty. Since the express aim of the science of statistics is to provide and develop means of describing and analysing situations involving variability and uncertainty it is clear that the statistician may have an important technical contribution to make in determining the best possible medical care for individual patients.

To be a successful consultant the statistician must first and foremost take steps to become familiar with the real medical problem of interest. This can be a slow and time-consuming part of the consultative process in which patience, understanding and determination are often required to overcome a communication gap between the two disciplines of medicine and statistics. The statistician must therefore be prepared not only to listen carefully to the medical aspects of the problem but also to suggest in simple language how the problem is being translated and formulated in statistical terms and so to search, by trial and error and by question and dialogue, towards a sensible formulation of the problem. This formulation will involve abstracting from the real medical problem the essential relevant components, recognising their possible interdependence and expressing this interdependence in the construction of a statistical model which may describe the clinical variability observed. The next task is, through the tools of statistics and mathematics, to develop the model in such a direction that there is a hope of answering the questions initially posed by the clinician. Once the statistical development and analysis of the model have been completed the answer obtained must be translated back into terms of the real world, into a language that the clinician, and possibly even the patient, can understand. Moreover the answers obtained must constantly be under review to ensure that the statistical methodology is adequate. When it is possible to compare the answer provided by the model, for example a suggested disease category for the patient, with an eventually emerging 'true' answer, for example the actual disease category determined by post mortem examination, then the reason for any discrepancy must be fully probed and, if necessary, the model must be modified either by complication or simplification to attain greater realism and effectiveness in application.

Throughout the presentation of medical statistics in this book we shall use real medical problems as the motivating source for the development of concepts, principles and techniques. A consequence of this problem-oriented approach is that our subdivisions of the subject will be arrived at from medical considerations. To obtain an early view of what these subdivisions may sensibly be we record here a consultative problem as first presented and focus interest on the problem of management of a particular patient.

1.2 A challenging problem in differential diagnosis

In the presentation of this first problem, as with all applications in this book, we shall attempt to express it in terms as similar as possible to those of its first referral to a statistician. Such an approach has the great advantage of allowing the reader to experience to some extent the immediacy of the original problem and to gain some idea of the nature of consultative work. The reader will thus be placed in the position of posing many necessary questions. Have I fully understood the problem? Is it really a problem for a statistician? How relevant and reliable are the data? Have they been collected from past patients in such a way that they may give a biased view of the pattern of variability we are likely to encounter in new patients? Have I been given all the information I need to formulate the problem in statistical terms? Have enough relevant data been collected? Is this one of the standard statistical problems I am already familiar with or does it involve considerable adaptation of current methodology or even research? And so on. The advantage almost certainly arises from the autobiographical nature of the material, mostly at first hand from the authors' consultative diaries. The one disadvantage is that some of the problems must inevitably come from diaries of some years ago and may therefore not be of immediate medical interest. We hope, however, that awareness of their interest to the clinician at the original time of study may offset any old-fashioned or outmoded look in the medical findings as assessed today.

We hope that the appropriateness of the statistical analyses of the problems recounted in this volume, whether a decade or a day old, may prove equally interesting and encourage the reader to tackle new problems with the same spirit of adventure and patience. The fact that our first problem, dating back over thirty years, has been used repeatedly as a teaching example and has never failed to rouse a vigorous response encourages us to believe that problems, presented and accepted as consultative challenges, provide an adequate stimulus to the acquisition of statistical skills. All problems will therefore be introduced as if the clinician were conveying the problem for the first time to a statistician.

Differential diagnosis in Conn's syndrome

The following is a paraphrase of a clinician's introduction of his problem to a consulting statistician in 1969.

You probably know that at the Medical Research Council Blood Pressure Research Unit at the Western Infirmary here in Glasgow our work is concerned not only with trying to unravel the various physiological, biochemical and psychological factors that influence blood pressure but also with the management of patients with blood pressure problems, mainly, of course, problems of high blood pressure. One of these hypertensive conditions is Conn's syndrome, so called because it was first described by Conn (1955); if you would like an easily-read description have a look in the book on hypertension by Pickering (1968, Chapter 28). At the Unit we have a special interest in this syndrome, not just because its features throw considerable light on the regulatory mechanism of blood pressure, but more importantly because one of our specialities is the treatment of Conn's patients.

We now have a reasonable means of detecting when a patient has Conn's syndrome: there is hypertension, a high concentration of plasma aldosterone, with low plasma potassium and low plasma renin. You probably don't know what these are but don't worry for the moment. Anyway, there was a time when we thought that the single cause of Conn's syndrome was an aldosterone-secreting adrenocortical adenoma – a benign lump somewhere on the 'skin' of one of your two adrenal glands, a lump that secretes too much of the hormone aldosterone and causes the abnormalities in these other plasma concentrations. We also thought that treatment was straightforward if not trivial: operate, find the tumour, remove it possibly with most of one adrenal gland and the patient is virtually cured. We have had 31 patients with Conn's syndrome over a number of years – you can see it is a relatively rare condition – and all of these patients have been operated on. Unfortunately in 11 of the cases the surgeon could find no adenoma; instead both adrenal glands were found to be slightly enlarged and to contain nodules, a condition we call bilateral hyperplasia. Knowing your mathematical inclinations we could call adenoma form A and bilateral hyperplasia form B of Conn's syndrome.

Well, to cut a long story short I can sum up our state of knowledge like this. If the patient has form A we want to operate, remove the adenoma and so provide the patient with a permanent cure. If the patient has form B then the operation is mostly ineffective, not without dangers, and it therefore seems much more sensible to try to reduce blood pressure by a drug therapy such as the use of spironolactone despite the possible side effects. So you can see our problem. A new patient has been referred to us because of his very high blood pressures and we know that he has Conn's syndrome because of his elevated

Table 1.1 *Preoperative information on 31 cases of Conn's syndrome of known form and on one case of unknown form. A1–A20 are of form A (adenoma) and B1–B11 are of form B (bilateral hyperplasia)*

Case	Age	Na	K	CO2	Renin	Aldo	Syst	Diast
A1	40	140.6	2.3	30.3	4.6	121.0	192	107
A2	37	143.0	3.1	27.1	4.5	15.0	230	150
A3	34	140.0	3.0	27.0	0.7	19.5	200	130
A4	48	146.0	2.8	33.0	3.3	30.0	213	125
A5	41	138.7	3.6	24.1	4.9	20.1	163	106
A6	22	143.7	3.1	28.0	4.2	33.0	190	130
A7	27	137.3	2.5	29.6	5.4	52.1	220	140
A8	18	141.0	2.5	30.0	2.5	50.2	210	135
A9	53	143.8	2.4	32.2	1.5	68.9	160	105
A10	54	114.6	2.9	29.5	3.0	144.7	213	135
A11	50	139.5	2.3	26.0	2.6	31.2	205	125
A12	44	144.0	2.2	33.7	3.9	65.1	263	133
A13	44	145.0	2.7	33.0	4.1	38.0	203	115
A14	66	140.2	3.1	29.1	4.7	43.1	195	115
A15	39	144.7	2.9	27.4	0.9	65.1	180	120
A16	46	139.0	3.1	31.4	2.8	192.7	228	133
A17	48	144.8	1.9	33.5	3.8	103.5	205	132
A18	38	145.7	3.7	27.4	2.8	42.6	203	117
A19	60	144.0	2.2	33.0	3.2	92.0	220	120
A20	44	143.5	2.7	27.5	3.6	74.5	210	114
B1	46	140.3	4.3	23.4	6.4	27.0	270	160
B2	35	141.0	3.2	25.0	8.8	26.3	210	130
B3	50	141.2	3.6	25.8	4.1	20.9	181	113
B4	41	142.0	3.0	22.0	4.7	20.4	260	160
B5	57	143.5	4.2	27.8	4.3	23.7	185	125
B6	57	139.7	3.4	28.0	5.2	46.0	240	130
B7	48	141.1	3.6	25.0	2.5	37.3	197	120
B8	60	141.0	3.8	26.0	6.5	23.4	211	118
B9	52	140.4	3.3	27.0	4.2	24.0	168	104
B10	49	140.0	3.6	26.0	6.3	39.8	220	120
B11	49	140.0	4.4	25.6	5.1	47.0	190	125
New	50	143.3	3.2	27.0	8.5	51.0	210	130

aldosterone and lowered potassium and renin concentrations. But has he form A, in which case we want to operate; or has he form B, in which case it is highly undesirable, even dangerous, to operate, and drugs are advisable? Oh, I've nearly forgotten to tell you the crucial point. The only way we can tell for sure whether it is A or B is to operate and provide our pathologists with part of the adrenal glands. But since an operation for a patient with form B is dangerous you can see that we need some means of making our differential diagnosis between A and B pre-operatively, on the basis of pre-operative information.

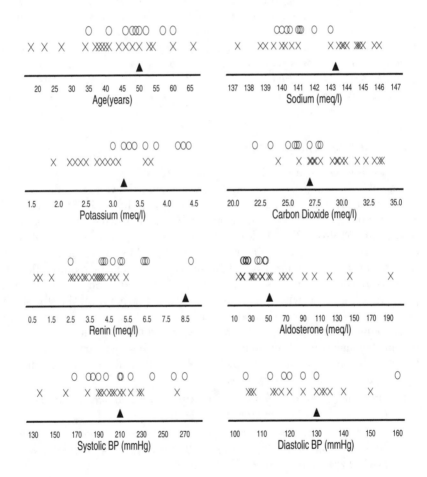

Figure 1.1 *Eight recorded features of Conn's syndrome for the 20 cases of form A (crosses) and 11 cases of form B (circles) and a referred new patient (triangle).*

*For the 31 cases who were operated on and whose form is therefore known,
20 of form A and 11 of form B, we do have information on each of eight features: age, plasma concentrations of sodium, potassium, carbon dioxide, renin
and aldosterone, and systolic and diastolic blood pressures. I have brought the
data (Table 1.1) along for you to see. Our problem is to find out whether this
information has any value in differentiating between forms A and B. For instance, I've also brought along the data for a Conn's syndrome patient who is
currently under investigation. If you look at his renin value of 8.5 meq/l you
will see that it falls within the range of B values but well outside the range of A
values so that on the basis of this feature alone the patient seems to have form
B. On the other hand his aldosterone measurement of 51.0 meq/l is above the
largest value of 47 meq/l experienced in form B patients and is nicely placed
in the range of A values, so that there seems to be evidence in this feature for
form A. We've drawn out separate scales for each of the eight features and
on each scale have shown the positions of the past 31 cases and this new case
(Figure 1.1). You can see that at least some of the features do seem to separate
out a bit for the two forms. Our question to you must now be obvious. Is there
any way that mathematics or statistics can help us to assess pre-operatively
whether our new patient has form A or form B?*

1.3 Identifying the problem

Some experienced statistical readers may already have classified the problem
as one of discriminant analysis and be visualizing the construction, from the
data of the 31 cases of known form, of a linear discriminant, some linear
combination of the features which can conveniently be called a score and used
to separate A's from B's. The score for any new patient can then be calculated
and the patient allocated either to A or to B. Moreover some reasonable
estimate of the misclassification rate of such a process can be readily calculated
to measure the effectiveness of the allocation rule; and so on. Let us, however,
pause to ask if this is what the clinician is really wanting from the statistician.
We must surely recognize that whatever inference or decision we communicate
to the clinician about this patient is not the end of the clinical problem of
patient management. Only by further discussion between the clinician C and
the statistician S does a clearer picture of the problem emerge. The dialogue
continued along the following lines.

S. *What will happen to your new patient if, for example, I can assure you
that he has almost certainly form A?*

C. *As I have already said we would operate and hope to remove the adenoma.*

S. *What will you do if all I can say is that the evidence favours form A but
form B can by no means be ruled out?*

C. *Well, there is actually another diagnostic investigative technique, an
adrenal venogram, which can give us a kind of X-ray picture of the
adrenal glands. Unfortunately in the current (1969) stage of development the picture does not always show an adenoma, sometimes it shows*

what looks like a lump where none is, and even more unfortunately the investigation can occasionally cause serious damage to an adrenal gland. But it is a technique which sometimes helps and if there was a suspicion of an adenoma we might decide that it was reasonable to use it. Everything, of course, depends on the patient's general state of health. As you must be realizing by now, patient management in this area can be very complex.

After further similar exchanges, the statistician begins to visualize expressing the investigative and treatment possibilities for a Conn's syndrome patient in terms of a tentative decision tree. The statistician then asks whether the clinician can perhaps supply information about the loss structure. Not unreasonably the clinician says that he cannot quantify this and that if the statistician can somehow or other provide some comprehensible assessment of the patient's diagnostic position on the basis of the eight measurements it is then the clinician's responsibility to make the decisions. It thus seems that what the clinician wants from the statistician is some assessment of what might be realistic probabilities to assign to forms A and B on the basis of all the information available. Further discussion reveals that the clinician fully appreciates the notion of odds on and odds against and so it is agreed that the statistician will attempt to do this in as realistic a way as possible.

In arriving at such diagnostic probabilities or odds, the statistician will inevitably have to make a number of assumptions. For example, in the present problem assumptions may have to be adopted concerning the following aspects.

(i) The effect of the referral and selection of cases at blood pressure clinics on the pattern of variability of the features in the 31 cases of known type.

(ii) The relationship of the referral process of the new patient to that of the 31 cases in the basic data set.

(iii) The nature of the pattern of variability of the data. For example, is it reasonable to assume that the variability of the features for a given form is stable over time?

(iv) The form of any parametric class of distributions chosen to describe patterns of variability.

(v) The deliberate exclusion of available features, such as the sex of the patient, supposed to have no diagnostic value.

(vi) The degree of precision in observation and measurement, such as in the determination of the plasma concentrations of renin and aldosterone.

(vii) Where more than one clinic is involved the extent of any differences in their data collection processes.

All such assumptions form part of the modelling process and should be as clearly stated as possible. In any problem we shall denote the collection of all modelling assumptions generically as M, and indeed often refer to the model

M. Later we shall consider in much more detail processes of investigation of assumptions towards the formulation of such a model M. For the moment, let us suppose that such processes have been completed for the differential diagnosis of Conn's syndrome. If D denotes the given data set of 31 past cases of known type in Table 1.1, if v denotes the vector of eight measurements for our new patient and u his unknown form of Conn's syndrome, then what is required is an assessment of the two conditional probabilities

$$\Pr(u|v, D, M) \qquad (u = \text{A}, \text{B}),$$

so that the odds on A, namely

$$\frac{\Pr(u = \text{A}|v, D, M)}{\Pr(u = \text{B}|v, D, M)},$$

can be quoted.

We shall certainly retain the M behind the conditioning vertical bar in this chapter as a constant reminder that all statistical analysis, as indeed all applied mathematics, depends to some extent, and sometimes crucially, on the statistical model adopted. Arriving at a sensible model M is not always a trivial exercise and we shall spend some effort in the following chapters in discussing this aspect and in attempting to lay down some guidelines for arriving at a reasonable M.

1.4 Communication with practitioners

Now that we have seen a typical consultancy process the following set of pointers and reminders may be of some help to inexperienced statistical consultants in their communication with clinicians.

First, you must realise that clinicians will probably have virtually no statistical training or, sometimes even worse, have had some minimum and poor instruction which has left them with misconceptions not easily eradicated and fears difficult to subdue. Like any other expert they have their own jargon and will inevitably use it regardless of how much they try not to, in an attempt to make the communication of their problem easier for you. Careful listening to the problem is essential, with questioning and re-questioning until you are sure that you understand the problem. Never be afraid or ashamed to appear simple-minded. You are more likely to get to the heart of the matter by such a process than by assuming that you will be able to disentangle the remaining problems in the quiet of your office or study. To say this is not to suggest that everything about the problem must be resolved at the first encounter. By all means go into retreat with uncertainties about the problem but only with the intention of meeting again to check whether your studied interpretation is really what the problem is or to ask further questions. The process is an iterative one, and sometimes requires a substantial number of iterations before convergence to an appropriate formulation.

Do not fall into the trap of simply verifying an analysis suggested by the clinician without really discovering the problem. To do so is sloppy consultation, which you would never tolerate in a doctor's surgery. You would regard it as ridiculous for a doctor to confirm a diagnosis suggested by a patient without carrying out a sufficiently detailed investigation. Equally, just because a clinician has collected data into a two-way table and has carried out a chi-squared test, it does not mean that this is necessarily the most efficient or even an appropriate analysis of the data.

In your discussions use diagrams wherever possible, and do not hesitate to use a situation simpler than that being considered in order to illustrate a concept or a method and in order to verify whether an interpretation by you of the clinician's problem is a valid one. You and the clinician are equals in a collaborative effort to help patients and you will probably find that the more insights you gain into each other's expertise the more fruitful the joint venture. Thus it often pays to get over to the clinician the idea that you are model-building, to show in as simple terms as you can the ingredients of the model and to encourage the clinician to appreciate the steps at which translation from the real world to the model and back again are taking place, and where mathematics and statistical analysis are taking place.

Above all, when you meet to explain and interpret your statistical analysis of the clinical problem, be as simple as you can without withholding necessary caveats, and be as forbearing with the clinician's questions, which you should encourage, as the clinician has been with yours.

The greater the rapport between clinician client and statistical consultant the more hope there is of helping patients

1.5 Components of the medical process

We shall later examine in some detail a number of the statistical problems associated with the differential diagnosis of Conn's syndrome as described in Sections 1.2–1.3, but our present purpose is simply to use this consultative problem to identify useful subdivisions of the complete process of patient management so that we may isolate them for more intensive separate study. Readers may find it useful to try to identify these subdivisions in their own experience with clinicians.

Experience

In the assessment of a patient's condition and in anticipating what will happen if a certain course of action is adopted, a clinician is continually referring back to past experience, gained either personally or through communication with others. A simple example of this is in the notion of the normal range of some measurement or characteristic. For instance, in our discussion of Conn's syndrome the fact that plasma concentration of aldosterone was high and so of significance in assessing the patient's state was due to a comparison with the variability that had been experienced in the aldosterone concentrations in apparently normal and healthy persons. How can such experience most effectively be summarized, particularly when there is a whole variety of different measurements made on one individual? A common expression used by clinicians is that a case is completely outside previous experience of a condition. Can this notion be quantified in any objective way?

Again, in our case of Conn's syndrome we spoke of the blood pressure readings as being well outside the normal range for the patient's age. Does experience justify the implication that blood pressure varies in some systematic way with age and if so what is the most convenient way of describing this aspect of experience?

In situations where clinicians apparently require to take a great variety of measurements on cases to describe experience is it possible that there are interdependencies in the measurements such that fewer of them would be as effective in describing experience? Some further consultative problems illustrating the need for medical statisticians to be concerned with modelling and quantifying clinical experience are presented in Section 1.6.

The characterization and harnessing of experience to the clinician's aid are discussed in detail in Chapter 5.

Observation and measurement

Because of some discomfort or abnormality which a patient experiences a doctor is consulted, or some screening process may suggest a need for further investigation of the patient, and the process of observation and measurement is formally started. The pattern is familiar. The patient is 'under observation'.

Items of the patient's history may be recorded: How old are you? What is your occupation? Have you ever had rheumatic fever? Have you ever suffered from a nervous disorder?

The patient may be questioned about current symptoms: Do you suffer from indigestion? Are you sleeping well? Do you ever have any headaches? Do these headaches always happen at the same time of day?

The clinician may then elicit signs by carrying out a routine clinical examination: What is the patient's pulse rate? What is the patient's temperature? What are the systolic and diastolic blood pressures? Is there any sugar being excreted in the urine? Further investigative observation and measurement may be called for in the form of more specific tests: Does a heart X-ray show any irregularities? Does a 24-hour I^{131} uptake test give any evidence of over-activity of the thyroid gland? What is the plasma concentration of aldosterone?

Parts of this process are simple and straightforward. For example, in our case of Conn's syndrome the patient's age is easily and accurately obtained. Other parts of the observation and measurement process are more complicated. The use of the sphygmometer in the recording of blood pressures depends on subjective judgements by the clinician, and so questions arise about the objectivity of the measurement. Would two clinicians get the same reading? If there is some observer variability is it sufficient to influence decisions? Is there any point in one clinician passing on a blood pressure reading to another clinician if the measurement is personal to each clinician? Moreover the patient's blood pressure is itself a very variable quantity, and this variability raises the whole question of the definability of the concept of a single measurement of blood pressure. Such difficulties are not removed by automatic measurement, such as the autoanalyser determination of plasma concentrations of the electrolytes Na, K and CO_2 for the case of Conn's syndrome. How communicable are such results? Could determinations made in the autoanalyser in one hospital be communicated to another hospital and used as if they had been determined on that hospital's autoanalyser?

Some measurements have to be made in a very indirect way. For example, the direct isolation of aldosterone in blood plasma is not a feasible technique of measurement and so it has to be measured by an assay technique, that is by comparison of the effect of the unknown concentration of aldosterone on some substance with which aldosterone interacts against the corresponding effects of known concentrations of standard aldosterone samples. The fact that two samples at the same concentration of aldosterone do not necessarily produce the same effect in the other substance suggests that some statistical analysis may be required to produce a satisfactory estimation technique and to assess its reliability.

Some further introductory consultative problems will be considered in this chapter: a problem of observation and observer variability in Section 1.7, direct measurement problems in Section 1.8 and indirect measurement problems of assay and calibration in Section 1.9. The modelling and analysis of the processes of observation and direct measurement in clinical medicine form the subject matter of Chapter 6; the problems of indirect measurement including assay and calibration are studied in Chapter 7.

Diagnosis

In the process of tackling any problem, the human mind seems to find it a help to try to place the problem in some category. Thus politicians can be heard to say that our national problem is simply a balance of payments problem. Mathematicians say that a particular problem is one of linear algebra or of topology. A motor mechanic may trace the lack of response in your car to a carburettor fault. This narrowing of the possible area of investigation is also the spirit and nature of the diagnostic process in medicine. Hopefully the clinician may assign the disturbance from normal in a patient to some specific cause or diagnosis, such as a streptococcus infection or gallstones, and take appropriate action to overcome or remove the cause. But the aetiology of a disorder may be largely obscure. The diagnosis of benign hypertension, for example, simply denotes moderately raised blood pressure, with no traceable cause. The list of possible medical diagnoses is large and constantly changing and indeed it is clear that from the patient's point of view the concept is an unnecessary one. The patient is not strictly interested in what the condition is called, although some innocuous name may allay his or her anxieties, but is more interested in some treatment which will speedily move him or her from the current diseased state to some more comfortable or tolerable state.

Yet, in the current decision-making processes of medicine, diagnosis or the categorization of the problem certainly still plays an important role.

In our illustrative example of the medical process, diagnosis is clearly a useful tool. The initial observation of very high blood pressure immediately concentrates the clinician's mind on a limited set of possibilities. The fact that the patient is referred to a specialist blood pressure clinic is an indication of a step forward in the detection process. The observation of high plasma aldosterone and low plasma renin concentrations is in effect synonymous with the labelling of the patient's condition as Conn's syndrome. Although this diagnosis has greatly reduced the field of possibilities there still remains at this stage a further diagnostic problem, that of differentiating between the two possible forms, adenoma and bilateral hyperplasia, of Conn's syndrome. Thus after a primary diagnosis has been clearly established there may remain problems of differential diagnosis.

In the presence of diagnostic tests which display variability and uncertainty how can this diagnostic part of the process be defined, and what contribution can the statistician make to the understanding and the effectiveness of the diagnostic process?

The medical statistician will find that diagnostic problems come in many shapes and sizes, and we present briefly two further consultative problems in Section 1.10. We turn our attention to these problems in much greater detail in Chapters 8 and 9.

Prognosis and treatment allocation

Once the clinicians had made a diagnosis of Conn's syndrome for our patient they had to consider what it was possible to do to alleviate the patient's condition. Part of the kind of reasoning that took place then ran along the following lines. If the patient is left untreated then future prospects are likely to be poor. If the patient has an adenoma and we operate, locate and remove it then the chances are that there will be no further problems of Conn's syndrome type. If the patient has bilateral hyperplasia and is placed on a spironolactone drug therapy we should be able to get reasonable control of blood pressure though there might be some side effects. And so on. We notice in the form of reasoning here two new concepts, those of treatment allocation and of prognosis. Moreover the two concepts are very much involved with each other. In order to choose rationally between alternative treatments we clearly have to be able, for each of the possible treatments, to visualize, however informally, what the responses and effects of the treatment are likely to be. In other words we must formulate a prognosis for each possible treatment.

Since these two parts of the medical process are undoubtedly interlinked we shall find it convenient to study them together. The statistical problems involved in prognostic and treatment allocation aspects of medicine are treated in Chapter 10, but we present briefly in Section 1.11 a consultative problem to indicate the statistical nature of these aspects of clinical medicine.

Assessment

Any trade, profession or business must always be reviewing the performance of its procedures, skills and techniques, and so it is important to have methods for assessing the effectiveness of such procedures as diagnosis and treatment. Such techniques may focus attention on inconsistencies and irregularities so that steps may be taken to reduce or remove them.

In Chapter 11 we shall discuss some recent techniques which allow for such assessments and which can in fact throw considerable light on current practices in medicine.

Illustrative medical problems

In the remaining sections of this chapter we present a series of actual problems in medical practice and research in the terms in which they were first met by the authors. They are set out as a stimulus and challenge to the reader, and to motivate much of the subsequent modelling and analysis, although many other examples will be introduced as necessary to illustrate further points. It should be emphasized here that the reader is not expected to make any appreciable attempt to resolve these problems at this stage. Indeed the first step in resolving some of them may be to pose to the consultee further questions which have not been covered by the description of the situation so far. The importance of these examples is to define the proper perspective for applied statistical analysis, with the real problem motivating and dominating all.

These illustrative problems have been arranged as far as possible according to the medical subdivisions we have arrived at in this section. Since these and other problems will be repeatedly referred to in different parts of the book it is convenient to have a simple system by which the reader may refer to the data sets. We have therefore collected together all the data sets used in this book in an appendix – see Appendix A.

1.6 Experience

The problem of describing and quantifying previous experience of some phenomenon where there is variability and uncertainty is a recurrent one in medicine.

Normal ranges of steroids

Our problem here concerns part, cases N1–N37, of data set `cush`; the remainder of the data set will be required in the study of later problems.

For each of 37 normal healthy adults 14 steroid metabolites in a 24-hour urine collection were separated and measured by a paper-chromatographic method. These urine excretion rates (mg/24 hr) are shown in rows N1–N37 of data set `cush`. From these data there had been constructed, as is common practice in clinical medicine, a table of 'normal ranges', here identified with the actual ranges of the 37 cases, of urinary excretion rates of the 14 steroid metabolites. The purpose of these normal ranges, shown in Tables 1.2-3, is to attempt to communicate in some summary way the experience so far obtained

Table 1.2 *Normal ranges of urine excretion rates (mg/24h) of 14 steroid metabolites based on 37 normal healthy adults and and data on four new individuals* I1–I4

Steroid metabolite	I1	I2	I3	I4	Normal Range
1	4.79	1.58	4.50	3.60	0.30–2.80
2	0.60	1.00	0.80	2.50	0.10–2.40
3	12.88	2.09	3.80	5.10	0.80–4.90
4	0.32	0.08	0.03	0.10	0.00–0.05
5	0.79	0.11	0.07	0.22	0.01–0.10
6	0.51	0.11	0.12	0.14	0.02–0.13
7	2.19	0.06	0.11	0.05	0.00–0.09
8	0.20	0.25	0.42	0.14	0.02–0.22
9	3.24	0.26	0.32	0.28	0.05–0.68
10	0.65	0.10	0.16	0.00	0.03–0.20
11	0.01	0.01	0.00	0.00	0.00–0.04
12	0.01	0.02	0.00	0.01	0.00–0.02
13	1.58	0.30	0.80	1.20	0.20–2.80
14	15.49	0.03	0.18	0.10	0.00–0.50

Table 1.3 *Names of steroid metabolites*

Steroid metabolite	Name
1	Tetra hydrocortisol
2	Allo-tetrahydrocortisol
3	Tetra hydrocortisone
4	Reichstein's compound U
5	Cortisol
6	Cortisone
7	Tetra hydro-11-desoxycortisol
8	Tetra hydrocorticosteron
9	Allo-tetrahydrocorticosteron
10	Tetra hydro11dehydrocorticosteron
11	Corticosteron
12	11-dehydrocorticosteron
13	Pregnanetriol
14	Pregnenetriol

in this particular area. The table also shows the urinary excretion rates of four new individuals. The questions that are then posed are the following. Are these cases 'outside previous experience' of normal persons? More generally, is the normal range approach a valid and useful one?

The facts that I1 with nine features greatly in excess of the upper limits of the normal ranges is seriously ill and that I2 with only three features slightly above these upper limits is healthy may seem fairly obvious. But what would your judgment be about the normality or otherwise of I3 and I4? Our ability to quantify subjectively the extent of abnormality of a case when several features are involved is obviously in question. Readers who do not appreciate the difficulty may wish to attempt to identify which of the individuals I3 and I4 is seriously ill and to attempt to quantify the degree of abnormality in the identified patient.

Here then is an area of clinical medicine which presents a challenge to the statistician, namely to provide tools for the construction of appropriate normal regions for multivariate measurements and, equally importantly, to make the concepts clear to the clinician. To achieve this a main first aim must be to describe in some realistic and usable way the pattern of variability that has already been experienced in these past cases.

If we denote our previous experience, here cases N1–N37 of data set `cush`, simply by D, then in quantifying that experience for the purpose of assessing a new case with feature vector v we shall find ourselves interested in the conditional probability density function

$$p(v|D, M) \qquad (v \in V),$$

where V is the set of possible feature vectors and M is retained to emphasize that our answer will depend on what modelling assumptions are made. This tool for describing patterns of variability in past experience and for discussing the status of a new case will be considered in detail in Chapter 3 and in Section 5.3.

In describing previous experience the clinician may often wish to make allowances for other known measurements or characteristics. The following problem illustrates this type of situation.

Normal range of anti-diuretic hormone

An elevated plasma concentration of anti-diuretic hormone can give an early indication of a hormone-secreting tumour. It is therefore of some importance to define in some suitable way the values of plasma concentrations of anti-diuretic hormone to be expected in normal individuals. This may be complicated because the plasma concentration of anti-diuretic hormone in a normal individual may vary from time to time because of different urine osmolarity values. Moreover, this variation may depend on the sex of the individual. In order to investigate whether these other factors do indeed influence the plasma concentration of anti-diuretic hormone and, if so, in what way, a study was made of 61 males and 14 females, for whom urine osmolarity and plasma concentration of anti-diuretic hormone were determined. These are given in data set `adhorm`.

If we denote the data set here by D, sex by v_1, urine osmolarity by v_2, plasma concentration of anti-diuretic hormone by u, and our model assumptions by

M then it appears that a first useful step in quantifying experience for the above situation is to arrive at an assessment of

$$p(u|v, D, M) \qquad (u \in U),$$

for the given $v = (v_1, v_2)$ of the new case, where U is the set of possible concentrations of anti-diuretic hormone. This problem is investigated in Section 5.4.1.

1.7 Observation

It is well known that different observers, presented with essentially the same situation, may make different observations and arrive at different results. Such problems of observer error and measurement difference abound in medicine. The following is one such example.

Miniturization of X-ray films

This problem was first presented in the form of a letter received a week before the date, 19 October, referred to in the letter.

Dear ...

The storage of standard large X-ray films is now becoming a serious problem in many hospitals and, as an alternative, some people are suggesting that only small copies of the originals should be stored. We have recently carried out a study in which three radiologists were each asked to make diagnoses from a random sequence of large X-ray films for 100 cases and also from a different random sequence of the 100 small copies of these films. The correct diagnosis for each of the 100 cases is known from other tests. You will find the results set out in the attached sheets.

I think myself that these results show that those who advocate the storage of the small copies only are on a very sticky wicket but I can't see how to express this as a statistical 'significance'.

I would be very grateful for any comments you can give me on the results. Unfortunately I have to give a talk at the ... Conference on the 19 October. Is there any hope that you can complete your calculations by then?

Yours sincerely,

The results referred to are to be found in data set **xrays**. A glance at them will show the source of the difficulty of the problems. A radiologist may reach different conclusions with small and large films but these conclusions do not invariably support one particular size. Moreover radiologists can reach different conclusions even on the basis of the same film. How can we describe such variability in performance and how does it relate to the basic problem of the relative effectiveness of the large and small X-ray films as a diagnostic aid to radiologists?

This problem is further analysed in Section 6.6.

1.8 Direct measurement

Even the most direct methods of measurement may show annoying variability
which for its understanding requires some form of statistical analysis. The
following two examples are typical.

Table 1.4 *Counts of bacterial colonies on 20 sedimentation plates*

Plate no.	Observer no.		
	1	2	3
1	768	847	1010
2	583	641	713
3	386	389	413
4	332	354	373
5	230	236	244
6	148	152	158
7	149	129	155
8	118	104	125
9	90	85	96
10	83	83	91
11	81	80	81
12	63	59	71
13	54	51	55
14	42	43	46
15	29	30	33
16	24	27	26
17	23	23	23
18	15	13	16
19	13	16	16
20	8	8	8

Bacterial colony counting

A research group involved in designing efficient air conditioning in hospitals,
in the course of its investigations, has to conduct many air-sampling experiments with the subsequent assessment of infestations based on the counting
by human eye of the numbers of bacteria colonies cultivated on exposed petri
plates. The group is concerned about the reliability of the counting process
and has run a trial study to investigate sources of variability. In the study
three different observers obtained counts on each of 20 plates, the sequence
of presentation of plates being a different random ordering for different observers. The 60 counts are recorded in data set `bact` and shown in Table 1.4.

It is obvious to the naked eye that a large part of the variability in the complete set of data is due to differences between the infestations of plates, but there is also some variability between observers. How can we quantify this variability and how can we decide whether any such observer variation is of practical importance? Do we have to ask more questions of the research group? Do we need more information before we can start to formulate the problem in statistical terms?

This problem is further developed in Section 6.7.

Measurement of a diagnostic ratio from heart X-rays

In the examination of heart X-rays radiologists regard the ratio of the transverse diameter of the heart to the transverse diameter of the thorax as a useful diagnostic index. Traditionally the magnitude of this diagnostic ratio is judged visually without any direct measurement being recorded. The question now being posed is whether this ratio could be quantified in the sense that its computation from measurements made by one radiologist would be conformable with that from measurements made by another radiologist. Only in such circumstances would such a quantitative index be reliably objective.

To investigate the feasibility of this index as a worthwhile recordable measurement an observer error study had been carried out as part of a larger-scale assessment of the measurability of heart X-rays. Five consultant radiologists were each presented with 65 heart X-rays on a standard displaying screen in randomized order and asked to measure with a ruler and record certain lengths and angles whose definitions all had agreed. For the moment we shall confine our attention to the diagnostic ratio which is defined as $(v_1 + v_2)/v_3$ which is the ratio heart width to thorax width. For two of the radiologists 15 of the heart X-rays were presented once again in a randomized order without the radiologist's knowledge that these were repeats. The complete set of measurements is to be found in data set `dratio`.

The immediate question of the reliability of the diagnostic ratio and other aspects of the larger study are considered in detail later in Section 6.3.

1.9 Indirect measurement

Radioimmunoassay of angiotensin II

The direct measurement of the concentration of angiotensin II in a blood plasma specimen would require the isolation of this biochemical, an awkward and costly technique. Assay techniques exist whereby such an unknown concentration may be assessed by comparing the measurable effect the specimen has on some physical or biological system with the effects produced by specimens of known concentration on similar systems. In the radioimmunoassay of angiotensin II the measurable effect is the percentage bound of radioactive tritium when the specimen is allowed to interact with tritium saturated antigen.

The data set `angio` shows the information obtained from a particular radioimmunoassay. In the particular system in operation in the MRC Blood

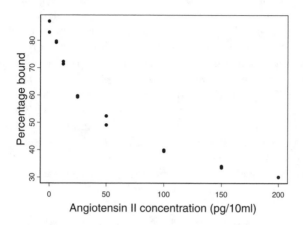

Figure 1.2 *Plot of the percentage bound against the concentration of angiotensin II.*

Pressure Unit in the Western Infirmary Glasgow the data were recorded on paper tape direct from a scintillator counter. The percentage bounds corresponding to standard preparations of volume 10 ml were recorded at a range of concentrations of angiotensin II. For each such concentration two separate preparations were used so that two replicates are available at each concentration. Figure 1.2 shows the scattergram of percentage bound against concentration for these standard preparations. For each of the new specimens of unknown concentration duplicate determinations of percentage bound were obtained for aliquots of blood plasma.

The questions posed by the steroid chemist are straightforwardly stated. Can you suggest an efficient method of estimating the concentrations of the new specimens, and how reliable are the estimates? Are we making the most of the facilities available to us in the design of these radioimmunoassays?

Here if we denote by D the data containing concentration and corresponding percentage bound response for the standards and by v the percentage bound measurements for the specimen of unknown concentration u then ideally we would like a realistic assessment of the conditional probability density function

$$p(u|v, D, M) \qquad (u \in U),$$

where U is the set of possible concentrations and the inclusion of M after the vertical bar reminds us that our assessment may well depend on the model assumptions adopted.

We shall investigate this problem in full detail in Section 7.5.

Foetal age from crown rump length of foetus
It is often difficult from information obtained from pregnant women to

estimate with any great accuracy the foetal age. Some estimate of the foetal age is important for a number of reasons. What is an approximate date of birth? If an abortion is being requested, is the foetal age greater than some minimum period beyond which a legal abortion is impossible? If we do not know the foetal age how can we assess whether the foetus is growing normally?

Sonar screening has now provided a safe method of making measurements on the foetus, and one such measurement is of the crown rump length. In a study of the interrelationship of crown rump length and foetal age 194 pregnant women for whom foetal ages were reliable to within 3 days were screened, some on a number of different occasions, and the crown rump lengths determined. Altogether the study provided 339 pairs of observations for the 194 women according to the schedule recorded in data set `foetal`. A recent referral to the clinic is a pregnant woman whose conception date is uncertain. Sonar screening reveals a crown rump length of 35 mm for the foetus. What can be deduced about the age of the foetus?

This is obviously a problem of indirect measurement, because we are trying to infer the foetal age u of the new case from information about the crown rump length v of her foetus and the data D contained in the data set `foetal`. One such form of inference would be to attempt to provide some assessment of the conditional density function

$$p(u|v, D, M) \qquad (u \in U),$$

where U is the set of possible foetal ages and M is again retained to emphasize that model assumptions may have a central role to play in the evaluation. With this conditional density function available we would obviously be in a strong position to make inferential statements about foetal age.

We continue our analysis of this problem in Section 7.4.

1.10 Diagnosis

The problems that arise in medical diagnosis because of variability and uncertainty have already been well illustrated by the challenge of differential diagnosis of Conn's syndrome discussed in Sections 1.2 and 1.5. The following further examples are presented to indicate the varying nature of the problems in this area of medicine.

Differential diagnosis of Cushing's syndrome

Cushing's syndrome is due to the over-secretion of cortisol by the adrenal glands. There are, however, four different forms that this syndrome may take, namely:

a: adrenal adenoma,
b: bilateral hyperplasia,
c: adrenal carcinoma,
d: ectopic carcinoma.

Table 1.5 *Urinary excretion rates (mg/24h) of the four steroid metabolites: Tetrahy-drocortisone (v3), Reichstein's compound U (v4), Cortisol (v5) and Pregnenetriol (v14)*

Type	v3	v4	v5	v14	Type	v3	v4	v5	v14
a1	3.1	0.10	0.19	12.60	d5	20.5	0.00	1.30	0.10
a2	3.0	0.00	0.22	1.20	d6	30.7	6.80	13.40	0.40
a3	2.6	0.04	0.40	5.10	d7	23.2	0.00	5.10	0.08
a4	1.9	0.24	0.24	0.00	d8	25.9	0.00	10.30	0.20
a5	3.8	0.16	0.40	0.04	d9	16.1	0.00	10.20	0.12
a6	4.1	0.11	0.42	0.30	d10	3.2	0.16	3.80	0.00
a7	1.9	0.02	0.30	0.00	n1	1.5	0.01	0.02	0.00
b1	15.4	0.10	0.41	0.06	n2	1.5	0.00	0.03	0.30
b2	7.1	0.04	0.16	0.00	n3	2.7	0.01	0.03	0.10
b3	5.1	0.00	0.26	0.80	n4	1.8	0.00	0.03	0.10
b4	15.7	0.04	0.34	0.80	n5	1.0	0.02	0.05	0.20
b5	13.6	0.00	1.12	2.00	n6	2.1	0.05	0.08	0.20
b6	4.2	0.00	0.15	0.00	n7	1.9	0.00	0.03	0.20
b7	5.5	0.00	0.20	0.04	n8	2.0	0.04	0.05	0.20
b8	13.0	0.04	0.26	0.34	n9	1.8	0.01	0.03	0.20
b9	5.7	0.08	0.56	0.00	n10	2.0	0.01	0.04	0.10
b10	8.3	0.08	0.26	0.00	n11	1.7	0.00	0.03	0.20
b11	3.8	0.04	0.16	0.16	n12	2.7	0.02	0.03	0.08
b12	8.3	0.12	0.56	0.14	n13	2.2	0.02	0.03	0.00
b13	3.9	0.08	0.36	0.00	n14	1.9	0.01	0.03	0.10
b14	6.4	0.08	0.26	0.10	n15	1.2	0.01	0.03	0.20
b15	8.3	0.06	0.48	0.40	n16	2.0	0.02	0.04	0.10
b16	7.7	0.05	0.80	0.30	n17	1.8	0.02	0.04	0.10
b17	6.5	0.12	0.40	0.10	n18	1.6	0.02	0.03	0.00
b18	4.9	0.09	0.22	0.10	n19	1.2	0.02	0.04	0.20
b19	7.7	0.16	0.24	0.20	n20	1.8	0.02	0.05	0.20
b20	7.8	0.12	0.56	0.70	n21	1.7	0.01	0.04	0.20
b21	3.9	0.00	0.40	0.07	n22	3.0	0.03	0.04	0.30
b22	7.8	0.12	0.88	0.20	n23	2.1	0.00	0.03	0.10
b23	9.1	0.06	0.44	0.10	n24	2.0	0.02	0.03	0.30
b24	7.8	0.05	0.24	0.10	n25	4.9	0.05	0.10	0.20
b25	3.8	0.06	0.27	0.20	n26	3.6	0.01	0.05	0.30
b26	4.5	0.08	0.18	0.00	n27	2.2	0.04	0.04	0.40
b27	3.8	0.09	0.60	0.10	n28	3.0	0.03	0.03	0.20
c1	10.2	0.12	0.80	3.30	n29	3.2	0.01	0.04	0.20
c2	9.2	0.00	1.44	10.80	n30	4.4	0.01	0.07	0.50
c3	9.6	0.08	1.30	1.70	n31	2.6	0.00	0.01	0.20
c4	53.8	0.08	3.84	1.00	n32	3.6	0.03	0.04	0.30
c5	15.8	0.30	0.88	10.60	n33	4.0	0.03	0.06	0.40
d1	12.7	0.00	2.00	0.16	n34	3.0	0.00	0.03	0.20
d2	15.4	0.00	1.30	0.16	n35	0.9	0.00	0.02	0.10
d3	3.9	0.00	2.00	0.00	n36	0.8	0.00	0.01	0.00
d4	9.0	0.00	1.60	0.16	n37	2.9	0.01	0.05	0.10

Since choice of treatment depends crucially on this differential form it is important to obtain as precise a preoperative diagnostic opinion as possible. The question of the diagnostic value of the urinary excretion rates of the fourteen steroid metabolites already referred to in Section 1.6 then arises. The data on four of the steroid metabolites are shown in Table 1.5 and the full data set cush gives the excretion rates for 87 cases of the following composition, where n denotes normal cases:

$$
\begin{array}{rl}
\text{a:} & 8, \\
\text{b:} & 27, \\
\text{c:} & 5, \\
\text{d:} & 10, \\
\text{n:} & 37.
\end{array}
$$

A glance at the pregnenetriol column, for example, shows that for bilateral hyperplasia patients the levels are moderate whereas for ectopic carcinoma patients these are high, and so this diagnostic 'test' is of some value in distinguishing between hyperplasia and ectopic carcinoma. To what extent does this differential ability extend to the other tests and with respect to the other forms, and indeed to distinguishing between normal individuals and cases of Cushing's syndrome. Is it in fact necessary to use all the tests? Are there any features of these tests which could make a misleading diagnosis possible? Could we perhaps obtain as firm a diagnostic opinion with only a subset of the tests?

The reader may at this stage wish to attempt an intuitive diagnostic assessment for the four undiagnosed cases I1–I4 whose data are given in Table 1.2.

The problem here differs from that of Conn's syndrome. Obvious aspects are the larger number of disease types and the increased dimension of the feature vector. More substantial differences, however, exist in the fact that the abnormal cases comprise an aggregated set from different clinics with possible variation in clinic referral processes. The selection process for normal cases is yet again different. As indicated in Section 1.2 a question of considerable importance is then the extent to which these data constitute a viable basis for differential diagnosis.

Differential diagnosis of non-toxic goitre

Non-toxic goitre is a disease which may take one of three possible forms:

$$
\begin{array}{rl}
\text{a:} & \text{simple goitre,} \\
\text{b:} & \text{Hashimoto's disease,} \\
\text{c:} & \text{thyroid carcinoma.}
\end{array}
$$

The case records for past cases showing the results of 4 tests are set out in data set goitre. All the cases have been correctly diagnosed by histopathological examination. The questions to be asked are again of the same form as previously. Do the 4 tests provide an adequate diagnostic basis, and if so, what diagnosis do they provide for the as yet undiagnosed cases given in data set goitre? One new aspect of this diagnostic problem is that all the feature components are no longer continuous: some, such as presence or absence of headache, are binary; some, such as consistency of gland (hard, medium, soft), are ordinal; others, such as 24-hour I^{131} uptake, are continuous. Another new aspect is that there is not a complete feature vector for every patient in the data set nor in some of the new cases. Discussion of how these aspects complicate the statistical analysis is deferred until Section 9.5.

Genetic counselling for possible haemophilia carriers

Haemophilia is a sex-linked genetic disease carried only by females and affecting only males. The son of a carrier has probability 0.5 of being a haemophiliac; the daughter of a carrier has a probability 0.5 of being a carrier. Any offspring of a non-carrying mother is normal with respect to the disease, that is, is not affected if a son and is a non-carrier if a daughter. There is no known test which will distinguish clearly whether a childless woman is a carrier or not, but there are two blood tests which measure coagulation properties (Factors I and IV) of the blood and which do seem to display some ability, albeit imperfect, to distinguish women who are carriers from non-carriers. The test results for 20 known carriers and 23 non-carriers are given in data set haemo.

The problem is then how to devise a system of genetic counselling which will incorporate a woman's family history (her genetic pedigree) and her coagulation test results into a realistic assessment of the chance of her being a carrier. The following case with a very simple family history is sufficient to give the flavour of the problem.

A married woman knows that her maternal grandmother was a carrier. She also has two brothers who are not haemophiliacs. She agrees to take the coagulation tests and her results are recorded. What advice can she be given about her chances of having a child who is normal with respect to haemophilia?

If D denotes the data from the blood tests of the 43 past cases, v the test results of the married woman, w her family history, and u her unknown category, carrier ($u = 1$) or non-carrier ($u = 2$), then we are searching for a means of arriving at a realistic assessment of the conditional probabilities

$$\Pr(u|v, w, D, M) \qquad (u = 1, 2),$$

where M denotes the model assumptions adopted.

We undertake a full analysis of this case and study the problem in general in Section 8.4.

1.11 Prognosis

Cutaneous malignant melanoma

Details of melanoma patients have been drawn from the records of the West of Scotland section of the Scottish Melanoma Group, which records details of all patients presenting with primary cutaneous malignant melanoma (CMM) in Scotland. The data are available in data set malmel. A total of 4332 patients, diagnosed as having invasive primary cutaneous malignant melanoma, were identified starting in 1979 and followed up until December 31st 1998. During this period there were 971 deaths due to CMM, 672 deaths due to other causes and 2775 patients were still alive. The survival times of patients in the last two categories were taken as censored. The effects of five factors – deprivation status, Breslow thickness, age group, histogenetic type and sex – are of interest and this information was recorded at the initial presentation. A deprivation 'score' was derived for each patient, giving seven categories from the most affluent (1) to the most deprived (7). There were five histogenetic types, type 1 to type 5, which are superficial spreading melanoma, nodular/polyploid, lentigo maligna melanoma, acral/mucosal and other/unspecified. Ages were grouped into six categories: <35, 35-44, 45-54, 55-64, 65-74 and >75 years. The Breslow factor had six categories. The first five were defined in terms of the thickness of the tumour, namely <1.5, 1.5-2.49, 2.5-3.49, 3.5-4.99 and >5.0, in millimetres, while the sixth category indicated the presence of stage 2 spreading of the tumour. In the statistical analysis these variables are treated as being of categorical type.

An individual referred patient presents with primary CMM and a given profile of the five factors. What are her survival prospects in the future? We will discuss this in Section 10.5.

1.12 Bibliographic notes

Many of the clinical problems introduced in this chapter and for which the statistical analyses were reported to the client have never been published and so we confine ourselves to citing only those for which further published information is available. For clinical details of Conn's sydrome see the original identification in Conn (1955) and for further information see Pickering (1968). Details of the specific problem of differential diagnosis between adenoma and bilateral hyperplasia are contained in Brown et al. (1968, 1969) and an early statistical analysis is presented in Aitchison and Dunsmore (1975). Clinical details of Cushing's syndrome are described in Pickering (1968). For details of the paper chromatography measurement of steroid metabolites in urine see, for example, Damkjaer Nielsen, Binder and Starup (1969) and Damkjaer Nielsen, Lund and Munch (1972). For information on the use of ultrasound in foetal scanning and, in particular, for crown rump length, see the excellent history of the subject at

www.ob-ultrasound.net/history2.

Details of the background of studies in the differential diagnosis of non-toxic goitre can be found in Boyle et al. (1965) and Taylor, Aitchison and McGirr (1971).

The melanoma data were kindly provided by Professor David Hole and further discussion is available in MacKie et al. (2002).

1.13 Problems

The following problems are designed to widen the range of experience of typical situations arising in clinical medicine. At this stage the reader should not attempt to answer the questions posed in any detail, but merely try to identify the particular aspects of uncertainty and variability which make the problems statistical in nature. These aspects will be examined in further detail in end-of-chapter problems in later chapters.

Problem 1.1 In an early assay technique the immune responsiveness of an infected patient with a bacterial infection was measured by an index computed in the following way. On examination of the blood of a patient R under the microscope the total number n_R of bacteria captured by 100 leucocytes was counted. Under similar conditions a similar count n_S was made of a person, known to be non-infected. The index used was then the responsive ratio n_R/n_S. Doubts were cast at the time about the reliability of this index as an indication of the natural response of such patients. The table below gives the results of the counts of four observers A,...,D on 10 infected persons R1,..., R10 and their uninfected comparisons. How might you advise on the reliability of the index?

Observers	A		B		C		D	
Cases	n_R	n_S	n_R	n_S	n_R	n_S	n_R	n_S
R1	93	100	86	94	97	94	101	93
R2	88	99	84	96	96	105	79	113
R3	90	103	85	110	94	99	97	93
R4	104	128	107	121	94	137	96	117
R5	107	99	110	93	104	97	112	104
R6	107	115	110	116	117	106	103	103
R7	101	135	98	137	96	146	110	131
R8	113	100	110	109	105	106	102	90
R9	82	121	84	125	86	125	91	130
R10	118	137	118	132	108	140	116	129

Problem 1.2 The assay department of a clinic has consulted you about problems concerning a possible assay procedure. The objective is to find a reasonably reliable means of determining the dosage of drug in a patient's blood. The idea is to compare two responses of the patient against the two responses recorded for standard known doses of the drug. The set of twenty standards and their responses are set out in the table below. Specific questions being asked by the department are the following. Which response is more reliable as a means of measuring the dosage? If both responses are used do we obtain a much more reliable assessment of the dosage?

How would you assess the dosages of two patients with values (i) 9.50 and 3.92 and (ii) 12.64 and 3.08 for responses 1 and 2?

Standard	Response 1	Response 2
20	7.14	4.46
40	8.29	4.25
60	9.77	3.77
80	9.79	3.75
100	10.42	3.49
120	10.88	3.54
140	10.96	3.58
160	11.06	3.47
180	10.98	3.40
200	11.37	3.42
220	11.61	3.26
240	12.30	3.13
260	12.11	3.22
280	12.19	3.22
300	12.32	3.06
320	12.21	3.21
340	12.26	3.16
360	12.47	3.05
380	12.34	3.12
400	12.92	3.01

Problem 1.3 A clinic with a differential diagnostic problem in distinguishing between two forms A and B of a newly identified blood disorder seeks your advice. For appropriate treatment it is important for the clinic to distinguish between these forms and this can be eventually done but often much later than desirable for the good of the patient. There is a possibility of speeding up the differential diagnostic process through the use of a set of three symptoms a_1, a_2, a_3 (1=present, 0 = absent) and the composition of a blood sample in terms of the proportions of four constituents c_1, c_2, c_3, c_4. For all the 40 cases, 15 of form A and 25 of form B, so far referred to the clinic, these symptoms and compositions have been recorded in Table 1.6.

You have been asked to investigate the possibility of using these data as a means of obtaining an early and reasonably reliable diagnosis of new patients. How would you report?

Problem 1.4 A dispute about the relative efficacy of rival treatments for the enhancement of low hormone level has given rise to a study of thirty patients, each suffering from low hormone levels. The patients have been allocated to one of the two treatments 1 and 2 at random and the enhanced level of hormone at the end of the treatment has been recorded. Table 1.7 shows the assignment of treatment and the initial and final hormone levels in standard units for each of the thirty patients.

You are consulted for an opinion on which, if any of the two treatments, is the more effective.

Table 1.6 *Data for Problem 1.3*

Type	a1	a2	a3	c1	c2	c3	c4
Form A	0	1	0	0.08	0.13	0.44	0.35
	0	1	0	0.06	0.11	0.45	0.38
	0	1	1	0.07	0.10	0.53	0.30
	0	0	1	0.08	0.13	0.31	0.48
	1	1	0	0.07	0.13	0.51	0.29
	1	1	0	0.08	0.13	0.34	0.45
	1	0	0	0.12	0.19	0.15	0.54
	1	1	1	0.11	0.18	0.27	0.44
	1	1	0	0.11	0.14	0.28	0.47
	1	0	0	0.12	0.19	0.13	0.56
	1	1	1	0.10	0.15	0.25	0.50
	1	0	0	0.11	0.17	0.22	0.50
	1	1	0	0.07	0.11	0.44	0.38
	1	1	1	0.08	0.13	0.34	0.45
	1	0	0	0.08	0.11	0.44	0.37
Form B	0	1	0	0.09	0.19	0.52	0.20
	0	1	1	0.12	0.23	0.37	0.28
	1	1	1	0.16	0.32	0.19	0.33
	0	1	1	0.14	0.31	0.28	0.27
	1	0	1	0.16	0.31	0.25	0.28
	0	1	1	0.17	0.34	0.17	0.32
	0	0	1	0.14	0.28	0.28	0.30
	0	1	0	0.14	0.31	0.26	0.29
	0	0	1	0.17	0.34	0.14	0.35
	0	1	0	0.17	0.30	0.21	0.32
	0	1	0	0.15	0.28	0.25	0.32
	1	0	0	0.15	0.28	0.33	0.24
	0	1	0	0.17	0.33	0.15	0.35
	0	1	0	0.14	0.31	0.20	0.35
	1	0	0	0.17	0.31	0.23	0.29
	1	1	0	0.12	0.25	0.40	0.23
	0	1	1	0.09	0.19	0.52	0.20
	0	1	1	0.10	0.22	0.47	0.21
	0	0	1	0.12	0.22	0.43	0.23
	0	1	1	0.12	0.25	0.31	0.32
	0	1	0	0.15	0.31	0.27	0.27
	1	0	0	0.18	0.33	0.13	0.36
	0	1	1	0.14	0.28	0.23	0.35
	1	1	1	0.14	0.26	0.28	0.32
	0	0	1	0.16	0.30	0.26	0.28

Table 1.7 *Data for Problem 1.4*

Initial level	Treatment	Final level
332	1	798
301	1	739
343	2	846
252	1	650
196	2	570
290	2	745
286	2	734
83	2	336
242	1	655
324	2	794
404	2	970
377	2	975
450	2	1116
272	1	707
118	2	366
268	1	658
122	2	434
99	1	431
246	1	663
248	1	704
240	1	673
307	2	807
305	2	774
263	1	716
127	1	495
415	1	933
344	2	857
135	1	514
512	1	1086
488	2	1151

Problem 1.5 A clinic has developed a new technique of measuring the concentration of five recently discovered enzymes, labelled e1,..., e5, and hopes to devise a means of determining whether new patients referred to the clinic are within normal experience of these enzymes. Forty normal individuals, 20 female and 20 male, have been used to obtain a data base on normal levels of these enzymes. The recorded values (in meq/l) are given in Table 1.8.

Table 1.8 *Data for Problem 1.5*

	e1	e2	e3	e4	e5
Females	25	30	17	69	93
	26	54	23	28	65
	17	55	26	31	46
	27	79	21	26	76
	35	24	17	43	122
	59	18	11	28	71
	28	49	14	60	23
	53	25	15	35	112
	23	29	22	68	70
	16	44	28	93	28
	20	42	48	40	46
	22	40	20	39	119
	35	50	17	49	49
	16	52	19	30	83
	26	21	16	56	90
	17	42	25	45	73
	9	32	25	55	83
	30	22	27	35	55
	19	37	30	29	105
	43	31	11	46	101
Males	35	31	32	31	14
	67	33	34	18	47
	26	42	14	42	62
	25	26	51	13	38
	37	47	21	32	24
	25	29	22	62	47
	44	34	40	31	22
	51	12	33	39	31
	35	27	20	23	72
	39	21	21	27	48
	29	20	20	61	73
	27	11	20	36	43
	18	14	40	19	49
	25	27	25	23	85
	16	28	9	70	42
	54	15	22	33	24
	23	20	33	39	30
	18	42	32	37	35
	16	27	25	77	39
	36	25	18	44	39

Two questions have been asked of you as consultant. Is there any evidence that females and males differ in normal enzyme levels? Whatever your answer to this question devise a means of detecting enzyme abnormality for the clinic.

Problem 1.6 SLGD is a sex-linked genetic disease carried only by females and affecting only males. The son of a carrier has probability 0.25 of being SGLD; the daughter of a carrier has a probability 0.75 of being a carrier. Any offspring of a non-carrying mother is normal with respect to the disease. There is no foolproof test for determining whether a woman is a carrier or not, but there are two independent tests which may be helpful. Past experience has shown that with test 1, 75 per cent of carriers give a positive result whereas only 10 per cent of non-carriers test positive: for test 2, 80 per cent of carriers test positive while 18 per cent of non-carriers test positive.

A married woman knows that her maternal grandmother was a carrier. She has a brother who is not SLGD and a sister who has two sons who are not SLGD. She has undergone the two tests and has had a negative result in test 1 but a positive result in test 2. You are asked to assess her status as a carrier of SLGD.

CHAPTER 2

Relating the Present Patient to Past Experience

2.1 Introduction

This chapter and the following two chapters are not intended to be a concise textbook of statistical theory. We assume that the reader has a sound grounding in basic statistical theory and we therefore concentrate on relating this knowledge to the particular requirements of the field of application described in Chapter 1. This will lead us to introduce aspects of statistical methodology not usually presented in standard texts and courses but essential for attaining confidence in medical statistical consultation. The emphasis will be on encouraging an open-minded approach to the formulation of models, on providing a succinct account of general methods which will withstand the attack of non-standard problems and on directing further, more-detailed study of particular areas. The more flexible and adaptable to new situations a statistician can become and remain the more successful and satisfying the consulting experience is likely to be.

Our main aim is to collect for easy reference in later chapters a substantial body of statistical concepts and methodology. Although much will be taken for granted and no proofs will be given the aim is to give an overall picture in sufficient detail to allow applications. Adequate references are supplied in the bibliographic notes of Chapters 2-4 for readers wishing to pursue particular techniques in greater detail. In presenting all of this material we must always remain aware of the direction of our study towards solving problems in the practice of clinical medicine such as those presented in Chapter 1. Thus we attempt to obtain a balance between developing too much detailed methodology before the practical problem provides the motivation and leaving too much of the technical development until consideration of the practical problem with the danger that the narrative then becomes broken. To achieve such a balance requires at the outset a clear view of what the basic statistical modelling problem is – a view which leads to a framework within which the various aspects of the clinical process can be more clearly formulated and studied. The starting point for any investigation of the role of statistical expertise in a medical problem is that central character, the present or referred patient, and consideration of the methodological problems of relating this patient to past experience.

2.2 The referred patient

In problems of medical statistics, no less than in the actual practice of medicine, the individual patient presently referred to us is of paramount importance and this point must be immediately brought out in our approach to statistical methodology in this chapter.

At a specific stage in the management of referred patient R there will usually be available a vector v of data specific to R: possibly personal information such as age, sex; presenting symptoms such as cough, nausea; results of investigation such as systolic and diastolic blood pressures, plasma concentration of potassium; current treatment. Before proceeding further in the management of R we are involved in making some inference from this information v, and hopefully also from relevant past experience, about some unknown aspect u of the individual patient R. For example in Section 1.2 we know the vector v of eight measurements on the referred patient awaiting differential diagnosis of Conn's syndrome but we do not know the disease category u: adenoma or bilateral hyperplasia. Given v we wish to make some inference about u, and a substantial step would be the assessment of the conditional probabilities of u for given v, namely

$$p_R(u|v). \tag{2.1}$$

Even when there is no immediate patient in view we can still see more clearly the nature of the problem through an imagined referred patient. For example, in a clinical trial comparing two different treatments for cancer of the uterus there might be no immediate patient. In any use of the experience of the clinical trial we imagine a typical present patient referred to us with information about the treatment she is undergoing but do not know what the survival time u will be.

2.3 Data set of past experience

Having formulated the nature of the required inference $p_R(u|v)$ for the present patient R referred to us we have to examine the relevant information available in a set of selected past cases $S_1, \ldots, S_n$. Ideally we would hope to have the following assumptions satisfied.

Assumption 2.1 For the past case S_i we know both u_i and v_i, defined similarly as u and v for the referred patient R, so that the data set is

$$D = \{(u_i, v_i) : i = 1, \ldots, n\}.$$

Assumption 2.2 The observation or measurement processes for u_i and v_i are identical to those for u and v.

Assumption 2.3 The process of referral of the patient R is identical to the process of selection of the past cases $S_1, \ldots, S_n$.

In the example of differential diagnosis of Conn's syndrome in Section 1.2 we have n = 31 with $S_1, \ldots, S_n$ the past cases A1, ... , A20, B1, ... , B11. The data set conn is complete in the sense that we have recorded for each past case the feature vectors $v_1, \ldots, v_n$ of the same nature as the feature vector v for the present case. Moreover the disease category, the unknown u for the present case, is recorded for each of the past cases. Hence Assumption 1 is satisfied. We also know that the methods of measurement of the eight features in v and vectors $v_1, \ldots, v_n$ are identical so that Assumption 2 is satisfied. Further, since we know that the 31 cases selected form the complete set of past cases referred to the clinic and that this present patient has been referred to the clinic in a similar way we are assured that Assumption 3 holds.

When Assumptions 1-3 are satisfied we refer to the data set as complete. We can, however, envisage circumstances under which each of these assumptions is violated.

2.4 Incomplete data sets

First suppose that the clinic dealing with Conn's syndrome now records a ninth feature, plasma concentration of angiotensin, and that the present patient's concentration is 179 meq/l. It is quite clear that Assumption 1 is not valid. Three possibilities arise.

(i) It may be possible to make the data set complete. For example, if there are still available plasma samples from the 31 past cases it may be possible to use them to obtain plasma concentrations of angiotensin and hence the required 9-dimensional vectors to allow full conditioning.

(ii) If the data set D cannot be made complete all we can hope to provide is an inference about u for the given 8-dimensional vector of features. We can make use only of our relevant experience.

(iii) If we feel that (ii) is inadequate we must consider building up prospectively a complete data set D^*, including plasma concentration of angiotensin, from the present and future patients with Conn's syndrome. A question that will then arise is the extent to which we may use the current incomplete data set D to supplement the complete prospective data set D^*. Clearly the combined data set (D, D^*) has missing values in some of the v vectors and this raises the question of missing data.

2.5 Measurement problems

Now suppose that the clinic has switched its measurement process for plasma concentration of aldosterone from double isotope assay, used for the data set conn, to a radioimmunoassay, used for the present patient. Two possibilities arise.

(i) There may be the possibility of calibrating the radioimmunoassay against the double isotope method of measurement. For example, data set aldo shows the results of such a calibration experiment in which two aliquots were taken from each of 72 plasma samples, one being assigned to double isotope assay and the other to radioimmunoassay. We then have to consider how the combined data sets conn and aldo and the patient's feature vector v may be used to obtain an inference about the unknown disease category u.

(ii) If no such calibration is possible then all we can do is to delete the plasma concentrations of aldosterone from the present patient vector v and all the past case vectors $v_1, \ldots, v_{31}$ and make our inference about u on the basis of these reduced vectors.

2.6 Referral and selection

In order to make any valid inference about the referred patient R from the patient's feature vector v and the past experience embodied in the data set D of the selected cases $S_1, \ldots, S_n$ we must examine the consequences of any differences in the processes of referral of the present patient and the selection of past cases. Failure to address the precise nature of the relationship between referral and selection is, in our view, the source of much confusion and misapplication in medical statistics. From our discussion so far we have seen that a common aim in many problems is to obtain an assessment of $p_R(u|v)$, the conditional probability function or probability density function of u for given v for the referred patient. Note that we have introduced the subscript R so that we shall be able to distinguish clearly between probabilistic statements relating to the referred patient R and those related to a typical selected patient S. As a first step in statistical modelling the consultant statistician, after arriving at an understanding of the clinical problem, must derive from knowledge of the referral and selection processes a specific relationship of $p_R(u|v)$ to assessable distributions associated with S.

There is a whole range of relationships between referral and selection but it is not sensible to attempt to catalogue these here. Rather we shall use a few of the practical problems from Chapter 1 to motivate and illustrate the process of connecting R to S. An underlying concept is the ability to visualize a common, background population Π for which the joint distribution of u and v has probability density function $\pi(u, v)$. We shall never need to assess $\pi(u, v)$: the sole purpose of its introduction is to provide a link between R and S.

2.7 Referral of the present patient R

For the referred patient R we do not know u and so referral can depend only on v. We shall assume that v contains all the information on which referral is based and that the probability of referral of an individual with v from the population Π is $\rho(v)$. For example, referral of patients to a regional blood pressure clinic may be based on general practitioners' determinations of systolic and diastolic blood pressures v_1 and v_2, with high v_1 and v_2 indicating referral. Consider all individuals in Π with specific values v_1 and v_2. Not all of these will consult their general practitioners, who may vary in their judgement of 'high'. The net effect is that some proportion of these individuals will be referred to the clinic. Our referral probability $\rho(v)$ is our model counterpart of this proportion, and it must be clear that this is in general unknown. With such a referral process the joint variability of u and v will differ from that in Π with density function

$$p_R(u,v) = \rho(v)\pi(u|v) = \frac{\rho(v)}{\pi(v)}\pi(u,v). \tag{2.2}$$

We note that the effect of referral on the basis of v is simply to alter the population joint distribution $\pi(u,v)$ by a factor $r(v) = \rho(v)/\pi(v)$, which depends only on v, to produce the relevant $p_R(u,v)$ for the referred patient R. In our study of referral and selection we shall use this multiplier $r(v)$ rather than the referral or selection probability.

We recall that our objective is to assess $p_R(u|v)$ and we have from (2.2) and simple conditional probability properties that

$$p_R(u|v) = \frac{r(v)\pi(u,v)}{r(v)\sum_U \pi(u,v)} = \frac{\pi(u,v)}{\pi(v)},$$

where U is the set of all possible u. (Note that the summation sign would be replaced by an integration sign if the set U is continuous.) Hence

$$p_R(u|v) = \pi(u|v). \tag{2.3}$$

Since the population conditional distribution does not depend on $r(v)$ we see that we shall make the same assessment of the conditional probability for every referred patient with given v, whatever the nature of the referral process.

2.8 Selection on the basis of v

Let us consider the 31 past cases of Conn's syndrome as recorded in data set conn, the complete experience of the clinic over a period of time. Each of these cases, selected as our past experience, was sent to the clinic not on the basis of disease type but on information contained in the feature vector v. We can allow for the possibility of a change in the clinic referral process between past and present cases by taking the probability that an individual with vector v is selected from Π to be different from the referral probability of the present patient. With such a selection process the joint variability of u and v in a selected case S will be influenced by a factor $s(v)$ different from $r(v)$ and have density function

$$p_S(u,v) = s(v)\pi(u,v). \tag{2.4}$$

By the same argument as led from (2.2) to (2.3) we have

$$p_S(u|v) = \pi(u|v). \tag{2.5}$$

From (2.3) and (2.5) we have immediately the simple relationship

$$p_R(u|v) = p_S(u|v) \tag{2.6}$$

between the assessment we require for our referred patient and those of selected cases. The implication for statistical analysis is that we should attempt
to model the conditional probability of u for given v for selected cases, use
the selected cases in conn to 'fit' this model to obtain an assessment or 'fit-
ted model' for $p_S(u|v)$ and transfer this directly to obtain an assessment of
$p_R(u|v)$.

In this diagnostic situation it is interesting to note that the incidence probabilities $p_R(u)$ and $p_S(u)$ for referred and selected patients and the prevalence
probability $\pi(u)$ in the underlying population Π are in general different. More
specifically,

$$p_R(u) = \sum_V r(v)\pi(u,v), \tag{2.7}$$

$$p_S(u) = \sum_V s(v)\pi(u,v), \tag{2.8}$$

$$\pi(u) = \sum_V \pi(u,v), \tag{2.9}$$

where V is the set of possible feature vectors v.

All of the above may seem obvious in the context of a simple diagnostic
problem and we may seem to be using a statistical sledgehammer to crack an
already exposed nut. The stability of $p_S(u|v)$ with respect to changes in the
selection process is, however, a crucial consideration in the modelling process.
This stability is not enjoyed by the conditional distribution of $p_S(v|u)$ which
forms the basis of a form of modelling commonly used in statistical diagnosis in
medicine, for example discriminant analysis based on assumptions of different
patterns of variability of vector v for each given type u. From (2.4) we have

$$p_S(v|u) = \frac{s(v)\pi(u,v)}{\sum_V s(v)\pi(u,v)} \tag{2.10}$$

showing clearly the dependence of $p_S(v|u)$ on the selection process $s(v)$. Thus
modelling of $p_S(v|u)$ is of doubtful value in such a situation.

The difficulties in the use of $p_S(v|u)$ as a basis of modelling in this simple
diagnostic problem can be more fully appreciated if we consider the convoluted
argument required to overcome this dependence on the unknown $s(v)$. If for
Conn's syndrome we let u denote adenoma and u^* bilateral hyperplasia then
we have, from (2.8) and (2.10),

$$\frac{p_S(v|u)}{p_S(v|u^*)} = \frac{\pi(u,v)/p_S(u)}{\pi(u^*,v)/p_S(u^*)} = \frac{\pi(u|v)}{\pi(u^*|v)} \Big/ \frac{p_S(u)}{p_S(u^*)}. \tag{2.11}$$

In our assessment of the referred patient R we may, instead of aiming for
$p_R(u|v)$, concentrate on the odds

$$\frac{p_R(u|v)}{p_R(u^*|v)} = \frac{\pi(u|v)}{\pi(u^*|v)} \tag{2.12}$$

from (2.3). From (2.11) and (2.12) we obtain

$$\frac{p_R(u|v)}{p_R(u^*|v)} = \frac{p_S(u)}{p_S(u^*)} \frac{p_S(v|u)}{p_S(v|u^*)}, \tag{2.13}$$

a relationship which is tantalizingly similar to the odds version of Bayes's formula:

$$\text{Posterior odds} = \text{Prior odds} \times \text{Likelihood ratio}.$$

Notice, however, that the 'prior odds' on the right refer to incidence probabilities in the selected group and not those associated with a referred patient. In applications it is quite common practice to multiply the likelihood ratio, estimated from the selected past cases, by a factor $p_R(u)/p_R(u^*)$ which is an assessment of the prior odds for a referred patient. It is clear that this is incorrect unless the referral factor $r(v)$ and the selection factor $s(v)$ on the basis of v are identical: the correct factor is $p_S(u)/p_S(u^*)$, which can, of course, be estimated from the numbers n_u and n_{u^*} of selected cases of type u and u^*.

The instability of $p_S(v|u)$ with respect to changes in the selection process and the complexity of the argument required to counteract our lack of information on $s(v)$ should warn us to avoid modelling based on $p_S(v|u)$. The stability of $p_S(u|v)$, in the sense of its independence of the selection process, makes it the obvious candidate in any sensible modelling under selection dependent on v. The question of how we should model $p_S(u|v)$, parametrically or non-parametrically, in any particular situation will be considered later.

2.9 Selection independently with respect to v and u

Although past cases may have been referred to a clinic on the basis of v, their subsequent selection for study as a summary of past experience may then be made independently on the basis of u. For example in a diagnostic situation where one of the disease types is rare the clinician may decide to use all cases of the rare type while selecting a random sample of the other disease types. In such a situation selection from the underlying population Π takes place in two independent stages, the first being essentially referral to the clinic with a factor $s_1(v)$ dependent on feature vector v and the second selection for further study with a factor $s_2(u)$ dependent on disease type u. For the referred patient we of course still have the relationship

$$p_R(u|v) = \pi(u|v). \tag{2.14}$$

For a selected patient we have

$$p_S(u,v) = s_1(v)s_2(u)\pi(u,v) \tag{2.15}$$

from which we obtain

$$p_S(u|v) = \frac{s_2(u)\pi(u,v)}{\sum_U s_2(u)\pi(u,v)} \tag{2.16}$$

and

$$p_S(v|u) = \frac{s_1(v)\pi(u,v)}{\sum_V s_1(v)\pi(u,v)} \tag{2.17}$$

as the two forms of conditional distribution. Each of these forms is dependent on one stage of the referral process and we can simplify our subsequent discussion if we aim to find a relationship between the odds

$$\frac{p_R(u|v)}{p_R(u^*|v)} = \frac{\pi(u|v)}{\pi(u^*|v)} \tag{2.18}$$

for the referred patient and ratios involving S. From (2.16) we have

$$\frac{p_S(u|v)}{p_S(u^*|v)} = \frac{s_2(u)}{s_2(u^*)} \frac{\pi(u|v)}{\pi(u^*|v)}, \tag{2.19}$$

so that

$$\frac{p_R(u|v)}{p_R(u^*|v)} = \frac{p_S(u|v)}{p_S(u^*|v)} \Big/ \frac{s_2(u)}{s_2(u^*)}. \tag{2.20}$$

If therefore we know $s_2(u)$, the sampling fractions of selection of the various disease types from the clinic's experience, we see that it is appropriate to model $p_S(u|v)$. In comparison with (2.18) the modification by the ratio $s_2(u)/s_2(u^*)$ is then seen simply as the price we have to pay for interference with a selection process based solely on v. Now let us examine the possibility of using the other conditional model of v for given u. The incidence probabilities $p_S(u)$ for the selected experience are given by

$$p_S(u) = \sum_V p_S(u,v) = s_2(u) \sum_V s_1(v)\pi(u,v). \tag{2.21}$$

From (2.17) and (2.21) we have

$$\begin{aligned}
\frac{p_S(v|u)}{p_S(v|u^*)} &= \frac{\pi(u|v)}{\pi(u^*|v)} \Big/ \frac{\sum_V s_1(v)\pi(u,v)}{\sum_V s_1(v)\pi(u^*,v)} \\
&= \frac{\pi(u|v)s_2(u)}{\pi(u^*|v)s_2(u^*)} \Big/ \frac{p_S(u)}{p_S(u^*)}
\end{aligned}$$

so that

$$\frac{p_R(u|v)}{p_R(u^*|v)} = \frac{p_S(v|u)}{p_S(v|u^*)} \frac{s_2(u)}{s_2(u^*)} \Big/ \frac{p_S(u)}{p_S(u^*)}.$$

Here $p_S(u)/p_S(u^*)$ could be estimated by the ratio n_u/n_{u^*} of the numbers of selected cases in the various disease types but again we require knowledge of the sampling fractions $s_2(u)$ of disease types to complete the inference process for the referred patient. In view of the extra complexity we would be well advised to base modelling again on the more direct form $p_S(u|v)$, recalling also its advantage of stability with respect to selection on v.

2.10 Referral and selection for assay

Suppose that we wish to assess the unknown concentration u of some substance in the blood sample of a referred patient R by an assay technique. To achieve this we have to compare some observed response v in the patient to this unknown concentration with the responses $v_1, \ldots, v_n$ to selected, standard, known concentrations $u_1, \ldots, u_n$. In this situation since u and v are both unknown at the time of referral we must suppose that referral has been based on some other aspect w, say, with referral factor $r(w)$. Starting with an imagined population Π with joint distribution $\pi(u, v, w)$ we then have

$$p_R(u, v, w) = r(w)\pi(u, v, w). \tag{2.22}$$

Since we do not know $r(w)$ our aim is again to attempt to assess $p_R(u|v)$ so that a summation over w is required. We may also reasonably assume that, for given u, the variability of v does not depend on w: more specifically,

$$\pi(v|u, w) = \pi(v|u). \tag{2.23}$$

Since $\pi(u, v, w) = \pi(u, w)\pi(v|u, w)$ we can then easily arrive at the following form:

$$p_R(u, v) = p_R(u)\pi(v|u), \tag{2.24}$$

where

$$p_R(u) = \sum_W r(w)\pi(u, w) \tag{2.25}$$

can be considered the 'incidence' probability for u, in other words the probability, prior to assay, with which a referred person has concentration u.

In the assay situation the standard concentrations are deliberately selected and we may suppose that $s(u)$ is the rate or probability with which a standard with concentration u is selected. For assay to be possible the conditional distribution of response v for given u must be the same as in the population Π, namely $\pi(v|u)$. Since

$$p_S(u, v) = s(u)\pi(u, v) \tag{2.26}$$

we indeed have

$$p_S(v|u) = \pi(v|u). \tag{2.27}$$

From (2.24) and (2.27) we then arrive at the relationship

$$p_R(u|v) = \frac{p_R(u)p_S(v|u)}{\sum_U p_R(u)p_S(v|u)}. \tag{2.28}$$

In this application we would thus be directed towards modelling the experience in the standards through the conditional distribution $p_S(v|u)$. To arrive at the required inference we note the important fact that we require to have some means of assessing $p_R(u)$.

2.11 Referral and selection for genetic counselling

For the genetic counselling problem described in Section 1.10 the unknown aspect u of the referred patient R is whether or not she is a carrier. Referral has clearly been made on the family history w with referral factor $r(w)$, say, and the feature vector v, consisting of her coagulation measurements, is determined after referral. Starting from an underlying population Π with joint distribution $\pi(u, v, w)$ we have the following referral process,

$$p_R(u, v, w) = r(w)\pi(u, v, w), \tag{2.29}$$

so that

$$p_R(u|v, w) = \pi(u|v, w). \tag{2.30}$$

A novel aspect now enters our argument: our knowledge of the genetics of the disease transmission. Before we have any information about v we can, given the family history w, compute $\pi(u|w)$. To exploit this knowledge in (2.30) we make use of simple properties of conditional probabilities:

$$\pi(u|v, w) = \frac{\pi(u|w)\pi(v|u, w)}{\sum_U \pi(u|w)\pi(v|u, w)}. \tag{2.31}$$

We can next make use of a further realistic clinical assumption, namely that the coagulation measurements depend only on whether a person is a carrier or not and not on the particular family history: more specifically,

$$\pi(v|u, w) = \pi(v|u). \tag{2.32}$$

Thus, combining (2.30)–(2.32) we have

$$p_R(u|v, w) = \frac{\pi(u|w)\pi(v|u)}{\sum_U \pi(u|w)\pi(v|u)} \tag{2.33}$$

as the vehicle for assessing the status, carrier or non-carrier, of the referred patient.

For a typical selected case we know the disease status, carrier or non-carrier, and the feature vector v, but not the family history w, so that we can confine our attention to $\pi(u, v)$ for Π. Selection has been directed towards obtaining a group of carriers and non-carriers and so is on the basis of some selection factor $s(u)$ based on u. Then

$$p_S(u, v) = s(u)\pi(u, v) \tag{2.34}$$

from which we easily obtain

$$p_S(v|u) = \pi(v|u) \tag{2.35}$$

which is stable relative to any change of selection policy. Hence assessment of the referred patient R may proceed through the relationship

$$p_R(u|v, w) = \frac{\pi(u|w)p_S(v|u)}{\sum_U \pi(u|w)p_S(v|u)}, \tag{2.36}$$

relying on our genetics-based assessment of $\pi(u|w)$ and our modelling of the selection-stable $p_S(v|u)$.

2.12 Bibliographic notes

The ideas used in this chapter require essentially only familiarity with properties of conditional probabilities, including Bayes's formula, and have been used implicitly in medical statistics over a number of years. The intention of the chapter has been to clarify the arguments so that the reader may avoid relating the referred patient to the selected experience in an incorrect way.

An early paper connecting different views of referral and their consequences is Day and Kerridge (1967). For two clear expositions of these aspects we recommend Anderson (1972) and Dawid (1976). The latter gives an exceptionally clear exposition of all the concepts involved. The main difference in our approach is that we have preferred to keep the development in terms of conditional probabilities rather than the special notation of Dawid (1976).

2.13 Problems

Problem 2.1 In a large sample survey of a population, each person was classified into one of two types A and B and for each person two simple binary tests, each with a positive or negative result, were carried out. The table below gives the estimated probability $p(u, v)$ of a person being of type u and giving test result v.

Test Results		Type u	
		A	B
−	−	0.05	0.16
−	+	0.13	0.12
+	−	0.17	0.09
+	+	0.25	0.03

Construct the two sets of conditional probabilities $p(u|v)$ and $p(v|u)$. Which would you regard as more appropriate for diagnoses of new cases if referral is to be on the basis of the diagnostic tests?

As a consulting statistician you are asked to suggest suitable methods for the following two situations.

(i) Experience in one clinic has suggested that different probabilities of referral attach to different test results at the preclinic referral stage, as follows:

Test Results		Probability of referral
−	−	0.1
−	+	0.2
+	−	0.3
+	+	0.4

How should the clinic use the test results for diagnostic purposes?

(ii) Experience at a second clinic has shown that the incidence of type A and type B cases that are referred to it are in the ratio 3 : 7. How should this clinic use the test results for diagnostic purposes?

Problem 2.2 A certain genetic disease is carried only by females and affects only males. There is no direct test which can ascertain whether a female is a carrier, but affected males can be immediately recognised. The daughter of a carrier has probability 0.5 of herself becoming a carrier; the son of a carrier has probability 0.5 of having the disease. The offspring of a non-carrying mother are normal.

(i) A woman knows that her maternal grandmother was a carrier. What is the chance that the woman is a carrier?

(ii) The woman's mother gives birth to two normal sons. How does this affect the chance that the woman is a carrier?

(iii) The woman herself subsequently gives birth to a normal son. What now is the chance that she is a carrier?

Problem 2.3 A clinic has conducted a trial in which a typical patient S referred to it on the basis of information v, and who has subsequently been diagnosed to have disease type u, is allocated treatment t (from among a set of trial treatments) and the outcome y of the treatment recorded. The clinic has therefore been able to obtain a reasonable assessment of $p_S(y|u, v, t)$. A new patient R with information vector v_R but with unknown disease type u_R has now been referred to the clinic which is naturally interested in how the patient will respond to treatment t, in other words to evaluate $p_R(y_R|v_R, t)$. The clinic has already carried out an independent investigation into the use of the information v for diagnostic purposes and so can evaluate $p_R(u_R|v_R)$. Can you provide the clinic with a means of evaluating the effect of treatment for this new patient?

Problem 2.4 A clinic has already carried out a trial to see how a typical treatment t may be able to control a hormone level v to a lower level y and so from the selected patients has produced an assessed conditional probability $p_S(y|v, t)$. Unfortunately it has been necessary to switch to a more efficient and less costly method of determining hormone level. A large number of blood samples from patients has been used and for each sample both hormone level v by the old method and hormone level w by the new method have been determined so that assessments of both can be obtained. For a new patient R with hormone level w_R, determined by the new method, how would you assess the required conditional probability $p(y_R|w_R, t)$?

Problem 2.5 In a simple case-control study to investigate the effect of exposure v or non-exposure v^* to a chemical on the possibility of developing (u) or not developing (u^*) a certain disease, a random sample of patients suffering from the disease and another random sample of individuals not suffering from the disease were selected and for each case it was determined whether the individual had been exposed to the chemical or not. Use the technique of the background population – with joint probability density function $\pi(u, v)$, selection into the study by factors $s(u), s(u^*)$ and referral of a generic 'new patient' R by factors $r(v), r(v^*)$ – to show that it is possible to assess the 'odds ratio'

$$\frac{p_R(u|v)}{p_R(u^*|v)} \bigg/ \frac{p_R(u|v^*)}{p_R(u^*|v^*)}$$

without knowledge of $s(u), s(u^*), r(v), r(v^*)$. Consider how you might explain the use of this odds ratio to a clinician.

Problem 2.6 Is the form of argument you have used in Problem 2.4 in any way altered if further information w (for example sex) is available on each individual in the study? In particular does such information alter in any way the assessment of an odds ratio built on the further conditioning $p_R(u|w, t)$?

CHAPTER 3

A Review of Statistical Methodology

3.1 Introduction

We have seen in Chapter 2 that in attempting to assess the relevant conditional distribution such as $p_R(u|v)$ for a referred patient R we are led to the problem of modelling one or other of the conditional distributions $p_S(u|v)$ and $p_S(v|u)$ for a typical selected case S. Once this modelling problem has been resolved our subsequent task is to use the data set

$$D = \{(u_i, v_i) : i = 1, \ldots, n\}$$

of the selected cases $S_1, \ldots, S_n$ to fit the model as a step towards arriving at an assessment of the appropriate conditional p_S distribution. To fix ideas for the moment we shall concentrate on the modelling and fitting of $p_S(u|v)$.

In our role of consulting statistician we must assume that the clinician has identified in u and v all that is possibly relevant to the referred patient's problem. In general u and v will be vectors and in our modelling we shall start with these complete vectors. Our first aim is to find a framework within which we can discuss the nature of the variability of the full vector u for any given value of the full vector v. It is in this sense that we describe this initial modelling stage as maximal: it envisages the extraction of the greatest possible information about u obtainable from knowledge of v. One of the aims of this maximal modelling is to provide a framework within which we can pose searching questions about whether the whole of u or v are really relevant to the modelling. Such questions take us into the area of hypothesis testing and this will be the focus of Section 3.10. For the moment we confine our attention to maximal modelling.

3.2 Maximal parametric modelling

Since the conditional distribution appropriate to the practical problem will sometimes be $p_S(u|v)$ and sometimes be $p_S(v|u)$ it will be sensible in our study of maximal modelling to use a neutral notation (x, y) for the two entities involved in the conditioning process and concentrate on the modelling of the conditional distribution $p(y|x)$. In applications (x, y) will sometimes be identified with (u, v) and sometimes with (v, u). Then the data set associated with the selected cases is denoted by

$$D = \{(x_i, y_i) : i = 1, \ldots, n\}.$$

Within statistical methodology there are two fundamentally different approaches to the modelling of a conditional distribution $p(y|x)$. We may adopt a parametric approach by specifying some mathematical form $p(y|x, \theta)$ for $p(y|x)$, where θ is some, possibly vector, parameter which acts essentially as an index in identifying the specific member of a class of distributions generated by varying the parameter over some set Θ. A familiar example is the class of normal regression models with $p(y|x, \theta)$ of univariate normal form with mean $\alpha + \beta x$ and variance σ^2 with the parameter space Θ defined as the set of all vectors (α, β, σ) in R^3, three-dimensional real space, with $\sigma > 0$. An alternative non-parametric approach might consider, for example, a method of kernel density estimation for $p(y|x)$. We shall consider such a non-parametric approach in Section 4.8.

There are three main classes of parametric models that serve the requirements of many applications: the multivariate normal regression model, the categorical regression model and the compositional regression model. These are associated with three different sample spaces for the dependent vector or variable y. After establishing some necessary notation and terminology for standard distributions in Section 3.3, we recall the main properties of the first two of these classes and the associated techniques of estimation in Sections 3.4–3.8. For convenience of reference we also collect in these sections some simple, useful and little known recursive formulae which make it easy either to remove a selected case from, or add a new selected case to, $S_1, \ldots, S_n$, the original set of selected cases. We discuss the compositional regression model in Section 4.2.

3.3 Standard distributions

Seven classes of distribution, the gamma, beta, normal, lognormal, Student, logStudent and Wishart, will play a central role in our analysis, and for convenience of reference we collect here their definitions in terms of their density functions. In the specification of their sample spaces we have used R^d to denote d-dimensional real space, R^d_+ its positive orthant and M^d the space of all positive definite matrices of order d. Note that in considering vectors in such d-dimensional spaces we adopt the convention that the vectors are row vectors of dimension $1 \times d$.

Definition 3.1 The distribution of $x \in R^1_+$ is said to be *gamma*, written $\text{Ga}(\alpha)$, where $\alpha > 0$, when its density function is

$$p(x|\alpha) = \frac{x^{\alpha-1} \exp(-x)}{\Gamma(\alpha)} \qquad (x > 0). \qquad (3.1)$$

The corresponding distribution function $I(t|\alpha)$ is given by

$$I(t|\alpha) = \Pr(x \leq t) = \int_0^t p(x|\alpha)dx \qquad (t > 0) \qquad (3.2)$$

and is the well-known incomplete gamma function.

Definition 3.2 The distribution of $x \in (0, 1)$ is said to be $\text{Be}(\alpha, \beta)$, where

$\alpha > 0, \beta > 0$, when its density function is

$$\frac{x^{\alpha-1}(1-x)^{\beta-1}}{B(\alpha, \beta)} \qquad (0 < x < 1). \qquad (3.3)$$

The corresponding distribution function $J(t|\alpha, \beta)$ is given by

$$J(t|\alpha, \beta) = \Pr(x \leq t) = \int_0^t p(x|\alpha, \beta)dx \qquad (0 < t < 1) \qquad (3.4)$$

and is the well-known incomplete beta function.

Definition 3.3 The distribution of the $1 \times d$ vector $x \in R^d$ is said to be multivariate normal, written $N^d(\mu, \Sigma)$, where the parameter μ is a $1 \times d$ vector and the parameter Σ is a $d \times d$ positive definite matrix, when its density function $\phi^d(x|\mu, \Sigma)$ is

$$(2\pi)^{-d/2}|\Sigma|^{-\frac{1}{2}} \exp\left\{-\tfrac{1}{2}(x-\mu)\Sigma^{-1}(x-\mu)^T\right\}. \qquad (3.5)$$

Definition 3.4 The distribution of the $1 \times d$ vector $x \in R_+^d$ is said to be multivariate lognormal, written $\Lambda^d(\mu, \Sigma)$, where the parameter μ is a $1 \times d$ vector and the parameter Σ is a $d \times d$ positive definite matrix, when its density function $\lambda^d(x|\mu, \Sigma)$ is

$$(2\pi)^{-d/2}|\Sigma|^{-\frac{1}{2}} \left(\prod_{i=1}^d x_i\right)^{-1} \exp\left\{-\tfrac{1}{2}(\log x - \mu)\Sigma^{-1}(\log x - \mu)^T\right\}. \qquad (3.6)$$

Definition 3.5 The distribution of the $1 \times d$ vector $x \in R^d$ is said to be multivariate Student, written $St^d(k, \mu, \Sigma)$, where the parameter μ is a $1 \times d$ vector and the parameter Σ is a $d \times d$ positive definite matrix, when its density function is

$$\frac{\Gamma\{\tfrac{1}{2}(k+1)\}}{\pi^{d/2}\Gamma\{\tfrac{1}{2}(k-d+1)\}|k\Sigma|^{1/2}} \frac{1}{\{1 + (x-\mu)(k\Sigma)^{-1}(x-\mu)^T\}^{(k+1)/2}}.$$

Definition 3.6 The distribution of the $1 \times d$ vector $x \in R_+^d$ is said to be multivariate logStudent, written $\Lambda St^d(k, \mu, \Sigma)$, where the parameter μ is a $1 \times d$ vector and the parameter Σ is a $d \times d$ positive definite matrix, when its density function is

$$\frac{\Gamma\{\tfrac{1}{2}(k+1)\}(\prod_{i=1}^d x_i)^{-1}}{\pi^{d/2}\Gamma\{\tfrac{1}{2}(k-d+1)\}|k\Sigma|^{1/2}} \frac{1}{\{1 + (\log x - \mu)(k\Sigma)^{-1}(\log x - \mu)^T\}^{(k+1)/2}}.$$

Definition 3.7 The distribution of a random positive definite matrix W of order $d \times d$ is said to be Wishart, written $Wi(k, \Sigma)$, where the parameter Σ is a $d \times d$ positive definite matrix, when its density function is

$$\frac{|W|^{(k-d+1)/2}\exp\{-\tfrac{1}{2}\mathrm{tr}(\Sigma^{-1}W)\}}{|\tfrac{1}{2}\Sigma|^{\pi d(d-1)/4}\Gamma(k)\Gamma(k-\tfrac{1}{2})\ldots\Gamma\{k-\tfrac{1}{2}(d-1)\}} \qquad (W \in M^d). \qquad (3.7)$$

We will require later the following distributional property.

Property 3.1 Let x and W be independently distributed as $N^d(0, \Sigma)$ and $Wi(k, \Sigma)$, respectively. Then

$$\frac{xW^{-1}x^T}{(xW^{-1}x^T + 1)}$$

is distributed as $Be\{\frac{1}{2}d, \frac{1}{2}(k - d + 1)\}$.

3.4 Multivariate normal regression model

Information about a patient often consists of measurements made on continuous scales, for example: weight in kg, systolic blood pressure in mm of Hg, quantity in ml of urine excreted in 24 hours, leading to a vector of real numbers. We now consider the problem of the parametric modelling of the conditional probability distribution $p(y|x)$ when y is a d-dimensional real row vector in R^d and when x is a c-dimensional row vector. To investigate this problem of describing the extent to which the variability in y is explainable by, or dependent on, x we make use of the familiar multivariate normal regression model.

Definition 3.8 If the conditional distribution of y for given x is of $N^d(x\mathrm{B}, \Sigma)$ form, where B is a $c \times d$ matrix parameter and Σ is a positive definite matrix parameter of order d, then we have a multivariate normal regression model for y with covariate x.

This type of modelling is often presented as a linear model in the following form

$$y = x\mathrm{B} + e, \tag{3.8}$$

where the random error d-dimensional row vector e is $N^d(0, \Sigma)$. For the selected cases $S_1, \ldots, S_n$ with data set

$$D = \{(x_i, y_i) : i = 1, \ldots, n\}$$

we can give a matrix expression to the combination of individual relationships of form

$$Y = XB + E, \tag{3.9}$$

where X, Y, E are $n \times c, n \times d, n \times d$ matrices formed from the row vectors x_i, y_i, e_i, respectively, and $e_1, \ldots, e_n$ are identically and independently distributed as $N^d(0, \Sigma)$. Note that each row of X, Y, E refers to an individual selected case whereas each column refers to an individual feature or covariate, including usually a vector of 1s corresponding to an intercept term. We shall refer to (3.9) as a multivariate linear model or more briefly as a linear model. Our next property records the essential maximum likelihood properties for this model.

Property 3.2 The maximum likelihood estimate $\hat{\mathrm{B}}$ of B under the linear model $Y = XB + E$ is

$$\hat{\mathrm{B}} = (X^T X)^{-1} X^T Y$$

and the residual sum of squares and cross products matrix is

$$\begin{aligned} R &= (Y - X\hat{B})^T(Y - X\hat{B}) & (3.10) \\ &= Y^TY - \hat{B}^TX^TY & (3.11) \\ &= Y^T\{I - X(X^TX)^{-1}X^T\}Y. & (3.12) \end{aligned}$$

Moreover an estimate of Σ, unbiased under the model defined in (3.9), is given by

$$\hat{\Sigma} = (n - c)^{-1}R.$$

Note. Two important assumptions have been made in the statement of Property 3.2, namely that $n > c$ and that X^TX is non-singular. We thus envisage more selected cases than the dimension of the covariate vector $(n > c)$ and that the $n \times c$ matrix X is of full rank c to ensure non-singularity of the $c \times c$ matrix X^TX. When this rank condition is not fulfilled it is still possible to establish results similar to those of Property 3.2, for example in terms of a pseudo-inverse of the now singular X^TX, but we shall have no need for such an elaboration.

We now record an important distributional property associated with the estimation process for the linear model.

Property 3.3 For the linear model of (3.9), and for any given covariate vector x, $x\hat{B}$ and R are distributed independently as

$$N^d(xB, x(X^TX)^{-1}x^T\Sigma) \quad \text{and} \quad Wi^d(n - c, \Sigma),$$

respectively.

Often we have to assess how closely a new case, either the referred patient R or a further selected case S, follows the linear model pattern fitted from the selected cases $S_1, \ldots, S_n$. For our discussion of this problem later in this chapter we shall require the technical result recorded in the following property.

Property 3.4 Suppose that a further case with covariate and feature vectors x and y also follows the linear model with conditional distribution of y for given x of $N^d(xB, \Sigma)$ form, independent of cases $S_1, \ldots, S_n$. Define the conditional quadratic form q of (x, y) relative to cases $S_1, \ldots, S_n$ by

$$q = (y - x\hat{B})\hat{\Sigma}^{-1}(y - x\hat{B})^T.$$

Then

$$\frac{q}{[q + (n - c)\{1 + x(X^TX)^{-1}x^T\}]}$$

is distributed as $Be\{\frac{1}{2}d, \frac{1}{2}(n - c - d + 1)\}$.

We can see this as an immediate use of Property 3.3 to give

$$(y - x\hat{B})/\{1 + x(X^TX)^{-1}x^T\}^{\frac{1}{2}} \quad \text{and} \quad (n - c)\hat{\Sigma}$$

distributed independently as $N^d(0, \Sigma)$ and $Wi^d(n-c, \Sigma)$, respectively, followed by a direct application of Property 3.1.

3.5 Recursive formulae

Suppose that we have carried out the linear model estimation procedure as described in Property 3.2 and based on the data set D of the n selected cases $S_1, \ldots, S_n$. It is often important to see how such estimation results are influenced by dropping out one of these selected cases or by including an extra case. Simple recursive relationships for such purposes can easily be derived. In deriving these relationships and others later we make repeated use of two useful matrix identities.

Property 3.5 Let A be a non-singular matrix of order d, b a $1 \times d$ vector and c a scalar. Then

$$\left(A + cb^T b\right)^{-1} = A^{-1} - \frac{cA^{-1}b^T bA^{-1}}{1 + cbA^{-1}b^T},$$

$$\left|A + cb^T b\right| = \{1 + cbA^{-1}b^T\}|A|.$$

We take as our starting point the linear model defined in (3.9) and the estimates $\hat{B}, \hat{\Sigma}$ and residual matrix R as determined in Property 3.2. Let us now consider the consequences of removing one pair (x, y) from D and denote this reduced data set by D_-. Then the linear model is reduced to

$$Y_- = X_- B + E_-,$$

where Y_-, X_-, E_- are simply Y, X, E with the rows appropriate to the (x, y) case deleted. Then

$$X_-^T Y_- = X^T Y - x^T y,$$
$$X_-^T X_- = X^T X - x^T x$$

and so, from Property 3.5,

$$(X_-^T X_-)^{-1} = (X^T X)^{-1} + \frac{(X^T X)^{-1} x^T x (X^T X)^{-1}}{1 - x(X^T X)^{-1} x^T}.$$

The maximum likelihood estimate $\hat{B}_-$ of B based on data set D_- is now readily obtained by Property 3.5 as

$$\hat{B}_- = (X^T X)^{-1} X^T Y - \frac{(X^T X)^{-1} x^T (y - x\hat{B})}{1 - x(X^T X)^{-1} x^T}$$

after some simplification. We can thus obtain $\hat{B}_-$ as a simple adjustment to $\hat{B}$ since $(X^T X)^{-1}$ will already have been determined as a step towards the computation of $\hat{B}$. Note also that the vector $r = y - x\hat{B}$ is the residual vector of (x, y) with respect to the fitted linear model based on D. The corresponding residual vector r_- based on D_- is easily related to r since

$$r_- = y - x\hat{B}_- = r/(1 - h),$$

where

$$h = x(X^T X)^{-1} x^T.$$

Similar recursive relationships can be easily obtained between other entities, such as $R_-, \hat{\Sigma}_-^{-1}$ and

$$q_- = (y - x\hat{B}_-)\hat{\Sigma}_-^{-1}(y - x\hat{B}_-)^T,$$

and $R, \hat{\Sigma}^{-1}$ and q, as defined in Properties 3.2 and 3.4 and based on D. For ease of reference we collect all of these relationships in Property 3.6.

Property 3.6 Let D_- denote the data set

$$D = \{(x_i, y_i) : i = 1, \ldots, n\}$$

with (x, y) deleted, and let subscript $-$ indicate that estimates and other factors associated with the linear model of Property 3.2 are based on D_- instead of the full data set D. The following recursive relationships then provide the adjustments to factors based on D to obtain the corresponding factors based on D_-.

$$\hat{B}_- = \hat{B} - (1-h)^{-1}(X^TX)^{-1}x^Tr,$$

$$r_- = (1-h)^{-1}r,$$

$$R_- = R - (1-h)^{-1}r^Tr,$$

$$\hat{\Sigma}_- = \frac{n-c}{n-c-1}\left\{\hat{\Sigma} - \frac{r^Tr}{(n-c)(1-h)}\right\},$$

$$\hat{\Sigma}_-^{-1} = \frac{n-c-1}{n-c}\left\{\hat{\Sigma}^{-1} + \frac{\hat{\Sigma}^{-1}r^Tr\hat{\Sigma}^{-1}}{(n-c)(1-h)-q}\right\},$$

$$|\hat{\Sigma}_-| = \left(\frac{n-c}{n-c-1}\right)^d\left\{1 - \frac{q}{(n-c)(1-h)}\right\}|\hat{\Sigma}|,$$

$$\text{trace}(\hat{\Sigma}_-) = \left(\frac{n-c}{n-c-1}\right)\text{trace}(\hat{\Sigma}) - \frac{rr^T}{(n-c-1)(1-h)},$$

$$q_- = \frac{(n-c-1)q}{(1-h)\{(n-c)(1-h)-q\}}.$$

We obtain similar relationship if, instead of removing a vector from D, we supplement D by adding a new vector (x, y) to obtain augmented data set D_+.

Property 3.7 Let D_+ denote the data set D with (x, y) added to the cases, and let subscript $+$ indicate that estimates and other factors associated with the linear model of Property 3.2 and based on D_+ instead of the original data set D. The following recursive relationships then provide the adjustments to factors based on D to obtain the corresponding factors based on D_+.

$$\hat{B}_+ = \hat{B} + (1+h)^{-1}(X^TX)^{-1}x^Tr,$$

$$r_+ = (1+h)^{-1}r,$$

$$R_+ = R + (1+h)^{-1}r^Tr,$$

$$\hat{\Sigma}_+ = \frac{n-c}{n-c+1}\left\{\hat{\Sigma} + \frac{r^Tr}{(n-c)(1+h)}\right\},$$

$$\hat{\Sigma}_+^{-1} = \frac{n-c+1}{n-c}\left\{\hat{\Sigma}^{-1} - \frac{\hat{\Sigma}^{-1}r^T r\hat{\Sigma}^{-1}}{(n-c)(1+h)+q}\right\},$$

$$|\hat{\Sigma}_+| = \left(\frac{n-c}{n-c+1}\right)^d\left\{1 + \frac{q}{(n-c)(1+h)}\right\}|\hat{\Sigma}|,$$

$$\text{trace}(\hat{\Sigma}) = \left(\frac{n-c}{n-c+1}\right)\text{trace}(\hat{\Sigma}) + \frac{rr^T}{(n-c+1)(1+h)},$$

$$q_+ = \frac{(n-c+1)q}{(1+h)\{(n-c)(1+h)+q\}}.$$

3.6 Categorical regression modelling

In a diagnostic problem the unknown u will belong to a set of disease types and so is categorical in nature. We have seen in Chapter 2 that we may wish to model $p_S(u|v)$ for such a diagnostic problem and so we require to consider parametric classes of conditional distribution for a categorical variable u given a covariate vector v. Fortunately there is such a versatile class, logistic regression models, and we collect here the important results which we shall require. We start with the simplest version with just two categories and then extend to any finite number of categories. Again we shall use the neutral notation of (x, y) for the covariate and categorical variable, respectively.

Binary regression models

In specifying a conditional model for a categorical variable y with two possible categories 1 and 2 we have to assign probabilities to the events $y = 1$ and $y = 2$. These probabilities depend on the $1 \times c$ covariate row vector x. In the interests of simplicity we might consider introducing linear combinations $x\beta^T$ of the components of x as in the multivariate normal regression model. Here β is a $1 \times c$ row vector and we adopt the usual convention that the first component of x may be a 'dummy variable' 1 to accommodate a constant in the linear expression. A constraint in our modelling here, however, is that probabilities have to be non-negative and indeed confined to the interval $(0, 1)$. Such non-negativity can, for example, be ensured by exploitation of the properties of the exponential function and use of $\exp(x\beta^T)$ rather than $x\beta^T$. Since we require two probabilities dependent on x and summing to 1 we may then consider

$$\Psi_1(x, \beta) = \frac{\exp(x\beta^T)}{\exp(x\beta^T) + 1}, \tag{3.13}$$

$$\Psi_2(x, \beta) = \frac{1}{\exp(x\beta^T) + 1} \tag{3.14}$$

as a basis for modelling.

Definition 3.9 The conditional distribution of a binary variable y for given covariate vector x is said to be of logistic regression form with vector parameter β when

$$p(y = j|x, \beta) = \Psi_j(x, \beta) \qquad (j = 1, 2),$$

where the Ψ_j are defined in (3.13) and (3.14).

For such a logistic regression model the logarithm λ of the odds on $y = 1$ against $y = 2$ is given by

$$\lambda = \log \frac{p(y = 1|x, \beta)}{p(y = 2|x, \beta)} = x\beta^T,$$

a linear combination of the components of the covariate vector x. We shall refer to λ briefly as the *logodds* for covariate vector x.

We now consider maximum likelihood estimation of β based on the data set $D = \{(x_i, y_i) : i = 1, \ldots, n\}$ of the selected cases $S_1, \ldots, S_n$. The loglikelihood l can be expressed as

$$l(\beta|D) = \sum_{i=1}^{n} \left[\delta_{y_i 1} x_i \beta^T - \log \left\{ \exp(x_i \beta^T) + 1 \right\} \right], \qquad (3.15)$$

where

$$\delta_{kj} = \begin{cases} 1 & (j = k) \\ 0 & (j \neq k) \end{cases}$$

is the Kronecker delta. The row vector l_1 of first partial derivatives of l with respect to the components of β can then be easily obtained in the following form:

$$l_1(\beta|D) = \sum_{i=1}^{n} \left\{ \delta_{y_i 1} - \Psi_1(x_i, \beta) \right\} x_i.$$

The likelihood derivative equations $l_1(\beta|D) = 0$ have no explicit solution for β and so recourse has to be made to a numerical method such as the Newton-Raphson iteration or one of its modifications. For this purpose the matrix l_2 of second derivatives is required:

$$l_2(\beta|D) = -\sum_{i=1}^{n} \Psi_1(x_i, \beta)\Psi_2(x_i, \beta)x_i^T x_i.$$

Dropping D from the notation and writing $M(\beta)$ for $\{-l_2(\beta|D)\}^{-1}$ the Newton-Raphson iterative step from present iterate $\beta^{(0)}$ to next iterate $\beta^{(1)}$ can be expressed as

$$\beta^{(1)} = \beta^{(0)} + l_1(\beta^{(0)})M(\beta^{(0)}). \qquad (3.16)$$

Since there is now adequate computer software for this iterative procedure we shall not consider this computational problem further. We may note, however, that if $\hat{\beta}$ denotes the converged vector, and so also the maximum likelihood estimate of β, we may then use $M(\hat{\beta})$ as an estimate of $V(\hat{\beta})$, the covariance matrix of $\hat{\beta}$. An immediate consequence is that for the estimate $\hat{\lambda} = x\hat{\beta}^T$ of the logodds associated with covariate vector x we have an estimated standard error

$$\text{ese}(\hat{\lambda}) = \left\{ x M(\hat{\beta}) x^T \right\}^{\frac{1}{2}}. \tag{3.17}$$

With no explicit formula available for $\hat{\beta}$ we cannot expect to obtain exact recursive relations for the leave-one-out and add-one-in effects as we did for the multivariate normal regression model. We can, however, obtain a useful first approximation by the following argument. Consider the deletion of (x, y) from the data set D to obtain D_-. Again we use a $-$ subscript to denote estimates and other factors associated with the use of D_- rather than D. Then dropping the dependence on D

$$l_-(\beta) = l(\beta) - [\delta_{y1} x \beta^T - \log\{\exp(x\beta^T) + 1\}], \tag{3.18}$$
$$l_{1-}(\beta) = l_1(\beta) - \{\delta_{y1} - \Psi_1(x, \beta)\} x. \tag{3.19}$$

One way to obtain a first approximation to $\hat{\beta}_-$ is to use the Newton-Raphson iterative step with $\beta^{(0)} = \hat{\beta}$ and consider the resulting $\beta^{(1)}$ as our $\hat{\beta}_-$. The matrix $M(\beta)$ in (3.17) is, of course, based on l and D instead of on l_- and D_- but this should not affect the iterative step too much; indeed it is common practice in some forms of Newton-Raphson iteration not to recompute the M matrix at each step. In the resulting iterative step, we can use the fact that $l_1(\hat{\beta}) = 0$ in (3.19) to obtain

$$\hat{\beta}_- = \hat{\beta} - \{\delta_{y1} - \Psi_1(x, \hat{\beta})\} x M(\hat{\beta}).$$

Postmultiplication by x^T and the use of (3.17) yields a corresponding result for the logodds:

$$\hat{\lambda}_- = \hat{\lambda} - \{\delta_{y1} - \Psi_1(x, \hat{\beta})\}\{\text{ese}(\hat{\lambda})\}^2.$$

Similar results hold for the addition of a case (x, y) to the data set D to obtain an augmented data set D_+ with the following approximate relationships:

$$\hat{\beta}_+ = \hat{\beta} + \{\delta_{y1} - \Psi_1(x, \hat{\beta})\} x M(\hat{\beta}), \tag{3.20}$$
$$\hat{\lambda}_+ = \hat{\lambda} + \{\delta_{y1} - \Psi_1(x, \hat{\beta})\}\{\text{ese}(\hat{\lambda})\}^2. \tag{3.21}$$

3.6.1 Alternative models

There is nothing intrinsically correct about the choice of the logistic functions $\Psi_j(x, \beta)$ as the functional forms for the categorical probabilities in the above discussion. They are on the whole used because of their simplicity in providing an appropriate model. Alternatives are possible. For example, for a binary regression model we could have equally set

$$p(y = 1|x, \beta) = \Phi(x\beta^T),$$
$$p(y = 2|x, \beta) = 1 - \Phi(x\beta^T).$$

Indeed in terms of inferences and probability assessments experience suggests that there is little, if any, practical difference between the logistic and normal forms for binary regression models. The explanation for this close agreement undoubtedly lies in the fact that there is a good normal approximation to the standard logistic distribution function $\Psi(t) = \exp(t)/(\exp(t) + 1)$ of the form

$$\Psi(t) = \Phi(0.59t).$$

Such an approximation ensures an error in the relative value of less than 1 percent over the range $t > 0$.

3.6.2 The d-category model

In our discussion above we have deliberately used a terminology and notation which easily extends to the situation where y may be one of d categories $1, 2, \ldots, d$. Instead of the $1 \times c$ parameter vector β of the 2-category model we now have $d - 1$ such $1 \times c$ vectors $\beta_1, \ldots, \beta_{d-1}$ and for subsequent analysis it is convenient to string these out to form an extended $1 \times c(d - 1)$ vector

$$\beta = [\beta_1 \cdots \beta_{d-1}]$$

with β_j as its jth partition. We can then present the d-category model in the following terms.

Definition 3.10 The conditional distribution of a d-category variable y for given covariate x is said to be of logistic regression form with parameter vector β of order $c(d - 1)$ when

$$p(y = j | x, \beta) = \Psi_j(x, \beta),$$

where

$$\Psi_j(x, \beta) = \exp(x\beta_j^T) / \left\{ \sum_{k=1}^{d-1} \exp(x\beta_k^T) + 1 \right\} \quad (j = 1, \ldots, d - 1),$$

$$\Psi_d(x, \beta) = 1 / \left\{ \sum_{k=1}^{d-1} \exp(x\beta_k^T) + 1 \right\}$$

and β_j are the $1 \times c$ partitions of β.

The convenient way to consider logodds for the d-category model is to compare each of the categories $1, \ldots, d - 1$ with category d. For example the logodds on category j against category d,

$$\lambda_j = \log \frac{p(y = j | x, \beta)}{p(y = d | x, \beta)} = x\beta_j^T,$$

is again a linear combination of the components of the covariate vector x.

The loglikelihood $l(\beta | D)$ is only a little more complicated than the loglikelihood of the 2-category model in (3.15):

$$l(\beta | D) = \sum_{i=1}^{n} \left[\sum_{j=1}^{d-1} \delta_{y_i j} x_j \beta_j^T - \log \left\{ \sum_{k=1}^{d-1} \exp(x_i \beta_k^T) + 1 \right\} \right].$$

The vector $l_1(\beta|D)$ of first derivatives of l is now of order $1 \times c(d-1)$ and the matrix $l_2(\beta|D)$ of second derivatives of order $c(d-1) \times c(d-1)$. In what follows we imagine these to be partitioned conformably with the partition of β. The jth partition of $l_1(\beta|D)$, corresponding to first order partial derivatives with respect to the components of β, is

$$\sum_{i=1}^{n} \{\delta_{yij} - \Psi_j(i_i, \beta_j)\}x_i.$$

The submatrices of $l_2(\beta|D)$ corresponding to the (j, j) and (j, k) partitions are

$$-\sum_{i=1}^{n} \Psi_j(x_i, \beta)\{1 - \Psi_j(x_i, \beta)\}x_i^T x_i \qquad (j = k)$$

and

$$-\sum_{i=1}^{n} \Psi_j(x_i, \beta)\Psi_k(x_i, \beta)x_i^T x_i \qquad (j \neq k),$$

respectively.

Again computer software is readily available and we present only the unfamiliar approximate recursive relationships corresponding to those in Properties 3.6 and 3.7. The matrix $M(\beta)$ again denotes the inverse of $-l_2(\beta|D)$. Denoting the submatrix in the (j, k) position of the partition of $M(\beta)$ by $M_{jk}(\beta)$ we know that, for estimates $\hat{\lambda}_j = x\hat{\beta}_j^T$ of the logodds, $\mathrm{cov}(\hat{\lambda}_j, \hat{\lambda}_j)$ is estimated by

$$\mathrm{estcov}(\hat{\lambda}_j, \hat{\lambda}_k) = x M_{jk}(\hat{\beta})x^T.$$

We then have the following approximate recursive relations associated with the removal of (x, y) from D to obtain D_-:

$$\hat{\beta}_- = \hat{\beta} - [\{\delta_{y1} - \Psi_1(x, \beta)\}x \cdots \{\delta_{y,d-1} - \Psi_{d-1}(x, \beta)\}x] M(\hat{\beta}),$$

$$\hat{\lambda}_{j-} = \hat{\lambda}_j - \sum_{k=1}^{d-1} \{\delta_{yk} - \Psi_k(x, \hat{\beta})\}\mathrm{estcov}(\hat{\lambda}_j, \hat{\lambda}_k).$$

For the d-category regression model there is no normal form directly comparable with the simple logistic form. We could, however, envisage a 3-category model of the following form:

$$\begin{aligned}
p(y = 1|x, \beta) &= \Phi(x\beta_1^T), \\
p(y = 2|x, \beta) &= \{1 - \Phi(x\beta_1^T)\}\Phi(x\beta_2^T), \qquad (3.22) \\
p(y = 3|x, \beta) &= \{1 - \Phi(x\beta_1^T)\}\{1 - \Phi(x\beta_2^T)\}.
\end{aligned}$$

This might be appropriate for example if category 1 referred to a normal patient and categories 2 and 3 referred to two different forms of a disease. Since

$$\begin{aligned}
p(y = 1|x, \beta) &= \Phi(x\beta_1^T), \\
p(y = 2 \text{ or } 3|x, \beta) &= \{1 - \Phi(x\beta_1^T)\}
\end{aligned}$$

and

$$p(y = 2|y = 2 \text{ or } 3, x, \beta) = \Phi(x\beta_2^T),$$
$$p(y = 3|y = 2 \text{ or } 3, x, \beta) = 1 - \Phi(x\beta_2^T)$$

we see that the model defined in (3.22) is equivalent to a two-stage model. At the first stage the separation is between normal and diseased patients with β_1 the relevant parameter. The parameter β_2 at stage 2 then refers to the differential diagnosis between categories 2 and 3.

3.7 Lattice testing towards a working model

In Section 3.2 we regarded the setting up of a maximal model for the conditional distribution $p_S(y|x)$ as the most complex description of the dependence of the pattern of variability of y on the covariate vector x we were prepared to envisage. To what extent, however, may this be too complex a model to describe variability in y? Would perhaps a subvector x_H of x provide as adequate a description of the pattern of variability of y as the complete vector x? For example, if our maximal model is the multivariate normal regression model of Definition 3.8

$$Y = XB + E, \tag{3.23}$$

with X of order $n \times c$, then consideration of only a subvector x_H of the covariate vector x is equivalent to consideration of the model

$$Y = X_H B_H + E, \tag{3.24}$$

where X_H is of order $n \times c_H$ and is constructed from the appropriate subvectors. Statistically, (3.24) provides a simpler explanation of the dependence of y on x and is a linear hypothesis within the model (3.23); it is, of course, equivalent to setting to zero the columns of B in (3.23) corresponding to the omitted covariate components. Later we shall have to consider several such hypotheses, but for the moment we confine our attention to the testing of a single hypothesis within the maximal model. If we reject such a hypothesis we conclude that the conditioning stated in the hypothesis does not provide an adequate explanation of the variability of y and we are justified in retaining the more complex explanation in the maximal model. If we cannot reject the hypothesis then we are not justified in using the maximal model: we may then consider use of the hypothesis as a working model on which to base subsequent assessments.

3.8 Testing a single hypothesis

We first provide the basic procedures for testing a hypothesis within our two forms of maximal model: the multivariate normal regression model and the logistic regression model. To make clear what refers to the hypothesis we have already introduced a subscript H as in (3.24); for further emphasis of the distinction between model and hypothesis we also introduce a subscript M when referring to the maximal model.

Property 3.8 For testing the linear hypothesis H,

$$Y = X_H B_H + E,$$

where X_H is $n \times c_H$ and of full rank c_H, within the multivariate normal regression model M,

$$Y = X_M B_M + E,$$

where X_M is $n \times c_M$ and of full rank c_M, let t be the computed value of the test statistic

$$T = 1 - (|R_M|/|R_H|)^a,$$

where R_M and R_H are the residual matrices under M and H respectively. Then the significance probability is

$$1 - J(t|b, c) = J(1 - t|c, b),$$

where a, b, c for special cases are given in Table 3.1, $k = c_M - c_H$ and J is the incomplete beta function given in Definition 3.2. The result is exact for the first four cases and approximate, for large n, in the final case.

Table 3.1 *Characteristics of lattice tests in the normal case*

d	k	n	a	b	c
1	any	$> k+1$	1	$\frac{1}{2}k$	$\frac{1}{2}(n-k-1)$
2	any	$> k+2$	$\frac{1}{2}$	k	$n-k-2$
any	1	$> d+1$	1	$\frac{1}{2}d$	$\frac{1}{2}(n-d-1)$
any	2	$> d+2$	$\frac{1}{2}$	d	$n-d-2$
any	any	'large'	$\left(\dfrac{d^2+k^2-5}{d^2k^2-4}\right)$	$\frac{1}{2}dk$	$\frac{1}{2}[\{n-1-\frac{1}{2}(d+k+1)\}a^{-1}$ $-\frac{1}{2}dk+1]$.

Property 3.9 For testing the hypothesis H,

$$p(y = j|x_H, \beta_H) = \Psi_j(x_H, \beta_H) \qquad (j = 1, \dots, d),$$

where x_H is a $1 \times c_H$ subvector of the $1 \times c_M$ covariate vector, within the logistic regression model M,

$$p(y = j|x_M, \beta_M) = \Psi_j(x_M, \beta_M) \qquad (j = 1, \dots, d),$$

let l_M and l_H be the maximized loglikelihoods under the model M and hypothesis H, respectively. Let t denote the computed value of the generalized likelihood ratio test statistic

$$T = 2(l_M - l_H).$$

Then the significance probability is approximately

$$1 - I(2t|k/2),$$

where $k = c_M - c_H$ and I is the incomplete gamma function from Definition 3.1.

3.9 The lattice of hypotheses

Seldom will our task be as simple as the testing of a single hypothesis within a maximal parametric model. For example, in a diagnostic problem with two disease types, we may be in some doubt as to which, if any, of the components of the covariate (x_1, x_2, x_3) have any diagnostic value. As our maximal model suppose we adopt a logistic regression model

$$p(y = j|x, \beta) = \Psi_j(x, \beta) \qquad (j = 1, 2)$$

as in Definition 3.9. We assume here that x includes a dummy covariate 1 with coefficient β_0. There are now many hypotheses of interest, for example H_2, that $\beta_2 = 0$ or that only x_1 and x_3 are of diagnostic value and not x_2; or again H_{23}, that $\beta_2 = \beta_3 = 0$ or that only x_1 has diagnostic value. Such hypotheses place constraints on the parameters of the maximal model. We can then show clearly the hypotheses of interest and their relations of implication with respect to each other and the maximal model in diagrammatic form in a lattice.

The lattice of Figure 3.1 displays all the possible hypotheses for our simple diagnostic problem. Note the following features of such a lattice. The hypotheses and maximal model have been arranged in a series of levels. At the highest level is the maximal model M with its four parameters $\beta_0, \beta_1, \beta_2, \beta_3$; at the lowest level is the hypothesis of no dependence of disease type on the covariate vector (x_1, x_2, x_3), of essentially unexplained variability of disease type, with only one parameter β_0 related with the incidence rates of the disease types. At intermediate levels are hypotheses of the same intermediate complexity such as H_{23} described above with two parameters β_0, β_1 at level 2, with similarly defined hypotheses H_{12} and H_{13}, and H_1 also described above at level 3 with similarly defined H_2 and H_3. When a hypothesis at a lower level implies one at a higher level the lattice shows a line joining the two hypotheses: for example, the hypothesis H_{23} that $\beta_2 = \beta_3 = 0$ at level 2 implies H_3 that $\beta_3 = 0$ at level 3 and so a join is made between H_{23} and H_3, whereas H_{23} does not imply H_1 that $\beta_1 = 0$ and so no join is made. In short, the lattice displays clearly the relative simplicities and the hierarchy of implication of the hypotheses and their relation to the model.

3.10 Testing within a lattice

Once the maximal model and relevant hypotheses have been set out in a lattice, how should we proceed to test the various hypotheses? The problem is

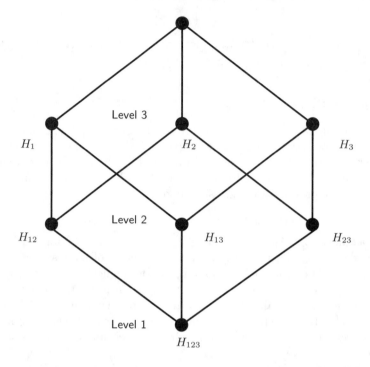

Maximal Model M

Level 3

H_1 H_2 H_3

Level 2

H_{12} H_{13} H_{23}

Level 1

H_{123}

Figure 3.1 *Lattice of hypotheses about the nature of disease type on components of a covariate vector* (x_1, x_2, x_3).

clearly one of testing multiple hypotheses with no optimum solution unless we can frame it as a decision problem with a complete loss structure, a situation seldom realized for such problems. Some more *ad hoc* procedure is usually adopted. In our approach here we adopt the simplicity postulate of Jeffreys (1961), which within our context may be expressed as follows: we prefer a simple explanation, with few parameters, to a more complicated explanation, with many parameters. In terms of the lattice of hypotheses, therefore, we will want to see positive evidence before we are prepared to move from a hypothesis at a lower level to one at a higher level. In terms of standard Neyman-Pearson testing, the setting of the significance level ε at some low value may be viewed as placing some kind of protection on the hypothesis under investigation: if the hypothesis is true our test has only a small probability, at most ε, of rejecting it. With this protection, rejection of a hypothesis is a fairly positive act: we believe that we really have evidence against it. This is ideal for our view of hypothesis testing within a lattice of hypotheses under the simplicity postulate. In moving from a lower level to a higher level we are seeking a mandate to complicate the explanation by introducing further parameters.

The rejection of a hypothesis gives us a positive reassurance that we have reasonable grounds for moving to this more complicated explanation.

Our lattice testing procedure can then be expressed in terms of the following rules.

1. In every test of a hypothesis within the lattice, regard the maximal model as the alternative hypothesis.

2. Start the testing procedure at the lowest level, by testing each hypothesis at that level within the maximal model.

3. Move from one level to the next higher level only if all hypotheses at the lower level have been rejected.

4. Stop testing at the level at which the first non-rejection of a hypothesis occurs. All non-rejected hypotheses at that level are acceptable as 'working models' on which further analysis such as assessment of conditional probabilities may be based.

Assessment of conditional distributions for the working model

Suppose that we have arrived by lattice testing at a working parametric model for the dependence of y on x for a selected case S, say $p_S(y|x, B, \Sigma)$ of $N^d(xB, \Sigma)$ form for multivariate normal regression modelling or $p_S(y|x, \beta)$ equal to $\Psi_y(x, \beta)$ for a logistic regression model. Suppose further that we have carried out the maximum likelihood estimation procedures described in Section 3.4 or 3.6 and have obtained $\hat{B}, \hat{\Sigma}$ or $\hat{\beta}$ whichever is appropriate. Hypothesis testing with the lattice and estimation are, however, not the end of the statistical analysis but only a means towards the solution of the problem as identified in Chapter 2, the assessment of the conditional density function of y for given x for a typical selected case S. Let us denote such an assessment based on the data set D of selected cases $S_1, \ldots, S_n$ by

$$p_S(y|x, D).$$

It is tempting to imagine that for the multivariate normal regression model all we require to do is to replace the parameters B and Σ in $p_S(y|x, B, \Sigma)$ by their estimates $\hat{B}$ and $\hat{\Sigma}$ to give

$$p_S(y|x, D) = p_S(y|x, \hat{B}, \hat{\Sigma}),$$

which is, of course, of $N^d(x\hat{B}, \hat{\Sigma})$ form. Such an estimative method, which uses the estimates as if they were the true values without taking any account of their sampling variabilities, is now known to be less reliable than what has come to be known as the predictive method. The predictive method recognizes that values of B and Σ other than $\hat{B}$ and $\hat{\Sigma}$ are possible by forming a weighted average of the possible $p_S(y|x, B, \Sigma)$ with weighting function $w(B, \Sigma|D)$. As its notation suggests the weights attaching to different (B, Σ) must depend on the data set D. A popular way of arriving at such a weighting function is through a Bayesian analysis with $w(B, \Sigma|D)$ the posterior distribution $p(B, \Sigma|D)$ based on a prior distribution for the parameters (B, Σ). Much argument can then centre on what is an appropriate prior distribution. We shall adopt here the pragmatic view that prior to observing D little is known about (B, Σ) and so a standard vague prior is reasonably appropriate. The issue here is not whether the approach should be Bayesian or otherwise but the practical necessity of adopting a predictive assessment in face of the inadequacies of the estimative assessment. The vague prior weighting function provides a reasonable means of arriving at a predictive assessment.

For ease of future application we state the required predictive assessment result for the multivariate normal regression model.

Property 3.10 For the multivariate normal regression model $p_S(y|x, B, \Sigma)$ of $N^d(xB, \Sigma)$ form for a typical selected case the vague prior predictive assessment $p_S(y|x, D)$ based on the data set $D = \{(x_i, y_i) : i = 1, \ldots, n\}$ of n selected cases $S_1, \ldots, S_n$ is of

$$St^d \left[n - c, x\hat{B}, \{1 + x(X^T X)^{-1} x^T\} \hat{\Sigma} \right] \qquad (3.25)$$

form, where $\hat{B}$ and $\hat{\Sigma}$ are the estimates described in Property 3.2.

In the special case in which there are no covariates, so that $c = 1$, $x = 1$ and $x(X^T X)^{-1} x^T = n^{-1}$, the vague prior predictive assessment has the form

$$St^d \left[n - 1, \bar{x}, \{1 + n^{-1}\} \hat{\sigma}^2 \right]. \qquad (3.26)$$

3.11 Measures of atypicality

We are now in a position to pose the following question for a referred patient R with associated information (x_R, y_R). How typical is (x_R, y_R) of the experience we have met in the data set $D = \{(x_i, y_i) : i = 1, \ldots, n\}$ of selected cases $S_1, \ldots, S_n$ or more specifically in relation to the working model we have obtained for the relevant conditional distribution $p_S(y|x, D)$. We can conveniently base our assessment on the following considerations. The predictive conditional distribution assigns a probability density to each possible y for the given covariate x_R of the referred patient. The smaller the density assigned to a y the more it inclines towards atypicality. First determine the conditional density associated with the actual y_R of the referred patient. Then compute the probability, on the basis of the conditional predictive distribution, that a case with covariate x_R has a conditional density greater than or equal to the conditional density of the referred patient and call this the *atypicality index* of the referred patient. Formally the definition of the atypicality index $A(y_R|x_R)$ of referred patient R is

$$A(y_R|x_R) = \int_{C(y_R|x_R)} p(y|x_R, D) dy, \qquad (3.27)$$

where $C(y_R|x_R)$ is the region

$$\{y : p(y|x_R, D) \geq p(y_R|x_R, D)\} \qquad (3.28)$$

of the space Y.

The atypicality index therefore ranges between 0 and 1 and the closer the index is to 1 the more atypical the referred patient is relative to the experience of the selected cases.

3.11.1 The multivariate normal model

Fortunately the atypicality indices associated with the predictive density function of Property 3.10 are easily computed. The result is contained in the following property.

Property 3.11 Under the conditional predictive assessment of the multivariate regression model of Property 3.2 the atypicality index $A(y_R|x_R)$ of a referred patient R with data (x_R, y_R) is given by

$$J\left[\frac{q_R}{\{q_R + (n-c)(1+h_R)\}} \mid \tfrac{1}{2}, \tfrac{1}{2}(n-c-d+1)\right],$$

where $q_R = (y_R - x_R\hat{B})\hat{\Sigma}^{-1}(y_R - x_R\hat{B})^T$ is the Mahalanobis distance, h_R is the 'hat' value $x_R(X^T X)^{-1}x_R^T$ of the referred patient and J is the incomplete beta function.

Note that the h_R value gives an indication of how typical the referred patient R is with respect to the covariate experience of the selected set of cases. Roughly speaking the larger the value of h_R the further the referred case is from the centre of the covariate cluster and the nearer we may be approaching extrapolation rather than interpolation in our analysis. We note how this is reflected in the atypicality index. For a given q_R value, the larger the value of h_R then we can say the less atypical is R.

3.11.2 Extrapolation index

In the above conditional analysis we have assumed that the covariate vector x_R of the referred patient R is within the previous experience of covariate vectors in the selected cases, and it is clearly important that this should be the case. For example, in a clinical trial on the effect of a particular drug therapy on patients with slightly raised systolic blood pressure, say in the range 110-130 mm Hg, we might record x as the covariate, current systolic blood pressure, say, and y as the response, the reduction in systolic blood pressure. We would surely be reluctant to apply any working model fitted to a new patient with very high systolic blood pressure, say 190 mm Hg. We would be in danger of a very risky form of extrapolation. It is therefore sensible to have some measure of the degree of extrapolation as a check on whether the covariate vector x of a referred patient is reasonably within previous experience.

We can construct such an extrapolation index $\text{ext}(x)$ in the following way. Let $\bar{x}$ and $\hat{\Sigma}$ be the sample mean vector and sample covariance matrix of the selected set of covariate vectors. Define the Mahalanobis distance of selected case S_i as

$$q_i = (x_i - \bar{x})\hat{\Sigma}^{-1}(x_i - \bar{x})^T \qquad (i = 1, \ldots, n)$$

and let q_{min} and q_{max} be the minimum and maximum of these Mahalanobis distances. For a referred case with covariate vector x_R let

$$q_R = (x_R - \bar{x})\hat{\Sigma}^{-1}(x_R - \bar{x})^T$$

and consider

$$\text{ext}(x_R) = \frac{q_R - q_{min}}{q_{max} - q_{min}}$$

as a possible indicator of extrapolation. If $\text{ext}(x_R) \leq 1$ then we can be reasonably sure that we are involved in interpolation. If $\text{ext}(x_R) \geq 1$ then we are involved in extrapolation and the amount of the excess over 1 will provide an indication of just how risky the extrapolation may be.

3.11.3 The logistic regression model

Assessment of conditional distributions for the logistic regression model is less tractable. We can, however, resolve the problem by numerical or approximate methods. To arrive at a predictive assessment we have to apply a weighting function $p(\beta|D)$ to $p_S(y|x, \beta)$ or $\Psi_y(x, \beta)$ to obtain

$$p_S(y|x, D) = \int_{R^{c(d-1)}} \Psi_y(x, \beta)p(\beta|D)d\beta. \tag{3.29}$$

We are thus apparently faced not only with the difficulty of finding a reasonable weighting function, but also with an integration over the whole of $c(d-1)$-dimensional real space. As a means of obtaining a reasonable weighting function we may adopt the Bayesian version of the asymptotic normality properties of maximum likelihood estimation by taking

$$p(\beta|D) = \phi^{c(d-1)}\{\beta|\hat{\beta}, M(\hat{\beta})\}, \tag{3.30}$$

using the notation of Definition 3.3. We may note, however, that $\Psi_y(x, \beta)$ depends on β only in the forms

$$\lambda_1 = x\beta_1^T, \ldots, \lambda_{d-1} = x\beta_{d-1}^T$$

and that the joint distribution of $\lambda = (\lambda_1, \ldots, \lambda_{d-1})$ is also normal with density function $\phi^{d-1}\{\lambda|\hat{\lambda}, \hat{\Lambda}\}$, where the (j, k)th element of $\hat{\Lambda}$ is $xM_{jk}(\hat{\beta})x^T$, as already discussed in Section 3.6.2. Hence the $c(d-1)$-dimensional integral can be dramatically reduced to a $(d-1)$-dimensional integral:

$$p_S(y|x, D) = \int_{R^{d-1}} \Psi_y(\lambda)\phi^{d-1}(\lambda|\hat{\lambda}, \hat{\Lambda})d\lambda, \tag{3.31}$$

where

$$\Psi_y(\lambda) = \frac{\exp(\lambda_y)}{\{\exp(\lambda_1) + \cdots + \exp(\lambda_{d-1}) + 1\}} \quad (y = 1, \ldots, d-1),$$

$$\Psi_d(\lambda) = \frac{1}{\{\exp(\lambda_1) + \cdots + \exp(\lambda_{d-1}) + 1\}}.$$

No explicit form for (3.31) is available and so recourse has to be made to some form of numerical integration or to an approximation. For d not too large the integral in (3.31) is ideally suited to Hermitian integration and, since we shall have recourse to this powerful technique in other problems, we append a note at the end of this section.

To obtain an approximate result for (3.31) consider the Taylor expansion of $\Psi_y(\lambda)$ about $\hat{\lambda}$ up to second order terms:

$$\Psi_y(\lambda) = \Psi_y(\hat{\lambda}) + (\lambda - \hat{\lambda})D\Psi_y(\hat{\lambda}) + \tfrac{1}{2}(\lambda - \hat{\lambda})D^2\Psi_y(\hat{\lambda})(\lambda - \hat{\lambda})^T,$$

where $D\Psi$ and $D^2\Psi$ denote the vector of first derivatives and matrix of second derivatives with respect to λ, respectively. Since $\hat{\lambda}$ is the mean of λ with respect to the $\phi^{d-1}(\lambda|\hat{\lambda}, \hat{\Lambda})$ density function the second term in the integration of (3.31) is zero. Also since

$$
\begin{aligned}
(\lambda - \hat{\lambda})D^2\Psi_y(\hat{\lambda})(\lambda - \hat{\lambda})^T &= \operatorname{trace}\{\lambda - \hat{\lambda})D^2\Psi_y(\hat{\lambda})(\lambda - \hat{\lambda})^T\} \\
&= \operatorname{trace}\{(\lambda - \hat{\lambda})^T(\lambda - \hat{\lambda})^T D^2\Psi_y(\hat{\lambda})\},
\end{aligned}
$$

we arrive at the following approximation:

$$p_S(y|x, D) = \Psi_y(\hat{\lambda}) + \tfrac{1}{2}\operatorname{trace}\{\hat{\Lambda}D^2\Psi_y(\hat{\lambda})\}.$$

We note that for the binary regression model a more satisfactory approximation may be obtained from the fact that a good normal approximation $\Phi(a\lambda)$ may be obtained to the logistic function $\Psi_1(\lambda)$, where $a = 0.59$. Thus when $\Psi_1(\lambda)$ and $\Psi_2(\lambda)$ in (3.13) and (3.14) are replaced by $\Phi_1(a\lambda)$ and $1-\Phi_1(a\lambda)$ we have one-dimensional convolution integrals so that the predictive assessments in (3.29) become

$$p_S(y = 1|x, D) = \Phi\left[a\hat{\lambda}/\{1 + xM(\hat{\beta})x^T\}^{\frac{1}{2}}\right], \qquad (3.32)$$

$$p_S(y = 2|x, D) = 1 - \Phi\left[a\hat{\lambda}/\{1 + xM(\hat{\beta})x^T\}^{\frac{1}{2}}\right]. \qquad (3.33)$$

The reliability distribution

The derivation of the predictive assessments in (3.32) and (3.33) above is simply the computation of the expectation of $p(y|x, \beta)$ with respect to the posterior distribution $p(\beta|D)$. In doing this we are looking at a single characteristic, namely the mean of a distribution over the interval $(0,1)$, namely that induced on $p(y|x, \beta)$ as a function of the parameter β by the distribution $p(\beta|D)$. Such a distribution provides some indication of the reliability of the predictive assessment in the sense that we hope that there is not a great variation about the mean value. We shall thus term this distribution the *reliability distribution* of the categorical regression model.

For the logistic binary regression model we can readily identify the form of the reliability distribution. The predictive assessment splits the unit of probability available between two parts $y = 1$ and $y = 2$ and so is mathematically a two-part composition as defined in Section 4.2. The corresponding logratio

$$\log \frac{p(y = 1|x, \beta)}{p(y = 2|x, \beta)} = x\beta^T = \lambda$$

is, from the above discussion, of the approximate $N(x\beta^T, xMx^T)$ form, from
(3.30), and we have $p(y = 1|x, \beta)$ distributed according to the logistic-normal
form $L^1(x\beta^T, xMx^T)$. Logistic-normal distributions will be discussed in more
detail in Section 4.2. For our purposes here we require only the density function
of $L^1(\mu, \sigma^2)$ which has the form

$$\frac{1}{\sigma\sqrt{2\pi}y(1-y)} \exp\left\{-\frac{1}{2\sigma^2}\left(\log\frac{y}{1-y} - \mu\right)^2\right\} \quad (0 < y < 1).$$

The idea clearly extends to the d-category case with the predictive assessment composition

$$\{p(y = 1|x, \beta), \dots, p(y = d|x, \beta)\}$$

of the $L^{d-1}(\lambda, \Lambda)$ form discussed in detail in Section 4.2.

We shall see in Chapter 8 how useful this concept of reliability distribution
can be. Figure 3.2 shows four examples (a)-(d) of reliability distributions, each
with the same predictive assessment $p(y = 1|x, D)$ of 0.75. It is clear from
the reliability distributions that these inferences are in descending order of
reliability and that for (d) the mean value of 0.75 emerges only as a confusion
between stronger possibilities that $p(y = 1|x, \beta)$ is more likely to be near 0 or
near 1 than near 0.75.

Extrapolation index in the logistic regression model

Investigation of atypicality for this model is not relevant but we can ask
as above whether the referred case R has a covariate x_R which ensures that
we are not in danger of extrapolating in our inferences about R. Thus we
may examine $\text{ext}(y_R|x_R)$ as above in the multivariate regression model to
give some indication of the extent to which we may be extrapolating rather
than interpolating from experience.

A note on multivariate Hermitian integration

Any integral of the form

$$\int_{R^d} g(z) \exp(-z^T z) dz, \tag{3.34}$$

where $g(z)$ is a reasonably smooth function on R^d, can be approximated by a
multiple sum

$$\sum_{i_1=1}^{k} \cdots \sum_{i_d=1}^{k} w_{i_1} \dots w_{i_d} g(z_1, \dots, z_d),$$

where $w_1, \dots, w_k$ and $z_1, \dots, z_k$ are the weights and points for Hermitian
integration of order k on R^1; see, for example, Abramowitz and Stegun (1972).

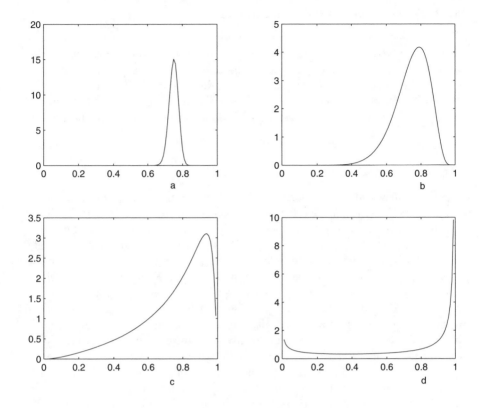

Figure 3.2 *Four reliability curves each with the same predictive diagnostic assessment.*

In our statistical applications in clinical medicine we shall encounter a number of integrals of the form

$$\int_{R^d} f(y)\phi^d(y|\mu, \Sigma)dy,$$

where μ and Σ are known. For such an integral we can always find a transformation

$$y = \mu + \sqrt{2}T\,z,$$

where $AA^T = \Sigma$, and application of this yields

$$\int_{R^d} \pi^{-d/2} f(\mu + \sqrt{2}T\,z) \exp(-z'z)dz,$$

which is of the form of (3.34) with

$$g(z) = \pi^{-d/2} f(\mu + \sqrt{2}T\,z).$$

3.12 Concordance of data and model

The process of arriving at a working model to describe the pattern of variability observed in a data set is a complex one and it is sensible to undertake a thorough review of how well working model and data are in agreement. Are any of the assumptions of the working model challenged by the data? Are there any cases which seem to be unduly influencing the choice of the working model? Methods of investigating such important questions are the subject matter of this section.

3.12.1 Tests of normality

For the multivariate regression model the underlying assumption is that the conditional distribution of y for given covariate vector x is $N^d(x\mathrm{B}, \Sigma)$. This assumption of the normal form, essentially for the distribution of the residual vector e in the linear form $y = x\mathrm{B} + e$, can be tested. From the battery of such tests we describe below the range of tests we have found most useful. All these tests are based on a similar idea. From the set of residuals $r_i = y_i - x_i\hat{\mathrm{B}}$ $(i = 1, \ldots, n)$ each test introduces some transformation $t = f(r)$ leading to t_i $(i = 1, \ldots, n)$ whose distribution, under the assumption of normality of e, is known, say with distribution function $G(t)$. Then each of $z_j = G(t_j)$ $(j = 1, \ldots, n)$ is uniformly distributed over the interval $(0,1)$ and, although not strictly independent because of their common dependence on the y_i, are considered so in the assessment of significance probabilities. The argument then continues that the set of (increasingly) ordered z_j, say $z_{[j]}$ $(j = 1, \ldots, n)$, should correspond approximately to quantiles of the uniform distribution over $(0,1)$. There is some element of choice about which particular set of quantiles are appropriate; in what follows we have chosen those given by $o_j = (j - 0.5)/n$ $(j = 1, \ldots, n)$.

From the variety of tests based on the order statistics $z_{[j]}$ $(j = 1, \ldots, n)$, each aimed at a different form of departure from normality, we have selected three test statistics, the Anderson-Darling Q_A, the Cramer-von Mises Q_C and the Watson Q_W, defined as follows:

$$Q_A = -(1/n) \sum_{i=1}^{n} (2i - 1)\{\log z_{[i]} + \log(1 - z_{[n+1-i]})\} - n,$$

$$Q_C = \sum_{i=1}^{n} \{z_{[i]} - (2i - 1)/(2n)\}^2 + 1/(12n),$$

$$Q_W = Q_C - n(\bar{z} - 1/2)^2.$$

Q-Q plots

Under the assumption of normality of the residuals r, if the ordered set of residuals is plotted against the corresponding theoretical quantiles obtained as $\bar{r} + s_r \Phi^{-1}(o_{[i]})$, where $\bar{r}$ and s_r denote the mean and standard deviation of the residuals, then the resulting points should lie approximately along the diagonal of the (square) plot. Such a diagram, often referred to as a Q-Q plot, provides a useful visual guide with curvature often providing a clear indication of the need to question the normality assumption and take remedial measures. See Chapter 5 for examples of this form of plot.

Marginal tests

Corresponding to each component r_j of a residual vector r we can obtain a marginal test of normality through the transformation $t_j = r_j/\sqrt{\sigma_{jj}}$ and by setting $G = \Phi$, the standard normal cumulative distribution function.

Bivariate tests

Since e has a $N^d(0, \Sigma)$ distribution we can find a transformation $w = Me$ such that w has a spherical normal distribution $N^d(0, I_d)$. The transformation matrix M will, of course, depend on Σ but can be approximated by M obtained from the estimate $\hat{\Sigma}$. Corresponding to each pair of components (r_j, r_k) of a residual vector r we can obtain a bivariate angle test based on the following considerations. Since the distribution of (w_j, w_k) is circular normal centred on the origin, the angle t_{jk} which the vector from $(0,0)$ to (w_j, w_k) makes with the w_j axis should be uniformly distributed over the range $(0, 2\pi)$. Then $z = G(t) = t/(2\pi)$ produces the necessary transformed residuals which should be approximately uniformly distributed over $(0,1)$.

Radius test

In this test $t = r\Sigma^{-1}r^T$, what we referred to as the Mahalanobis distance in Section 3.11. Then G is the distribution function of the $\chi^2(d)$ distribution or, equivalently, of the $Ga(\frac{1}{2}d)$ distribution.

The critical values for all these tests are based on slightly modified versions of the test statistics and are provided in Table 3.2.

3.12.2 Transformations to normality

When a data set fails tests of normality a question often posed is whether some transformation, say $y_j^{(c)}$ of the jth component of y, may yield residuals which are closer to multivariate normality. One useful class of transformations is the Box-Cox class, defined by

$$y_j^{(t_j)} = \begin{cases} (y_j^{t_j} - 1)/t_j & (t_j \neq 0), \\ \log(y_j) & (t_j = 0). \end{cases}$$

On the assumption that $y^{(t)}$ follows a multivariate normal regression model $N^d(xB, \Sigma)$, the loglikelihood $l(t, B, \Sigma)$ can be written as

Table 3.2 *Modified empirical distribution function test statistics and their critical values*

Significance level (per cent)	Anderson-Darling	Cramer-von-Mises	Watson
Marginal tests			
	$Q_A \left[1 + \frac{4}{n} - \frac{25}{n^2}\right]$	$Q_C \left[1 + \frac{1}{2n}\right]$	$Q_W \left[1 + \frac{1}{2n}\right]$
10	0.656	0.104	0.096
5	0.787	0.126	0.116
2.5	0.918	0.148	0.136
1	1.092	0.178	0.163
Bivariate angle and radius tests			
	Q_A	$\left[Q_C - \frac{0.4}{n} + \frac{0.6}{n^2}\right] \times \left[1 + \frac{1}{n}\right]$	$\left[Q_W - \frac{0.1}{n} + \frac{0.1}{n^2}\right] \times \left[1 + \frac{0.8}{n}\right]$
10	1.933	0.347	0.152
5	2.492	0.461	0.187
2.5	3.070	0.581	0.221
1	3.857	0.743	0.267

$$l(t, \mathrm{B}, \Sigma) = -\tfrac{1}{2}d\log(2\pi) - \tfrac{1}{2}\log(|\Sigma|) + \sum_{j=1}^{d}(t_j - 1)\sum_{i=1}^{n}y_{ij}$$
$$-\tfrac{1}{2}\mathrm{trace}\{(Y - X\mathrm{B})\Sigma^{-1}(Y - X\mathrm{B})^T\}. \qquad (3.35)$$

Choice of $t = (t_1, \ldots, t_d)$ is then determined by maximization of l with respect to t, B, Σ. Since for given t the corresponding maximizing values of B, Σ are simply

$$\hat{\mathrm{B}}_t = (X^T X)^{-1} X^T Y^{(t)},$$
$$\hat{\Sigma}_t = (Y^{(t)} - X\hat{\mathrm{B}}_t)^T (Y^{(t)} - X\hat{\mathrm{B}}_t)/(n - d)$$

those obtained from replacing Y by $Y^{(t)}$ in the standard linear model given in Definition 3.8, the usual maximization procedure is to program the easily computed profile loglikelihood given by

$$l_P(t) = \max_{\mathrm{B}, \Sigma} l(t, \mathrm{B}, \Sigma) = l(t, \hat{\mathrm{B}}_t, \hat{\Sigma}_t)$$

and to maximize this profile loglikelihood with respect to t.

As a test of whether the use of the corresponding maximizing t is justified we can carry out a test of the hypothesis $t = 1$ which corresponds to no transformation, with 1 denoting a d-vector of 1s. A simple approximate test here is to compare

$$2\{l(\hat{t}, \hat{B}_t, \hat{\Sigma}_t) - l(t = 1, \hat{B}, \hat{\Sigma})\} \tag{3.36}$$

against critical values of the $\chi^2(d)$ distribution.

3.12.3 Atypicality

In Section 3.11 we introduced the concept of the atypicality index of a referred patient R relative to the set $S_1, \ldots, S_n$ of selected cases. A useful way of checking whether any one of the selected cases, say S with corresponding vector (x, y), may be unduly influencing our inferences is to ask how typical it would appear relative to the reduced data set D_- consisting of D with the case S removed. A simple way of assessing this is to compute the atypicality index $A(y|x)$ of S with respect to D_-. The result is contained in the following property.

Property 3.12 Under the conditional predictive assessment of the multivariate regression model the atypicality index $A(y|x)$ of a selected case S with vector (x, y) with respect to the reduced data set D_- is given by

$$J\left[\frac{q_S}{q_S + \{(n - c)(1 - h_S)\}} \mid \tfrac{1}{2}d, \tfrac{1}{2}(n - c - d)\right],$$

where $q_S = (y - x\hat{B})\hat{\Sigma}^{-1}(y - x\hat{B})^T$ is the conditional Mahalanobis distance, $h_S = x(X^T X)^{-1}x^T$ is the 'hat' value of the selected case S relative to the full data set D and J is the incomplete beta function given in Definition 3.2.

The simplicity of this computation has exploited the recursive relationships of Property 3.6 and to examine all the selected cases in this way requires the q_S and h_S values to be computed only once relative to the full data set D. We may also note here that the value of the atypicality depends upon two aspects of the selected case, with h_S reflecting the extent to which the position of S in the covariate space is one of extrapolation and with q_S measuring the extent of the departure of S from the fitted regression model. We note particularly here the way in which h_S and q_S combine in the form $q_S/(1 - h_S)$ in the formula for the atypicality index. The larger either of those characteristics is the larger will be the atypicality index.

3.12.4 Regression diagnostics

We have seen above in the leave-one-out atypicality index one measure of the possible influence that a selected case may have on the inferences we make. We should certainly ask questions about any such case with a high atypicality index relative to the associated reduced data set. There is now a large literature under the general heading of regression diagnostics. In general these are h_S or q_S separately or in some combination of the two characteristics. For example h_S is often referred to as the leverage of S and since the average value of all the leverages in the selected set is $(1/n)\text{trace}\{X(X^TX)^{-1}X^T\}$ it is sometimes suggested that cases with leverage greater than $2c/n$ should be investigated carefully as possibly having undue influence on the statistical analysis. In the next subsection we consider one measure which seems particularly appropriate within the context of assessing the relevant conditional distributions required in clinical medicine.

3.12.5 Influence in terms of Kullback-Liebler divergences

In terms of the multivariate regression model if we were to leave out the selected case S from the data set we would arrive at the relevant conditional predictive density function $p(y|x, D_-)$ for describing the variability in the y of S for given x. On the other hand, if we were to regard S as a new case then the corresponding predictive density function would be $p(y|x, D)$. Clearly then in terms of the basic problem in clinical medicine of trying to assess conditional distributions some measure of how far $p(y|x, D)$ is from the target $p(y|x, D_-)$ will be sensible in determining the extent to which S is atypical or influential. Such a measure is provided by the Kullback-Liebler directed divergence measure

$$K(y|x) = \int_Y p(y|x, D_-) \log \frac{p(y|x, D_-)}{p(y|x, D)} dy.$$

With the use of the recursive relations of Property 3.6 this can readily be evaluated in terms of h_S and q_S as

$$
\begin{aligned}
K(y|x) = \ & -\tfrac{1}{2}(n-c)d - \tfrac{1}{2}d\log\frac{n-c}{n-c-1} + \tfrac{1}{2}\frac{h_S^2 q_S}{(1-h_S)^2} \\
& -\tfrac{1}{2}\log\left(1 - \frac{q_S}{(n-c)(1-h_S)}\right) \\
& +\tfrac{1}{2}\frac{n-c}{n-c-1}\left(d - \frac{q_S}{(n-c)(1-h_S)}\right).
\end{aligned}
$$

Note that this involves an expression $h_S^2/(1-h_S)$ in h_S alone which increases with h_S, with the remaining part involving the now familiar combination $q_S/(1-h_S)$.

3.13 Bibliographic notes

Much of the statistical modelling and methodology of this chapter is obtainable in standard texts. For example, the normal regression model has a long history and details can be found in such references as Anderson (1984), Rao (1965), Johnston and Wichern (1998), Mardia, Kent and Bibby (1979), Morrison (1976) and most statistical software supports the computational aspects of the methods. Less well known, perhaps, are such aspects as the recurrence formula of Section 3.5 which are an extended version of Clarke (1971) and Campbell (1985).

The categorical regression model dates back to probit analysis introduced by Gaddum (1933) and Bliss (1934) and developed by R.A. Fisher; for a detailed account and references see the monograph by Finney (1971). The simpler logistic analysis is based on the alternative first introduced by Berkson (1944). There was indeed a heated dispute over the relative merits of these approaches, neither party seeming to realise that the practical differences were negligible because of the closeness of the normal and logistic distribution functions. For modern accounts see McCullagh and Nelder (1989), Collett (2003a) and Agresti (2002).

Lattice testing is based on simplicity and parsimony concepts going back to William of Ockam and well expressed in Jeffreys (1961). In our view when faced with a multiple hypotheses situation the statistician is well advised to construct a lattice as in Section 3.9. Our own experience in working with these was developed in the 1970's in collaboration with A D McLaren in statistical laboratory work in the undergraduate classes in the University of Glasgow. These were partly developed to counteract confusion caused in the use of standard analysis of variance tables. The only text we are aware of which uses such an approach is Aitchison (1986).

The use of the predictive distribution is old though not well known and is traceable to Bayes (1763) for a very simple situation. Jeffreys (1961) also was a strong advocate of the concept. For a detailed account of uses of predictive distributions, see Aitchison and Dunsmore (1975).

Normal ranges, usually for univariate measurements, have been used in clinical medicine for many years. An early advocate of the consideration of multivariate measurements was Hamilton (1956) though no technique for implementation was considered. The extension to multivariate measurements through the use of the atypicality index seems relatively new with Aitchison and Kay (1975) providing a formal definition and means of computation; see also Aitchison and Dunsmore (1975).

The extrapolation index and reliability curve are, we believe, new to this book.

Much is available on tests of concordance of data and model. The normal tests are based on the expository article by Stephens (1982) and may be also found in Aitchison (1986). Regression diagnostics, in both its normal and categorical form, is a huge subject, covered in such texts and papers as Cook and Weisberg (1982) and Pregibon (1981).

We believe that the use of the K-L influence measure is an appropriate one in clinical problems and is, as far as we are aware, new.

3.14 Problems

Problem 3.1 Using the general form of the results in Property 3.2 establish for the simple univariate model of linear regression

$$y_i = \alpha + \beta x_i + e_i \quad (i = 1, \ldots, n),$$

where e_i $(i = 1, \ldots, n)$ are independent $N(0, \sigma^2)$ errors and the x_i are real numbers, that

$$\hat{\beta} = \sum_{i=1}^{n}(x_i - \bar{x})(y_i - \bar{y}) \Big/ \sum_{i=1}^{n}(x_i - \bar{x})^2 \,,$$

$$\hat{\alpha} = \bar{y} - \hat{\beta}\bar{x},$$

where $\bar{x}, \bar{y}$ are the means of the x_i, y_i observations.

Show that the h value corresponding to the last observation (x_n, y_n) is

$$h = \frac{1}{n} + \frac{(x_n - \bar{x})^2}{\sum_{i=1}^{n}(x_i - \bar{x})^2}$$

and hence find expressions for estimates of α and β formed from the data set diminished by the removal of (x_n, y_n).

Problem 3.2 Suppose that a clinic has devised a differential diagnostic system for two types $t = 1, 2$ and based on a $1 \times c$ feature vector x on the basis of a fitted binary normal model

$$\Pr(t = 1 | x, \beta) = 1 - \Pr(t = 2 | x, \beta) = \Phi(x\beta^T).$$

Suppose further that the referred patients have feature vectors which follow a $N^c(\mu, \Omega)$ distribution. Show that the clinic will diagnose a proportion

$$\Phi\left\{ \frac{\mu\beta^T}{(1 + \beta\Omega\beta^T)^{\frac{1}{2}}} \right\}$$

of referred patients as of type 1.

Suppose that an alternative system based on a binary logistic model with

$$\Pr(t = 1 | x, \gamma) = 1 - \Pr(t = 2 | x, \gamma) = \Psi(x\gamma^T)$$

is used. Find an approximation to the proportion of referred patients diagnosed as of type 1.

Problem 3.3 Identify some of the hypotheses of interest for problems 1.1, 1.3, 1.4, 1.5 and construct appropriate lattices for the investigation of these hypotheses.

Problem 3.4 In assessing the infectivity of a patient a clinic has decided that the variability of the total count of bacteria in 100 blood cells is well described by a Poisson distribution with probability function

$$p(y|\theta) = \exp(-\theta)\theta^y / y! \quad (y = 0, 1, 2, \ldots).$$

On the assumption that a Bayesian posterior distribution for θ of $Ga(\alpha, \beta)$ form has been obtained from a set of selected patients what predictive form for a patient count y would you suggest?

Problem 3.5 A clinic with large experience of the relationship of how a measurement y varies with age x has decided that a reasonable predictive conditional density function for the dependence of y on x is of lognormal form $\Lambda(\alpha + \beta x, \sigma^2)$. On the assumption that only large measurements are regarded as atypical what atypicality index would you assign to a patient aged x_R with measurement y_R ?

Problem 3.6 A study of the effects of a treatment for patients with a certain history of blood pressure problems has been carried out. Recorded below are the initial systolic and diastolic blood pressures in mm Hg of 15 patients in the study and their corresponding blood pressures at the end of treatment.

Before treatment		After treatment	
Systolic	Diastolic	Systolic	Diastolic
166	109	143	103
153	111	139	105
171	111	160	105
173	111	161	93
159	97	138	86
182	119	151	110
182	104	154	103
170	116	144	109
173	126	155	110
172	105	136	95
168	116	141	110
177	124	161	125
164	93	148	79
192	108	175	92
169	114	148	104

Compute the extrapolation indices of the patients in the study by the leave-one-out method.

Would you regard it as reasonable to predict the effect of this treatment for the following two patients with blood pressures as follows?

Patient	Systolic	Diastolic
1	160	120
2	185	95

Problem 3.7 In a study of the value of a diagnostic test result x for the differential diagnosis of two types $t = 1, 2$ a clinic has arrived at a logistic

regression model

$$\Pr(t = 1 | x, \alpha, \beta) = 1 - \Pr(t = 2 | x, \alpha, \beta) = \frac{\exp(\alpha + \beta x)}{1 + \exp(\alpha + \beta x)},$$

with information about α, β contained in a posterior normal distribution with mean vector $(1.5, -0.2)$ and covariance matrix

$$\begin{bmatrix} 0.12 & -0.05 \\ -0.05 & 0.20 \end{bmatrix}.$$

Sketch the reliability curves associated with the use of this system for patients with test results $x = 0.1, 2.0, 5.0$, respectively.

Problem 3.8 The following two data sets consist of two different test results (in standard units) on each of 20 normal patients. Draw the Q-Q plots for each of these data sets and comment on the possible nature of the underlying distributions.

Test 1	Test 2
99	702
73	1100
118	914
112	88
87	326
86	545
82	62
123	251
94	463
96	49
69	71
108	471
166	199
107	357
65	895
106	341
65	85
104	458
59	167
118	82

CHAPTER 4

Further Statistical Methodology

4.1 Introduction

We consider in this chapter some statistical methods that are a little more specialised. In Section 4.2 we present a discussion of regression analysis when the response vector is compositional in nature and describe a methodology for modelling such data. Following up on the material on binary logistic regression contained in Chapter 3, we then consider in Section 4.3 a Bayesian solution which overcomes the problem of complete separation. In Section 4.4 we discuss the challenge of statistical diagnosis when the types are naturally tree-structured. In our applications we have used mixed-effects models, which are briefly introduced in Section 4.5, and also Gibbs sampling, which is discussed in Section 4.6. Biplots often provide a useful summary of multivariate data and we discuss them in Section 4.7 in the contexts of unconstrained and compositional multivariate data. Finally in Section 4.8 we consider some kernel methods which are useful in non-parametric modelling.

4.2 Compositional regression analysis

4.2.1 The nature of compositional data

Compositional data consisting of vectors of positive components summing to unity, usually as proportions of some whole, arise in clinical medicine. For example the compositions of renal calculi may be set out as the proportions of occurrence of four different types of stone: calcium, struvite, uric acid or cystine. A less obvious example is in differential diagnostic assessments, where the available unit of probability is distributed among the set of mutually exclusive and exhaustive categories of disease. Such compositional data can be set out in a compositional data matrix $Z = [z_{ni}]$ with z_{ni} the ith component of the nth D-part composition. The typical vector $(z_1, \ldots, z_D)$ of such a D-part composition has components z_i $(i = 1, \ldots, D)$ subject to the unit-sum constraint $z_1 + \cdots + z_D = 1$. This unit-sum constraint reduces the effective dimension of D-part compositions to $d = D - 1$, and an appropriate sample space for the study of compositions is then the d-dimensional unit simplex S^d. There is now an extensive literature demonstrating the folly of applying standard statistical methodology such as product-moment correlation, which was designed for the analysis of unconstrained multivariate data, to such constrained vectors either by ignoring the constraint or by dropping out one of the components.

Particularly important in the study of compositions is the concept of a sub-composition, the counterpart of a marginal distribution in unconstrained multivariate analysis, and a requirement that any form of analysis must possess subcompositional coherence. This is best considered in terms of two scientists A and B, with A able to record all the D parts of the composition and so arrive at the full composition $(z_1, \ldots, z_D)$, whereas B is aware of, or can record, only some of the parts, say $1, \ldots, C$, and so arrives at the $(1, \ldots, C)$-subcomposition $(s_1, \ldots, s_c) = (z_1, \ldots, z_c)/(z_1 + \cdots + z_c)$.

The requirement of subcompositional coherence is then simply that any inference which scientist A makes about the parts $1, \ldots, C$ from the full compositions should coincide with the corresponding inference made about these parts by scientist B from the subcompositions. Simplistic ideas such as the product-moment correlation between raw components do not have this necessary subcompositional coherence. A simple illustrative example shows the folly of the use of product-moment correlation of the crude components, namely $\mathrm{corr}(z_1, z_2)$ for A and $\mathrm{corr}(s_1, s_2)$ for B, as a means of communication. For example, for the 4-part compositions

$$(0.1, 0.2, 0.1, 0.6), \quad (0.2, 0.1, 0.1, 0.6), \quad (0.3, 0.3, 0.2, 0.2)$$

and the 3-part subcompositions formed from parts 1, 2, 3, namely

$$(.25, .50, .25), \quad (.50, 0.25, 0.25), \quad (0.375, 0.375, 0.25),$$

we have $\mathrm{corr}(z_1, z_2) = 0.5$ and $\mathrm{corr}(s_1, s_2) = -1$.

4.2.2 Covariance structures for compositions

Our knowledge that any meaningful function of a composition must be expressible in terms of ratios of components and the obvious fact that ratios are unaltered in the process of forming subcompositions $(s_i/s_j = z_i/z_j)$ leads us inevitably to consideration of some form of covariance structure for compositions based upon ratios of components. We reiterate here that subcompositions play a central role in compositional data analysis, replacing the concept of marginals in unconstrained multivariate data analysis.

Recognition that the study of compositions is concerned with relative and not absolute magnitudes of the components has led to the advocacy of forms of analysis which involve logarithms of the ratios of components. Note that such a form of analysis meets the demands of subcompositional coherence, since ratios and, a fortiori, logratios of components are invariant under the operation of forming a subcomposition. There are three equivalent definitions of compositional covariance structure, the advantage of any particular form depending on the nature of the application. For a D-part composition $(z_1, \ldots, z_D)$ these are defined as the set of relative variances

$$\tau_{jk} = \mathrm{var}\{\log(z_j/z_k)\} \qquad (j = 1, \ldots, D - 1; \ k = j, \ldots, D), \qquad (4.1)$$

the logratio covariance matrix $\Sigma = [\sigma_{jk}]$ with

$$\sigma_{jk} = \text{cov}\{\log(z_j/z_D), \log(z_k/z_D)\} \qquad (j, k = 1, \ldots, D-1) \qquad (4.2)$$

and the centred logratio covariance matrix $\Gamma = [\gamma_{jk}]$ with

$$\gamma_{jk} = \text{cov}\{\log(z_j/g(z)), \log(z_k/g(z))\} \qquad (j, k = 1, \ldots, D), \qquad (4.3)$$

where $g(z)$ is the geometric mean of the components of z.

Note that in terms of the logratio vector

$$y = \{\log(z_1/z_D), \ldots, \log(z_{D-1}/z_D)\}$$

the covariance structure is being defined in terms of the covariance matrix of y with typical elements σ_{jk}. The relationship of the τ_{jk} to the basic logratio variances σ_{jk} is simply obtained as $\tau_{jk} = \sigma_{jj} + \sigma_{kk} - 2\sigma_{jk}$.

There appears to be some reluctance to change from the bad habits and meaningless consequences of ignoring the special nature of compositional data. In the unconstrained world the concept of product-moment correlation is so ingrained into statistical argument as a useful and straightforward tool for the description of dependence that it is difficult to conceive of other ways of describing dependence. For example, within logratio analysis the simplest construct of two components is the logratio variance $\tau_{jk} = \text{var}\{\log(z_j/z_k)\}$ and this can range over all non-negative values. The value zero, in which case z_j and z_k are in constant proportion, replaces the concept of 'perfect positive correlation' whereas large values, corresponding to the components departing substantially from constant proportionality, replace the concept of 'negative correlation'.

Despite the fact that the simplest of these covariance structure specifications, the set of relative variances, involves consideration of just two components at a time, the unfamiliarity of the concept of a covariance structure being defined by a set of variances and the additional complexity in the other forms seem to act as deterrents to potential users of the logratio methodology. Moreover, although it is obvious that any question concerning compositions must be expressible in terms of ratios, and hence of logratios, there seems to be misunderstanding as to the nature of logratio transformations in the statistical analysis of compositional data. It is therefore of some importance to attempt to provide insights into the nature of compositional data by as simple means as possible. We shall see in Section 5.5.2 that compositional biplots often provide such insights.

If we wish for a compositional data set something equivalent to the mean vector and the covariance matrix for a data set of unconstrained vectors then we can do no better than set out in a $D \times D$ variation array the obvious sample estimates of $\text{E}\{\log(z_j/z_k)\}$ below the diagonal and the sample estimates of $\text{var}\{\log(z_j/z_k)\}$ above the leading diagonal of the array.

4.2.3 Parametric classes of distributions on the simplex

The well-known Dirichlet class of distributions on the simplex with typical density function proportional to

$$z_1^{\alpha_1 - 1} \cdots z_D^{\alpha_D - 1}$$

is incapable of describing the vast majority of situations of compositional variability. The main reason for this is that the Dirichlet distribution has the maximum degree of independence available to compositions. For example, every subcomposition is independent of any other non-overlapping subcomposition. To describe real variability, and to allow the investigation of hypotheses of independence, some parametric class richer in dependence structure is required. An answer to this is to be found in the old idea of inducing a distribution (for example, the lognormal distribution) on an awkward space (the positive real line) from one (the normal distribution) on a more familiar space (the real line) by way of transformations (the exponential and logarithmic) between the two spaces. Our situation with awkward space S^d and familiar space R^d and its multivariate normal class is hardly more difficult than this early use of the transformation technique. Probably the simplest transformation from $y \in R^d$ to $z \in S^d$ is the 'additive' logistic transformation $z = \text{alg}(y)$, defined by

$$
\begin{aligned}
z_j &= \exp(y_j)/\{\exp(y_1) + \cdots + \exp(y_d) + 1\} \quad (j = 1, \ldots, d), \\
z_D &= 1/\{\exp(y_1) + \cdots + \exp(y_d) + 1\}
\end{aligned}
\tag{4.4}
$$

with inverse transformation from S^d to R^d given by the logratio transformation $y = \text{alr}(z)$, defined by

$$y_j = \log(z_j/z_D) \quad (j = 1, \ldots, d). \tag{4.5}$$

There are, of course, many other possible such transformations which may be of relevance to certain aspects of compositional data analysis but we shall confine attention here to the simple version above.

We provide a formal definition of the logistic-normal parametric class of distributions on the simplex

$$S^d = \{(z_1, \ldots, z_D) : z_i > 0 \, (i = 1, \ldots, D), z_1 + \cdots + z_D = 1\}.$$

Definition 4.1 A D-part composition z is said to be distributed with logistic-normal form $L^d(\mu, \Sigma)$ if

$$y = \text{alr}(z) = \{\log(z_1/z_D), \ldots, \log(z_d/z_D)\}$$

is distributed as $N^d(\mu, \Sigma)$ over R^d. The corresponding density function $p(z)$ is

$$\frac{1}{(2\pi)^{d/2} \left(\prod_{i=1}^{D} z_i \right) |\Sigma|^{\frac{1}{2}}} \exp[-\tfrac{1}{2}\{\text{alr}(z) - \mu\}\Sigma^{-1}\{\text{alr}(z) - \mu\}^T] \quad (z \in S^d).$$

4.2.4 A methodology for compositional data analysis

The above discussion suggests a simple methodology for compositional data analysis: transform each composition $(z_1, \ldots, z_D)$ to its logratio vector

$$y = \{\log(z_1/z_D), \ldots, \log(z_d/z_D)\}$$

and, after reformulating your problem about compositions in terms of the corresponding logratio vectors, apply the appropriate, standard multivariate procedures to the logratio vectors.

Since any meaningful function of a composition must always be expressible in terms of ratios, and therefore logratios, of components, the required reformulation can always be achieved. The fact that the final component is used as divisor raises the question of whether the choice of another divisor might lead to a different conclusion. It can readily be established that standard multivariate statistical procedures are invariant under the group of permutations of the parts $1, \ldots, D$ of the composition, in particular with respect to a common divisor z_j different from z_D.

4.2.5 Assessment of conditional distributions for the compositional
     regression model

As we have seen above an appropriate form of analysis of compositional data is to use the transformation from D-part composition $(z_1, \ldots, z_D)$ to logratio vector $y = \text{alr}(z)$ and then apply standard multivariate regression analysis to the set of logratio vectors. In particular, the method considered in Property 3.10 of assessing conditional distributions applies straightforwardly.

4.3 The complete separation problem

We present a Bayesian solution to the complete separation problem. The standard binary regression model seeks to explain the variability of a binary response y, labelled 1 or 2, in terms of some covariate, a $1 \times c$ vector x, through the use of the conditional linear model

$$\Pr(y = 1|x, \beta) = 1 - \Pr(y = 2|x, b) = F(x\beta^T), \qquad (4.6)$$

where β is a $1 \times c$ parameter and F is a cumulative distribution function, commonly taken to be either the standard normal distribution function Φ or the logistic distribution function Ψ defined by $\Psi(t) = \exp(t)/(1 + \exp(t))$. We allow the possibility of a constant in the linear predictor $x\beta^T$ by adopting the usual convention that the first element of the covariate vector x is 1. Occasionally we shall use $z = (z_1, \ldots, z_{c-1})$ to denote the true covariate, so that $x = (1, z)$. When, for the data set $D = \{(x_i, y_i) : i = 1, \ldots, n\}$ available for fitting the model, there exists a value of β, say β_s, such that $x_i\beta_s^T$ is positive for all i for which $y_i = 1$ and negative for all i for which $y_i = 2$ there is complete separation in the covariate space of the sets of covariate vectors associated with the two responses. The method of maximum likelihood then

produces estimates which are infinite. This is readily seen from the form of
the likelihood function

$$
\begin{aligned}
L(\beta|D) &= \prod_{\{i:y_i=1\}} F(x_i\beta^T) \prod_{\{i:y_i=2\}} \{1 - F(x_i\beta^T)\} \\
&= \prod_{\{i:y_i=1\}} F(x_i\beta^T) \prod_{\{i:y_i=2\}} F(-x_i\beta^T). \qquad (4.7)
\end{aligned}
$$

Since the arguments of the function F associated with β_s are positive in both
products it follows that $L(k\beta_s|D)$ is monotonic increasing in k and so the
maximum likelihood estimates are infinite with maximized likelihood equal
to 1. Any new cases would then be assigned to one of the categories with
certainty. While this may be reasonable for large data sets with complete separation the phenomenon often arises where the data set is modest in relation
to the dimension c of the covariate vector. For such situations common sense
dictates that there can be no certainty in the allocation of new cases and so
it is clear that there is a serious breakdown of maximum likelihood estimation. The explosive nature of maximum likelihood can indeed occur when the
configuration in the covariate space is nearly separate, though not completely
separate in the sense described above. We shall see practical examples of this
in our applications in Sections 8.5 and 9.7. Such a breakdown is, of course,
not unique. Other cases have been reported, notably in estimation problems
where there is a range parameter in the underlying distribution, as with the
three-parameter lognormal distribution, where the absolute maximum of the
likelihood function is shown not to be at the local maximum but at a point at
infinity. For this lognormal estimation problem the situation was resolved by
the introduction of a vague prior on the parameters which essentially forces the
maximum likelihood estimate back to its local maximum position. A similar
feature arises with maximum likelihood estimation of the skewness parameters of the recently introduced multivariate skew normal class where, for data
sets with substantial skewness, maximum likelihood tries to push the skewness estimates above the range of possibility of the skew normal class. For the
complete separation problem of binary regression there is no local maximum
but we shall argue that the covariate information in the sample provides an
appropriate prior distribution for the parameter β which not only prevents the
complete separation explosion but which seems to provide categorical probability assessments which match those based on maximum likelihood estimates
even in the case of no separation.

4.3.1 Construction of a fair prior

The controlling effect of introducing a prior density function for the parameter vector β is readily seen. Any sensible $p(\beta)$ will be such that $p(\beta)$ de-
creases monotonically towards 0 as $|\beta| \to \infty$. Moreover the likelihood $L(\beta|D)$
is bounded above by 1. If then we consider use of the posterior mode, the β
which maximizes $L(\beta|D)p(\beta)$ cannot be infinite. The question of what con-

stitutes a sensible $p(\beta)$ is readily addressed. Clearly the information in the covariate vectors may, indeed must, be used since, for example, any change in the scale of the measurements would clearly affect the scale of the components of β. Since binary regression is concerned with the modelling of the conditional distribution of the binary response y for given covariate vector x, the use of the covariate information in no way involves an implicit double use of the data. We assume that the selection process for the cases in the data set D has been on the basis of information, possibly including the covariate but not involving the type or category. This, of course, is the reason for favouring the binary regression model in the analysis, in our case describing the variability of y conditional on x. For simplicity of argument we suppose at this stage that the numbers of responses 1 and 2 in our sample of n are n_1 and n_2 with $n_1 = n_2$, It is well known that the differences between the use of the normal distribution function Φ and the logistic distribution function Ψ are seldom of any practical significance. Indeed each is well approximated by the other through the relationship

$$\Phi(t) = \Psi(0.59t), \tag{4.8}$$

as discussed in Section 3.6.1. Here we will concentrate on the normal version because it offers a more tractable argument. For convenience we set out the arguments for our fair prior in numerical sequence.

1. For reasons of tractability we consider it reasonable to adopt a c-dimensional normal distribution, say $N^c(b, B)$, for the prior density function.

2. The use of the prior density function $p(\beta)$ with the model $p(y|x, \beta)$ implies a prior diagnostic assessment

$$p(y|x) = \int p(y|x, \beta)p(\beta)d\beta = \Phi\left\{\frac{xb^T}{(1 + xBx^T)^{\frac{1}{2}}}\right\} \tag{4.9}$$

for every covariate vector x. Since we have no prior information on response associated with specific x this, as an expression of ignorance, should lead to a-priori odds 1 for every x. Obviously $b = 0$ is a necessary and sufficient condition for this expression of prior ignorance. We recall here that with the assumption that $n_1 = n_2$ we are effectively assuming an incidence rate $p(y = 1) = p(y = 2) = 1/2$.

3. As already mentioned binary regression is concerned with modelling the *conditional* distribution of y given x. With this in mind we see that as long as we do not connect specific responses with specific covariates we are acting fairly in the use of the existing data. Suppose that we retain the order of the cases in the response vector y but consider assigning the rows of the $n \times c$ covariate matrix by a random permutation P to the responses y. Then we create a permuted data set $D_P = (PX, y)$. Because of this random permutation there is little chance that there is now complete separation, so that we should be able to obtain the maximum likelihood estimate, say β_P, for β from the data set D_P. By generating a series of

random permutations of X we should then have a series of 'estimates' of β in the spirit of resampling techniques, and so be able to obtain a suitable prior distribution.

4. The substantial amount of computation inherent in such a resampling method is, however, unnecessary since we can discover the nature of such a prior distribution by simple analysis. From standard binary regression theory we know that the estimated covariance matrix of the estimator $\hat{\beta}$ is $\text{cov}(\hat{\beta}) = \{(PX)W(PX)^T\}^{-1}$, where W is a diagonal matrix whose elements are 'weights' associated with the different rows of X. Since, however, we have no reason for supposing these weights to vary in any specific way it seems quite reasonable to assume equality, in which case the covariance matrix takes the form $k(XX^T)^{-1}$ since P, being a permutation matrix, is orthogonal. Thus we are led to the conclusion that a fair prior distribution for β takes the form $N^c\{0, k(XX^T)^{-1}\}$.

5. The remaining task is to determine k in such a way as to express prior vagueness about the nature of the conditional distribution of response for given covariate. The implication of the adoption of the prior density function $p(\beta)$ for diagnostic assessments can be analyzed at a deeper level than in item (2) above. The type 1 response probability

$$p_x(\beta) = \Pr(y = 1|x, \beta) = \Phi(x\beta^T) \tag{4.10}$$

as a function of β is a random variable with a distribution induced by that of β. The requirement of item (2) above can then be interpreted as the limited constraint that, for every x, $E_\beta p_x(\beta) = 1/2$. We can ask the more detailed question of what requirement should be placed on the induced distribution of $p_x(\beta)$ to express prior vagueness. For given x we can obtain the distribution function of p_x as

$$\Pr(p_x \le t) = \Pr\{x\beta^T \le \Phi^{-1}(t)\} = \Phi\{\Phi^{-1}(t)/(h_x k)^{-\frac{1}{2}}\} \tag{4.11}$$

and consequently its density function as

$$(h_x k)^{-\frac{1}{2}}\phi\{\Phi^{-1}(t)/(h_x k)^{-\frac{1}{2}}\}/\phi\{\Phi^{-1}(t)\}, \tag{4.12}$$

where h_x is the well known 'hat' value $x(X^T X)^{-1}x^T$ corresponding to the covariate row vector x. The distribution thus depends only on the combination $h_x k$ and the density function can readily be graphed for any such combination. In Bayesian analysis, expression of increasing vagueness about a binomial probability such as p_x varies from the uniform distribution through beta density functions such as $t^{a-1}(1-t)^{b-1}$ to improper prior density functions proportional to $t^{-1}(1-t)^{-1}$. The question then arises: is it possible to choose k so that, whatever the covariate vector x may be, the prior distribution of β is never less vague than the uniform distribution? This can readily be achieved. First note from density function (4.12) that the uniform distribution corresponds to the case $h_x k = 1$. Moreover the more that $h_x k$ exceeds 1 the more the density function approaches the vaguer U-shaped density functions. We also know that for every covariate vector x in the covariate matrix X there are lower and upper bounds on the value of h_x, namely $1/n$ and 1. Thus if we take $k = n$ we can ensure that $h_x k \geq 1$ for every covariate vector x in the data matrix X and that the prior distribution on β is inducing extremely vague information on p_x. Thus the fair prior distribution that we recommend for β is of form $N^c(0, n(XX^T)^{-1})$. There is an intuitive appeal in this form of prior, most simply recognized if we make a reparametrizing transformation from β to γ implied by working with a centred form of the linear predictor

$$x\beta^T = \beta_0 + \beta_1 z_1 + \cdots + \beta_{c-1} z_{c-1} = \gamma_0 + \gamma_1(z_1 - \bar{z}_1) + \cdots + \gamma_{c-1}(z_{c-1} - \bar{z}_{c-1}),$$

where $\bar{z}_i$ is the mean of the ith covariate in the sample. The prior distribution on γ induced by the prior on β is easily derived as $N^c(0, C)$, where

$$C = \begin{bmatrix} 1 & 0 \\ 0 & S^{-1} \end{bmatrix}$$

and S is the estimated covariance matrix of the set of all true covariate vectors. A new feature here is that the prior distribution of γ_0 is independent of the prior distribution of $(\gamma_1, \ldots, \gamma_{c-1})$. This is sensible since it is well known that the primary role of γ_0 is the determination of the incidence rate. We note that at the mean covariate position the model assigns probability $\Phi(\gamma_0)$ to response 1 and $1 - \Phi(\gamma_0)$ to response 2, so that the $N(0, 1)$ prior on γ_0 allows a wide enough range of incidence rates for practical purposes. The role of S^{-1} is also appealing. If, for example, we change the scale of the covariates, for example from gm to kg, that is by a factor of 1000, we would expect the vector β to decrease by a factor $1/1000$. The variance of the prior, based on S^{-1}, would exactly reflect this rescaling.

4.4 Diagnosis with tree-structured types

We now take up the challenge of producing a diagnostic system in cases where the types are tree-structured. The motivating example for this analysis is given by the Cushing syndrome study, described in Section 1.10, which will be analysed later in Section 9.7. We discuss only the case of a binary tree; more general versions of the theory for cases in which there are branches into more than two nodes and/or when the types represented by these nodes are ordinal rather than nominal can be easily constructed. Consider the tree in Figure 4.1. Each terminal node in the tree corresponds to one of the types. Terminal nodes are denoted by squares, whereas a circle indicates a branch node. A terminal node at level m has $m - 1$ predecessor branch nodes in the tree. The total number of branch nodes is equal to $k - 1$, where k is the number of types. Let the parameter vector β_s be associated with the sth branch node and suppose that v represents a vector of values of explanatory variables, including a 1 to accommodate an intercept term, obtained from an individual patient. Suppose also that F is a cumulative distribution function, which in

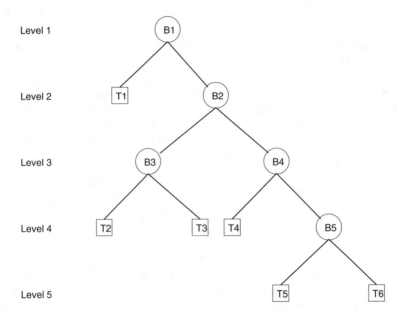

Figure 4.1 *An illustration of tree-structured types with six types represented by the six terminal nodes* T1-T6 *and 5 branch nodes* B1-B5.

special cases could be the logistic or normal. Without loss of generality we take the probability associated with a left branch at node s to be $F_s \equiv F(v; \beta_s)$ and that of a right branch $1 - F_s$; in particular, F_s might take the special form $F(v\beta_s^T)$. At the sth node let z_s be a binary variable which takes the value 1 for a left-branch and 0 otherwise. We may write a general formula for the unconditional probability that an individual belongs to type t as

$$\prod_{i=1}^{l_t-1} F_{s_{it}}^{z_{s_{it}}} (1 - F_{s_{it}})^{1-z_{s_{it}}} \tag{4.13}$$

where l_t denotes the level of the tree containing the terminal node for type t and s_{it} is the branch predecessor node for type t at level i in the tree. For example, in the illustrative tree in Figure 4.1 terminal node T4 has predecessor nodes 1,2 and 4 on levels 1,2 and 3, respectively. Thus $s_{14} = 1$, $s_{24} = 2$, $s_{34} = 4$ and $z_1 = 0$, $z_2 = 0$, $z_4 = 1$. Hence the unconditional probability associated with terminal node $T4$ is

$$[1 - F(v; \beta_1)][1 - F(v; \beta_2)]F(v; \beta_4).$$

Now suppose that there are n_t training cases of the tth type, with v_{rt} denoting the rth training case of type t. Then using (4.13) we may write the likelihood function of $\beta = (\beta_1, \beta_2, \ldots, \beta_{k-1})$ as

$$\prod_{t=1}^{k} \prod_{r=1}^{n_t} \prod_{i=1}^{l_t-1} F(v_{rt}; \beta_{s_{it}})^{z_{s_{it}}} [1 - F(v_{rt}; \beta_{s_{it}})]^{1-z_{s_{it}}}. \tag{4.14}$$

Clearly, this likelihood function factorises into a product of $k-1$ terms with each of them involving the beta parameter at each branch node. If we also assume that a priori the β_s are independent then it follows that the posterior distribution of β given the data will also factorise into a product of $k-1$ terms, one for each branch node. This has the advantage that the estimation process splits into separate processes for each branch node and so the unknown parameters associated with the different branch nodes can be estimated simultaneously, in parallel. It is perhaps simplest to grasp what is involved by using a simple example, and we consider the illustrative tree in Figure 4.1. There are six terminal nodes and five branch nodes. The likelihood (4.14) may then be written as a product of the following five terms.

$$\begin{array}{lll}
\text{Node 1} & \prod_{r=1}^{n_1} F(v_{r1}; \beta_1) & \times \quad \prod_{t=2}^{6} \prod_{r=1}^{n_t} [1 - F(v_{rt}; \beta_1)] \\[2ex]
\text{Node 2} & \prod_{t=2,3} \prod_{r=1}^{n_t} F(v_{rt}; \beta_2) & \times \quad \prod_{t=4,5,6} \prod_{r=1}^{n_t} [1 - F(v_{rt}; \beta_2)] \\[2ex]
\text{Node 3} & \prod_{r=1}^{n_2} F(v_{r2}; \beta_3) & \times \quad \prod_{r=1}^{n_3} [1 - F(v_{r3}; \beta_3)] \qquad (4.15) \\[2ex]
\text{Node 4} & \prod_{r=1}^{n_4} F(v_{r4}; \beta_4) & \times \quad \prod_{t=5,6} \prod_{r=1}^{n_t} [1 - F(v_{rt}; \beta_4)] \\[2ex]
\text{Node 5} & \prod_{r=1}^{n_5} F(v_{r5}; \beta_5) & \times \quad \prod_{r=1}^{n_6} [1 - F(v_{rt}; \beta_6)]
\end{array}$$

Examination of the terms in (4.15) shows that the analysis uncouples into five separate problems which can be tackled in parallel using, say, logistic regression. At node 1 we compute the probability that an individual is of type 1 against the alternative that he is one of types 2-6 using the training data for type 1 and the combined training data for types 2-6. At node 2, we divide the training data for types 2-6 into distinct sets for types 2-3 and 4-6, respectively, and compute the probability that an individual is either of type 2 or type 3 against the alternative that he is of types 4, 5 or 6, and similarly for the other nodes. The conditional diagnostic probability at node s that an individual patient with feature vector v is of type t is obtained from

$$\Pr(u = t | x, D) = \int F(v; \beta_2) p(\beta_s | D_s) d\beta_s, \tag{4.16}$$

where D_s denotes the training data relevant for the sth branch node. The uncoupling of the diagnostic problem into separate problems leads to the easy computation of the diagnostic probabilities for a new patient at each node in the tree and thus a diagnostic probability tree can be easily constructed for a new patient. The solution presented here could also have advantages in terms of feature selection. It could be that different subsets of the available features might be most relevant as discriminators at different nodes in the tree and this could be useful. This method developed here will be illustrated in the context of Cushing's syndrome in Section 9.7.

4.5 Mixed-effects models

In a few of the applications in Chapters 6 and 7 we make use of linear and non-linear mixed effects models. Given data from a univariate response together with p explanatory variables on n cases we may write a linear mixed-effects model in the form

$$y = X\phi^T + Zr^T + e, \qquad (4.17)$$

where $y = (y_1, \ldots, y_n)$ is a $n \times 1$ vector, ϕ is a $1 \times (p+1)$ vector containing the fixed effects, X is a $n \times (p+1)$ matrix containing a column of 1s and the values of the explanatory variables, r is a $1 \times q$ vector of random effects, Z is a $n \times q$ matrix of constants and e is a $n \times 1$ vector of random errors. We assume that the random vectors r and e are independent with $r \sim N(0, \Sigma_r)$ and $e \sim N(0, \Sigma)$. The covariance matrices Σ_r and Σ contain unknown fixed parameters, including variance components and covariances between random effects, collected together in the parameter θ. In cases where there are different independent sets of random effects the term Zr^T in (4.17) may be written as a sum of vectors, for example

$$Zr^T = Z_1 r_1^T + Z_2 r_2^T + Z_3 r_3^T$$

in the case of three sets of independent random effects.

From (4.17) and the above assumptions we have that the marginal distribution of y is

$$N(X\phi^T, \Sigma + Z\Sigma_r Z^T)$$

and so the log-likelihood of the parameters (ϕ, θ) is

$$l(\phi, \theta) = -\tfrac{1}{2}n \log(2\pi) - \tfrac{1}{2} \log |V| - \tfrac{1}{2}(y - X\phi^T)^T V^{-1}(y - X\phi^T), \quad (4.18)$$

where $V = \Sigma + Z\Sigma_r Z^T$. It follows from (4.18) by taking the partial derivative of (4.18) with respect to ϕ for fixed θ that the estimate $\hat{\phi}$ of ϕ is the solution of

$$\phi(X^T V^{-1} X^T) = y V^{-1} X^T. \qquad (4.19)$$

Substituting (4.19) into (4.18) we obtain the profile loglikelihood function for θ as

$$l_P(\theta) = -\tfrac{1}{2}n \log(2\pi) - \tfrac{1}{2} \log |V| - \tfrac{1}{2}(y - X\hat{\phi}^T)^T V^{-1}(y - X\hat{\phi}^T). \qquad (4.20)$$

The maximum likelihood estimates of ϕ and θ may be obtained by first maximising (4.20) with respect to θ and then substituting the answer into (4.19). Usually the solution process requires iterative methods. An alternative method for the estimation of the components of θ is to use restricted maximum likelihood estimates (REML) based on the profile restricted loglikelihood

$l_R(\theta)$, which is

$$-\tfrac{1}{2}(n-p-1)\log(2\pi)-\tfrac{1}{2}\log|V|-\tfrac{1}{2}\log|X^T V^{-1} X|-\tfrac{1}{2}(y-X\hat{\phi}^T)^T V^{-1}(y-X\hat{\phi}^T),$$
(4.21)

rather than (4.20). An advantage of the REML estimation is that that unbiased estimates of variance components can be obtained as opposed to the biased maximum likelihood estimates.

It is also possible to fit non-linear mixed-effects models and we will consider an example of this in Section 7.6. Given data on a univariate response and a single explanatory variable this type of model may be written as

$$y_i = g(x_i; \phi + r) + e_i,$$
(4.22)

where g is a non-linear function, the vector ϕ contains fixed effects, the vector r contains random effects and the random errors are mutually independent $N(0, \sigma^2)$ random variables and independent of the components of r, with $r \sim N(0, \Sigma_r)$. The estimates of the fixed effects and the unknown parameters in V are obtained using iterative methods. In our applications we have used the package *nlme*, written by Pinheiro and Bates (2000), to fit these models.

4.6 Gibbs sampling

In many of the applications considered in Chapters 7–10 we will adopt a Bayesian approach and perform the computation using Gibbs sampling in the package WinBUGS. These applications involve two main types of computation, namely (a) the computation of the posterior expectation of some smooth function $g(Z)$ of the parameters or variables $Z = (Z_1, Z_2, \ldots, Z_m)$ given data D and (b) the estimation of the posterior distribution of Z itself, from which highest posterior density intervals can be derived for the components of Z. If it were possible to sample independent realisations of Z from the posterior distribution $p(Z|D)$ then the posterior expectation of $g(Z)$ could be calculated as

$$E\{g(Z)|D\} = \frac{1}{N} \sum_{t=1}^{N} g(Z^{(t)}),$$
(4.23)

where $Z^{(t)}$ denotes the tth of the N realisations of Z. As $N \to \infty$ this empirical average converges to the required posterior expectation by the strong law of large numbers. However, in many important examples it is not possible to generate independent realisations from $p(Z|D)$ and recourse is made to Markov chain Monte Carlo (MCMC) methods. The basic idea of an MCMC method is to generate realisations from a Markov chain whose stationary distribution is $p(Z)$. While these realisations are no longer independent it is known under mild regularity conditions that, as $t \to \infty$, $Z^{(t)}$ converges in distribution to Z, where $Z \sim p(Z)$, and the empirical average in (4.23) converges almost surely to the theoretical posterior expectation.

We wish to generate a sequence of m-vectors $Z^{(t)} = (Z_1^{(t)}, Z_2^{(t)}, \ldots, Z_m^{(t)})$. Given a starting vector $Z^{(0)}$, and using a single-node updating procedure, at each iteration a realisation of each of the components of Z is generated from the full conditional distribution of that component given all the other components in Z. For example, a realisation of the ith component Z_i is generated from the conditional distribution $p(Z_i|Z_{-i})$, where Z_{-i} denotes the components of Z other than the ith one evaluated at their current values – an asynchronous updating procedure. The iterations proceed until the chain is in equilibrium and then computation of the required quantities is based on some further iterations; just how many iterations are required to reach equilibrium and for the estimation of the quantities of interest depends on the particular application, and in practice this is a matter of judgement.

The results of the initial iterations are discarded as 'burn-in'– at least 500 iterations and often more. Then a sequence of iterations is used to assess whether convergence to the stationary distribution has been attained. Much useful information is available by examining trace plots of the values of the quantities of interest as well as autocorrelation plots. Convergence may be assessed by running several chains in parallel, each from a different starting point, and then computing the Brooks-Gelman-Rubin (BGR) convergence statistics. Suppose that c chains are run in parallel and that we are interested in producing a $100(1 - \alpha)\%$ highest posterior density interval for Z_i computed from the empirical $100(\alpha/2)$ and $100(1 - \alpha/2)$ percentiles of the values of Z_i. We may monitor the width of this interval in two ways as the post-burn-in iterations proceed. First, we could pool all the values of Z_i over all c chains, form the interval and then compute its width, denoted by R_p. Secondly, we could compute the width of the interval separately from each of the c chains and then form the mean of these widths, denoted by R_w. Then the main BGR convergence statistic is the ratio $R = R_p/R_w$ of these widths. As the chains converge to their stationary distributions the statistics R_p and R_w will converge to stable values and R will converge to 1. If these checks are satisfied then it is reasonable to consider the chains to have converged and estimates of the quantities of interest can be based on a further set of iterations. The number of such iterations required depends on the autocorrelation in the successive values of Z_i. A simple rule-of-thumb suggested in the WinBUGS manual is that sampling be continued until the Monte Carlo error is within 5% of the standard deviation of the values of the node being monitored and this convention has been adopted in the applications we consider.

We consider the aldosterone data of data set `aldo`, which is discussed in Section 7.2, and use the regression analysis of the RIA value of the concentration of aldosterone on the DI value as a simple illustrative example of Gibbs sampling and the use of WinBUGS. We will also estimate the mean RIA concentration when the DI concentration is 40 mg/100ml. Assuming a normal linear regression model for the data, we have for $i = 1, \ldots, 72$

$$v_i \sim N(\alpha + \beta(u_i - \bar{u}), \sigma^2).$$

Note that in this model the DI values have been mean-centred in order to

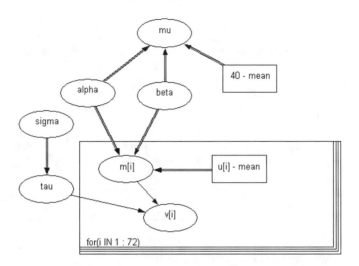

Figure 4.2 *Representation of the aldosterone model as a directed acyclic graph.*

improve the convergence of the iterations. There are four quantities of interest, namely the parameters α, β, σ and $\mu = \alpha + \beta(40 - \bar{u})$.

```
model
{
mean <- mean(u[])
for(i in 1:N)
  {
    v[i] ~ dnorm(m[i], tau)
    m[i] <- alpha + beta*(u[i]-mean)
  }
    tau <- 1/pow(sigma,2)
  alpha ~ dnorm(0, 1.0E-6)
   beta ~ dnorm(0,1.0E-6)
  sigma ~ dunif(0,1000)
     mu <- alpha+beta*(40-mean)
}
```

The full model assumed for the aldosterone data is represented in Figure 4.2 as a graphical model in the form of a directed acyclic graph. The graph indicates the conditional independence structure in the model; for instance, the $v[i]$ are conditionally independent given α, β and σ. The programme of instructions required to run this model in WinBUGS is given above. It is quite simple and follows closely the above model formulation.

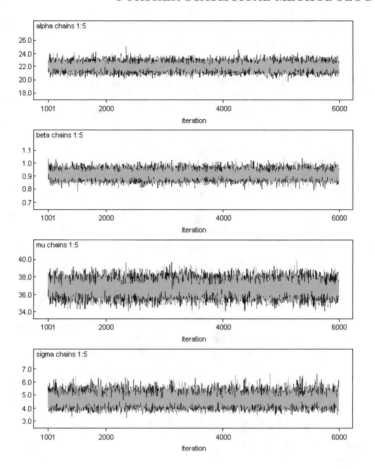

Figure 4.3 *Trace plots of five parallel chains from iteration 1,001 to 6,000 for the parameters α, β, μ and σ in sequence from top to bottom.*

We will assume independent 'non-informative' priors for the parameters α, β and σ:

$$\alpha \sim N(0, 10^6), \quad \beta \sim N(0, 10^6), \quad \sigma \sim U(0, 1000),$$

where U denotes the uniform distribution. Initial values for α, β and σ will be generated randomly from the prior distributions. This is alright in simple problems but usually, to avoid numerical overflow or very slow convergence, initial values would be specified. At each iteration the new values of α, β, σ are generated from the full conditional distributions as follows,

$$\begin{aligned} \alpha &\sim p(\alpha|\beta, \sigma, D), \\ \beta &\sim p(\beta|\alpha, \sigma, D), \\ \sigma &\sim p(\sigma|\alpha, \beta, D). \end{aligned}$$

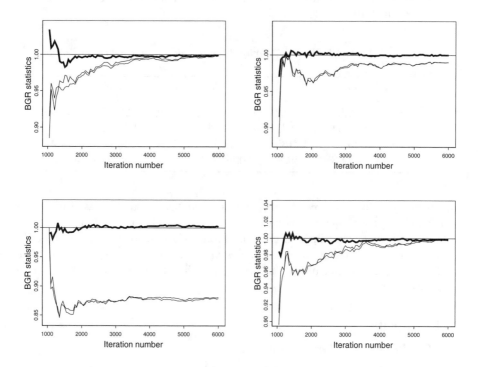

Figure 4.4 *Plots of the BGR convergence statistics R (in bold), R_p and R_w for the parameters α (top-left), β (top-right), σ (bottom-left) and μ (bottom-right).*

The normal distribution is specified in terms of precision τ ($=1/\text{variance}$) rather than variance. The nodes $v[i]$, α, β and σ are stochastic nodes and the τ and μ are logical nodes which define functions of the parameters in the model.

Five parallel chains were run and the results from the first 1,000 iterations were discarded as 'burn-in'. The chains were then run for a further 5,000 iterations in order to monitor convergence. The trace plots are shown in Figure 4.3 and indicate that the chains are stationary and well-mixed. The plots of the BGR statistics are shown in Figure 4.4. The default 80% intervals were used and the statistics were computed using the values from non-overlapping bins of size 50 (the default). For plotting purposes the statistics R_p and R_w were normalised to have a maximum value of unity. In all four cases the R statistic appears to be straddling 1 from about iteration 2,000. However, the stability of the other statistics is parameter-dependent, with σ being stable after about 1,000 iterations, β after 2,000, and μ and α stable after about 4,000 iterations.

Thus, overall, we would be reasonably safe in assuming that convergence has been reached after 4,000 iterations.

Table 4.1 *WinBUGS output for the aldosterone example*

node	mean	sd	MC error	2.5%	median	97.5%
α	22.05	0.5482	0.008438	20.99	22.05	23.13
β	0.9154	0.02931	4.234E-4	0.8581	0.9154	0.9739
μ	36.74	0.7189	0.009659	35.3	36.75	38.2
σ	4.63	0.3988	0.006391	3.922	4.604	5.482

Finally, we use the results obtained in a further 5,000 samples, 1,000 from each chain, to estimate the quantities of interest. The output is presented in Table 4.1. Note that in each case the Monte Carlo error is smaller than 5% of the standard deviation of the values of the node. Thus we may read off a 95% highest posterior density interval for each parameter from the 2.5% and 97.5% columns.

4.7 Biplots

4.7.1 Unconstrained multivariate data

The singular value decomposition of a data matrix has proved a very successful tool in exploratory analysis of unconstrained multivariate data and forms the basis of a variety of useful graphical aids to interpretation, such as principal component plots, biplots and correspondence analysis. The singular value decomposition property states that any $n \times d$ matrix M of rank r can be expressed as a product

$$M = G\text{diag}(s_1, \ldots, s_r)H^T,$$

where G and H are of orders $n \times r$ and $d \times r$, each with orthonormal columns, and the positive numbers $s_1, \ldots, s_r$, assumed here to be arranged in descending order of magnitude, are the singular values.

We start with the simplest situation of unconstrained multivariate data (vectors in R^d) with no covariate vector involvement. It is standard practice to centre such data at the mean vector by subtracting from each element of the $n \times d$ data matrix Y its corresponding column average; in matrix terms we consider the singular value decomposition of

$$M = \{I - (1/n)1^T1\}Y,$$

where 1 is a $1 \times n$ row vector of unit components. The relationship of this centred data matrix M and the singular value decomposition to aspects of multivariate statistical analysis of the data matrix Y can be readily established. For example, the sample estimate $\hat{\Sigma}$ of the covariance matrix Σ is given by

$$(n - 1)\hat{\Sigma} = M^T M.$$

From the relation

$$M^T M = H\text{diag}(s_1^2, \ldots, s_r^2)H^T,$$

we can identify $(n-1)^{-1}s_1^2, \ldots, (n-1)^{-1}s_r^2$ as the eigenvalues and the columns of H as the corresponding eigenvectors of a principal component analysis of the multivariate data. As a dual property we have that

$$MM^T = G\text{diag}(s_1^2, \ldots, s_r^2)G^T,$$

and so we can identify the principal coordinates as

$$MH = G\text{diag}(s_1, \ldots, s_r).$$

A further useful result is that the 'Mahalanobis distances' of the multivariate data vectors relative to the mean vector are given by the diagonal elements of

$$M\{M^T M/(n - 1)\}^{-1}M^T = (n - 1)GG^T,$$

so that the Mahalanobis distance of the ith case is easily obtained from the sum of squares in the ith row of G.

A hope of the decomposition is that the singular values $s_1, \ldots, s_r$ will decrease rapidly so that M will be well approximated by the ath order approximation

$$M^{(a)} = G_a\text{diag}(s_1, \ldots, s_a)H_a^T,$$

where G_a and H_a are the leading $n \times a$ and $d \times a$ submatrices of G and H respectively. The degree of approximation is usually measured in terms of the Frobenius norm $||M - M^{(a)}||$ of the difference between M and M_a, defined by

$$||M - M^{(a)}||^2 = \sum_{i=1}^{n}\sum_{j=1}^{d}(m_{ij} - M_{ij}^{(a)})^2$$

and the optimizing property is that, of all matrices of rank at most a, $M^{(a)}$ is that which minimizes this Frobenius norm with minimum value

$$||M - M^{(a)}||^2 = s_{a+1}^2 + \cdots + s_r^2.$$

As a measure of the quality of the approximation we can thus take the customary

$$(s_1^2 + \cdots + s_a^2)/(s_1^2 + \cdots + s_r^2),$$

which is the proportion of the total variability of the multivariate data set retained by $M^{(a)}$ or equivalently the first a principal components.

In order to obtain any useful graphical representation of the compositional data set we shall have to take $a = 2$ and in order to state the properties of the biplot clearly we shall assume that $r = 2$ so that the relationship $M = G_2\text{diag}(s_1, s_2)H_2$ is exact.

Suppose that with origin O in a two-dimensional diagram we plot the d points

$$(s_1 h_{j1}, s_2 h_{j2})/(n - 1)^{\frac{1}{2}} \qquad (j = 1, \ldots, d)$$

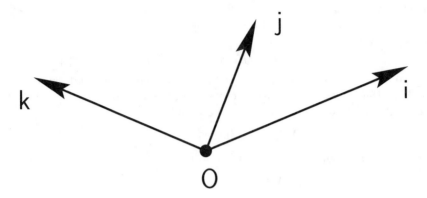

Figure 4.5 *Covariance diagram of the biplot showing the origin O and three rays corresponding to the three variables i, j and k.*

and regard these as the *vertices* j of the biplot for the multivariate data matrix Y; see, for example, Figure 4.5. Each vertex then corresponds to a component of the vector y. We then term $\overrightarrow{Oj}$ a ray of the diagram. It can then be shown that this diagram, consisting of the set of rays together with the various angles defined by rays, contains a complete quantitative picture of the covariance structure of the multivariate data set and can conveniently be termed the covariance diagram of the biplot. Specifically the representation is contained in the following property.

Property 4.1 The relation of the diagram to the covariance structure of the data matrix Y is provided by the following relationships:

$$
\begin{aligned}
|\overrightarrow{Oj}|^2 &= \text{estimate of var}(y_j), \\
\overrightarrow{Oj}.\overrightarrow{Ok} &= |Oj||Ok|\cos jOk \\
&= \text{estimate of cov}(y_j, y_k), \\
\cos(jOk) &= \text{estimate of corr}(y_j, y_k).
\end{aligned}
$$

A simple corollary is that an acute angle between two rays indicates positive correlation between the associated components whereas an obtuse angle indicates negative correlation. When two rays are at right angles then zero correlation is indicated.

The covariance diagram just described is only one aspect of a biplot, providing through the singular values s_1, s_2 and the H_2 matrix a view of the covariance structure of the data set. It provides no information about variability between the n individual cases which form the rows of Y. We can, however, introduce points in the diagram for each case which will allow us to see clearly this variability. To do this we use the ith row of G_2 to plot the point $(n-1)^{\frac{1}{2}}(g_{i1}, g_{i2})$ as the marker representing the ith case $(i = 1, \ldots, n)$, as in Figure 4.6.

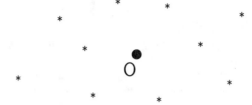

Figure 4.6 *Diagram showing the origin O and eleven markers of a biplot.*

Such markers have the following easily established property.

Property 4.2 The centred data matrix may be reconstructed through the following relationship between the case markers and the rays.

$$m_{ij} = \overrightarrow{Oi}.\overrightarrow{Oj}.$$

Thus $\overrightarrow{Oi}.\overrightarrow{Oj}$ represents the departure of y_{ij} from the average of this jth component over all the cases. Let P_i denote the projection of the ray Oi on the possibly extended ray Oj. Then $\overrightarrow{Oi}.\overrightarrow{Oj} = |OP_i||Oj|$, where the sign is taken to be positive or negative according to whether angle iOj is acute or obtuse. A simple interpretation can be obtained as follows. Consider the extended line Oj as divided into positive and negative parts by the centre O, the positive part being in the direction of Oj from O. If P_i falls on the positive (negative) side of this line then the jth component y_{ij} of the ith case exceeds (falls short of) the average value of this component over all cases and the further P_i is from O the greater is this exceedance (shortfall); if P_i coincides with O then the jth component coincides with the average. In Figure 4.7 the kth case clearly has a jth component y_{kj} which falls short of the overall average of this component.

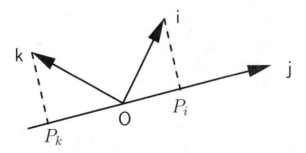

Figure 4.7 *Projection diagram of the biplot showing the origin O and the projections of the case markers i and k onto ray Oj. These projections are respectively positive and negative relative to the origin O.*

Although

$$|Oi|^2 = (n-1)(g_{i1}^2 + g_{i2}^2)$$

provides the Mahalanobis distance of the ith case when $s_3 = \cdots = s_r = 0$ we have found it as simple and more reliable to indicate possible outliers on the diagram by using the complete singular value decomposition and the exact Mahalanobis distance.

With this distance it is extremely simple to compute the atypicality index of any case. Recall from Section 3.11 that this is roughly the probability that a future case will be more typical or have a smaller Mahalanobis distance than the considered feature vector. To avoid resubstitution bias the standard leave-one-out technique is recommended and the atypicality index of a case with Mahalanobis distance q computed from the singular value decomposition for the full data set is, as already seen in Section 3.11,

$$J\left[\frac{qn}{(n-1)^2} \mid \tfrac{1}{2}(d-1), \tfrac{1}{2}(n-d)\right],$$

where J is the incomplete beta function given in Definition 3.2.

4.7.2 Compositional data

Before we do the required centering for a compositional data matrix X we require a preliminary transformation to ensure that we are working with logratio vectors. The simplest way of achieving this and of treating all the parts of each composition symmetrically is to use as common divisor the geometric mean of the composition components. This centering of both rows and columns produces a centred logratio data matrix $M = [m_{ij}]$ with

$$m_{ij} = \log x_{ij} - D^{-1}\sum_{j=1}^{D}\log x_{ij} - n^{-1}\sum_{i=1}^{n}\log x_{ij} + (nD)^{-1}\sum_{i=1}^{n}\sum_{j=1}^{D}\log x_{ij}$$

and with all row sums and column sums zero. This zero sum property carries over to the columns of G and of H in the singular value decomposition of M.

The relationship of this centred logratio data matrix M and the singular value decomposition to aspects of logratio analysis of the compositional data set X can be readily established. For example, the sample estimate $\hat{\Gamma}$ of the centred logratio covariance matrix Γ is given by

$$(n-1)\hat{\Gamma} = M^T M.$$

From the relation

$$M^T M = H\mathrm{diag}(s_1^2, \ldots, s_r^2)H^T$$

we can again identify $(n-1)^{-1}s_1^2, \ldots, (n-1)^{-1}s_r^2$ as the eigenvalues and the columns of H as the corresponding eigenvectors of a logcontrast principal component analysis of the compositional data. As a dual property we have that

$$MM^T = G\mathrm{diag}(s_1^2, \ldots, s_r^2)G^T$$

and so we can identify the logcontrast principal coordinates as

$$MH = G\mathrm{diag}(s_1, \ldots, s_r).$$

As for unconstrained multivariate data a further useful result is that the logratio 'Mahalanobis distances' of the compositions from the mean logratio vector are given by the diagonal elements of

$$M\{M^T M/(n-1)\}^- M^T = (n-1)GG^T,$$

where A^- denotes the Moore-Penrose inverse of A, so that the Mahalanobis distance of the ith case is easily obtained from the sum of squares in the ith row of G.

As for unconstrained multivariate data the quality of approximation attained by an ath order approximation, that M will be well approximated by $M^{(a)} = G_a\mathrm{diag}(s_1, \ldots, s_r)H_a^T$, is indicated by

$$(s_1^2 + \cdots + s_a^2)/(s_1^2 + \cdots + s_r^2),$$

which is the proportion of the total variability of the compositional data set retained by $M^{(a)}$ or equivalently the first a principal components.

In order to obtain any useful graphical representation of the compositional data set we shall have to take $a = 2$ and in order to state the properties of the biplot clearly we shall assume that $r = 2$ so that the relationship $M = G_2\mathrm{diag}(s_1, s_2)H_2$ is exact.

Suppose that with origin O in a two-dimensional diagram we plot the d points

$$(s_1 h_{j1}, s_2 h_{j2})/(n-1)^{\frac{1}{2}} \qquad (j = 1, \ldots, d)$$

and regard these as the *vertices* j of the biplot for the compositional data matrix X. Each vertex then corresponds to a component of the vector x. We then term Oj a ray of the diagram and the join jk between two vertices a link.

It can then be shown that the relative variation diagram of Figure 4.8, consisting of the set of vertices, rays and links, together with the various angles defined by rays and links, contains a complete quantitative picture of all the various covariance structures associated with the compositional data set X. We collect below the main properties of this relative variation diagram. The proofs of these properties depend simply on the relationships between the covariance structures and some simple properties of the cosine formula of elementary trigonometry and so are omitted.

Property 4.3 The origin O is the centroid of the vertices $1, \ldots, D$.

This consequence of the zero column sum property of H plays a central role in the use of the relative variation diagram for subcompositional analysis.

Property 4.4 The squared lengths of the links represent the set of estimated relative variances:

$$|jk|^2 = \text{estimate of var}\{\log(x_j/x_k)\}.$$

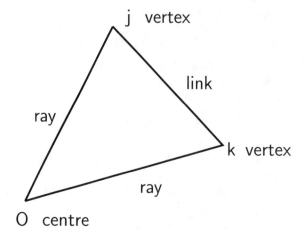

Figure 4.8 *Relative variation diagram.*

Property 4.5 Links and inter-link angles associated with part D represent the estimated logratio covariance matrix Σ:

$$|jD|^2 = \text{estimate of } \text{var}\{\log(x_j/x_D)\},$$

$$\overrightarrow{jD}.\overrightarrow{kD} = \text{estimate of } \text{cov}\{\log(x_j/x_D), \log(x_k/x_D)\}$$

so that

$$\cos(jDk) = \text{estimate of } \text{corr}\{\log(x_j/x_D), \log(x_k/x_D)\}.$$

Property 4.6 Rays and inter-ray angles represent the centred logratio covariance matrix Γ:

$$|Oj|^2 = \text{estimate of } \text{var}\{\log(x_j/g(x))\},$$

$$\overrightarrow{Oj}.\overrightarrow{Ok} = \text{estimate of } \text{cov}\{\log(x_j/g(x)), \log(x_k/g(x))\}$$

so that

$$\cos(jOk) = \text{estimate of } \text{corr}\{\log(x_j/g(x)), \log(x_k/g(x))\}.$$

A generalization of Property 4.6 involving four parts j, k, l, m is easily established and proves extremely useful in the exploration of independence properties of compositional data sets.

Property 4.7 If the links jk and lm intersect at P then

$$\cos(jPl) = \text{estimate of } \text{corr}\{\log(x_j/x_k), \log(x_l/x_m)\}.$$

Property 4.8 The measure of total compositional variability provided by the relative variation diagram can be expressed in terms of the lengths of either rays or links, as

$$(s_1^2 + s_2^2)/(n-1) = \sum_{j=1}^{D} |Oj|^2 = D^{-1} \sum_{j<k} |jk|^2.$$

Based on these properties we can now examine a number of aspects of the interpretation of relative variation diagrams so that their exploratory strengths may make more impact. Moreover we shall not bore the reader with pointing out obvious features such as the more expansive the diagram the more variable the compositional data set, but concentrate on four main ways in which interpretation differs from similar diagrams for unconstrained data sets.

4.7.3 Coincident vertices and proportionality

When two vertices j and k coincide or are close together then their link jk and, from Property 4.4, τ_{jk} = estimate of $\text{var}\{\log(x_j/x_k)\}$ is zero or small and so components x_j and x_k are in constant proportion or nearly so. While this is obvious it is not unimportant, particularly when we realise that the whole covariance structure is most simply defined in terms of relative variances and further that the concept of small relative variance with its associated high dependence of one component on another is essentially what is required to replace uninterpretable measures of dependence such as crude product-moment correlations $\text{corr}(x_j, x_k)$.

4.7.4 Subsets of vertices and subcompositional analysis

If we consider a subset, say $1, \ldots, C$, of parts of a D-part composition then the concept of the subcomposition $(w_1, \ldots, w_C)$ formed from these parts and defined by

$$(w_1, \ldots, w_C) = (x_1, \ldots, x_C)/(x_1 + \cdots + x_C)$$

plays a central role in compositional data analysis. One of the main reasons for claiming that relative variances provide the simplest specification of compositional covariance structure is that

$$\text{var}\{\log(w_j/w_k)\} = \text{var}\{\log(x_j/x_k)\} \qquad (j = 1, \ldots, C; \ k = j+1, \ldots, C).$$

The fact that the relative variance of two parts is the same within a subcomposition and within the full composition means that the relative variation diagram for any subcomposition is simply the subdiagram formed by the links of parts, or equivalently by the selection of vertices, associated with the subcomposition. Moreover the centre of the subcompositional diagram is, by Property 4.3, at the centroid, say O', of the subcompositional vertices. It is thus very simple to inspect visually within the full diagram the nature of any subcompositional variability. Indeed we could go further and estimate the proportion of the total compositional variability of the subcomposition. For example for the subcomposition formed from parts $1, \ldots, C$ this proportion is

$$\frac{\sum_{j=1}^{C} |O'j|^2}{\sum_{j=1}^{D} |Oj|^2}.$$

Collinear vertices and constant logcontrasts

If a subset, say $1, \ldots, C$, of vertices is approximately collinear then we know that the associated subcomposition has a relative variation diagram which is one-dimensional. Remembering the nature of the singular value decomposition we see that if we were to perform a principal component analysis on the set of such subcompositions we would find that only one eigenvalue was appreciably non-zero. An immediate implication therefore is that the subcompositional variability is one-dimensional and the nature of the one-dimensionality can be expressed as the constancy of $C - 2$ logcontrasts, of the form

$$\sum_{j=1}^{C} a_j \log x_j \qquad (a_1 + \cdots + a_C = 0).$$

4.7.5 Orthogonal links and subcompositional independence

If two links jk and lm intersect at right angles then we see from Property 4.7 that

$$\text{corr}\{\log(x_j/x_k), \log(x_l/x_m)\} = 0$$

and so the ratios x_j/x_k and x_l/x_m are uncorrelated and, within the context of additive logistic normality, independent. Thus in exploratory compositional data analysis the search for ratios which vary independently is associated with detecting orthogonal links. We may note that in this search for independent ratios j, k, l, m need not be different. It is for example meaningful to ask whether x_j/x_D and x_k/x_D are independent and in the relative variation diagram this would be associated with jDk being right-angled.

There is also no need to confine this search to a pair of ratios. If two subsets of vertices lie on two lines at right angles then the associated subcompositions are independent while showing a highly dependent structure within each subcomposition, because of the collinearity of vertices.

4.7.6 Composition markers

As for unconstrained multivariate data the relative variation diagram may be regarded as part of a biplot in that we may introduce composition markers which allow a visual inspection of the relationship of each composition to the covariance structure of the compositional data set. To do this we use the ith row of G_2 to plot the point $(n - 1)^{\frac{1}{2}}(g_{i1}, g_{i2})$ as the marker representing the ith composition $(i = 1, \ldots, n)$.

Such markers have the easily established property that $\overrightarrow{Oi.jk}$ represents the departure of $\log(x_{ij}/x_{ik})$ from the average of this logratio over all the

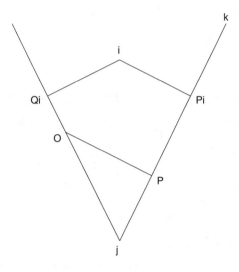

Figure 4.9 *Part of a biplot showing the relation of a case i composition to link jk and ray Oj.*

replicates. Let P and P_i denote the projections of the centre O and the compositional marker on the possibly extended link kj, as in Figure 4.9. Then $\overrightarrow{Oi}.\overrightarrow{kj} = \pm|PP_i||kj|$, where the positive sign is taken if the directions of PP_i and kj are the same and otherwise the negative sign is taken. A simple interpretation can be obtained as follows. Consider the extended line kj as divided into positive and negative parts by the point P, the positive part being in the direction of kj from P. If P_i falls on the positive (negative) side of this line then the logratio $\log(x_j/x_k)$ of the ith composition exceeds (falls short of) the average value of this logratio over all replicates and the further P_i is from P the greater is this exceedance (shortfall); if P_i coincides with P then the compositional logratio coincides with the average. In Figure 4.9 the ith composition clearly has a logratio $\log(x_j/x_k)$ which falls short of the overall average of this logratio.

A similar form of interpretation can be obtained from the fact that $\overrightarrow{Oi}.\overrightarrow{Oj}$ represents the departure of the centred logratio $\log\{x_j/g(x)\}$ of the ith composition from the average of this centred logratio over all replicates. Let Q_i be the projection of the composition marker i on the possibly extended ray Oj. Then $\overrightarrow{Oi}.\overrightarrow{Oj} = \pm|OQ_i||Oj|$, the positive or negative sign depending on whether Q_i and the vertex j lie on the same side or opposite sides from O. We then have the following simple interpretation. If Q_i lies on the same (opposite) side of the divided line as the vertex j then the centred logratio $\log\{x_j/g(x)\}$ of the ith composition exceeds (falls short of) the average of this logratio over all replicates, and so we can infer that the jth component of the ith composition is higher (lower) than average relative to the other components. Obviously also the further Q_i is from O the greater is the divergence from the average.

Remarks similar to those for unconstrained multivariate data apply in relation to Mahalanobis distance and atypicality for compositional data.

4.7.7 Differences between unconstrained and compositional biplots

It must be clear from the above aspects of interpretation that the fundamental elements of a relative variation diagram are the links, not the rays as in the case of variation diagrams for unconstrained multivariate data. The complete set of links, by specifying all the relative variances, determines the compositional covariance structure and provides direct information about subcompositional variability and independence. It is also obvious that interpretation of the relative variation diagram is concerned with its internal geometry and would, for example, be unaffected by any rotation or indeed mirror-imaging of the diagram.

Another fundamental difference between the practice of biplots for unconstrained and compositional data is in the use of data scaling. For unconstrained data if there are substantial differences in the variances of the components, biplot approximation may concentrate its effort on capturing the nature of the variability of the most variable components and fail to provide any picture of the pattern of variability within the less variable components. Since such differences in variances may simply arise because of scales of measurement a common technique in such biplot applications is to apply some form of individual scaling to the components of the unconstrained vectors prior to application of the singular value decomposition. No such individual scaling is necessary for compositional data when the analysis involves logratio transformations. Indeed, since

$$\operatorname{cov}\left[\log\{(c_j x_j)/(c_k x_k)\}, \log\{(c_l x_l)/(c_m x_m)\}\right] = \operatorname{cov}\{\log(x_j/x_k), \log(x_l/x_m)\},$$

it is obvious that the relative variation diagram is unchanged by any differential scaling of the parts. As long as we measure each individual part in a uniform set of units, the resulting biplot remains unaltered. Moreover any attempt at differential scaling of the logratios of the components would be equivalent to applying differential power transformations to the components of the compositions, a distortion which would prevent any compositional interpretation from the resulting diagram. It is perhaps worth pointing out here that even for unconstrained multivariate data consisting of positive vectors there is an advantage in the use of the logarithmic transformation, since biplots are then invariant to changes of scale because

$$\mathrm{cov}\{\log(c_j y_j), \log(c_k y_k)\} = \mathrm{cov}(\log y_j, \log y_k)$$

for any constants c_j, c_k.

4.8 Non-parametric modelling

4.8.1 Introduction

The methods so far discussed in this chapter have depended on the assumption that there is a reasonable class of parametric density functions available to model some conditional density function $p(y|x, \theta)$ of known form so that the statistical interest was in how to reduce or handle the uncertainty in the finite-dimensional parameter or index θ. In particular, attention was confined to three particular forms for $p(y|x, \theta)$. We have no parametric answer for the following situations.

(i) Continuous data resisting transformation to normality.

(ii) Discrete or categorical data.

(iii) Combinations of continuous and discrete data.

4.8.2 Kernel density estimation of an unconditional density function

Suppose that the task before us is to produce some estimate of an unconditional density function $p(y)$ on a sample spacè Y based on a data set $D = \{y_i : i = 1, \ldots, n\}$ of n replicates. If the sample space were the real line then a simple starting position might be to adopt the familiar histogram approach with the width of interval chosen not too small so as to avoid too peaked an appearance and not too large to avoid too flat an outline. The kernel density estimation approach is a slightly more sophisticated version of the histogram approach, whereby each little rectangle placed on an interval gives way to the placing on each sample point a fixed density function, termed a kernel, and the subsequent averaging of the overall picture. The kernel function contains a spread or width parameter λ, possibly a vector, analogous to the width of the histogram interval.

More specifically suppose that $K(y|\eta, \lambda)$ is a density function on Y, centred in some sense on $\eta \in Y$. For example, for $Y = R^1$, $K(y|\eta, \lambda)$ might be taken as the density function of the univariate normal distribution with mean η and standard deviation λ, and for $Y = R^d$ the density function of a d-dimensional normal distribution with mean vector η and covariance matrix $\lambda^2 I_d$. The technique is essentially to construct a density function on each of the observations y_i $(i = 1, \ldots, n)$ and then to average these to obtain a kernel density function $p(y|D, \lambda)$ given by

$$p(y|D, \lambda) = (1/n) \sum_{i=1}^{n} K(y|y_i, \lambda).$$

A well-tried method of determining a sensible value of the spread parameter λ is an adaptation of ideas of maximum likelihood. In the construction of a pseudo-likelihood here we must recognise that in estimating the density function at a point y_i in the data set we should avoid resubstitution bias and base the estimate on D_{-i}, the data set D depleted by the observation y_i so obtaining

$$p(y_i|D_{-i}, \lambda) = 1/(n-1) \sum_{j \neq i} K(y_i|y_j, \lambda).$$

The pseudo-likelihood $L(\lambda|D)$ to be maximized with respect to λ is then given by

$$L(\lambda, D) = \prod_{i=1}^{n} p(y_i|D_{-i}, \lambda).$$

If $\hat{\lambda}$ is the maximizing value of λ then the kernel density estimate of the underlying density function is $p(y|D, \hat{\lambda})$.

Examples of kernel density estimation of unconditional density functions will be found in Chapter 5.

4.8.3 Computation of atypicality indices

We consider two methods for estimating atypicality indices, namely the mesh technique and a Monte Carlo method.

First, consider the case where the sample space Y is the discrete set

$$\{y_i : i = 1, \ldots, n\}$$

and denote by $\hat{p}(y)$ the kernel estimate of the probability mass function $p(y)$ on Y. Then the atypicality index of a case with observed value y_R is

$$\Pr\{p(y) \geq p(y_R)\} = \sum_{y \in Y} p(y) I\{p(y) \geq p(y_R)\},$$

where $I(A)$ denotes the indicator function which takes the value 1 when event A happens and 0 otherwise. Thus the atypicality index is estimated by replacing $p(y)$ by $\hat{p}(y)$ in this formula. If we let z denote the random variable $\hat{p}(y)$, and let z have cumulative probability mass function F, then the atypicality may be estimated by computing $z = \hat{p}(y)$ for each $y \in Y$ and forming $F(y)$. Then the estimated atypicality is $1 - F\{\hat{p}(y_R)\}$.

In the case where the sample space Y is continuous the atypicality may be estimated by essentially discretising the sample space using a mesh technique. Suppose that the effective support of the density function $p(y)$ is divided into N equal intervals, each of width Δ and centred on the points

$$\{a_i : i = 1, \ldots, n\}.$$

Then form the probability elements $\Delta\hat{p}(a_i)$ $(i = 1, \ldots, n)$ and form their cumulative probability mass function as in the discrete case above. Then the estimated atypicality is $1 - F\{\hat{p}(y_R)\}$, where $\hat{p}(y_R)$ is the kernel estimate of the density function evaluated at y_R.

If the new value $y_R \notin D$ then the above calculations which are based on the whole data set D and which use a value of the bandwidth based on D may be used. However, if $y_R \in D$ then y_R should be removed from the data set D in the selection of the bandwidth and the formation of the kernel density estimate. To ease the computation some approximations can be considered: the bandwidth could be that obtained using the whole set D and perhaps also the kernel density estimate could be based on the whole data set D.

An alternative approach in the case of a continuous sample space is to use simulation to compute the atypicality index and we describe this method in the case in which the kernel is normal. For a given bandwidth the kernel density estimate is a mixture of n normal distributions, with the ith normal having mean y_i and standard deviation λ and the weights in the mixture being n^{-1} for each normal. Let $N = nk$ and simulate k values of y from each of the normal kernel distributions. For each simulated value of y compute $\hat{p}(y)$ and check whether it is greater than or equal to $\hat{p}(y_R)$; record a 1 if this is the case, and a 0 otherwise. Then estimate the atypicality of y_R as the proportion of 1s (and provide a confidence interval for the true atypicality). This method is simple to program and works effectively when, say, $N = 1000$, although a greater number of simulations could be required in cases of low atypicality.

Table 4.2 *Some typical kernel functions*

Data Type	Kernel Definition	Kernel formula $K(y\|x, \lambda)$	
Continuous	Normal	$(\lambda\sigma\sqrt{2\pi})^{-1} \exp\left\{-(y-x)^2/2\lambda^2\sigma^2\right\}$	
		$\sigma^2 = (n-1)^{-1} \sum(x - \bar{x})^2$	
Binary	Binary $\lambda \geq 1/2$	$K(y\|, x, \lambda) = \lambda$	$(y = x)$
		$K(y\|, x, \lambda) = 1 - \lambda$	$(y \neq x)$
Unordered Categorical	k-category unordered	$K(y\|, x, \lambda) = \lambda$	$(y = x)$
		$K(y\|, x, \lambda) = \frac{1-\lambda}{(k-1)}$	$(y \neq x)$
Ordered Categorical	k-category ordered	$K(y\|, x, \lambda) = \lambda$	$(y = x)$
		$K(y\|, x, \lambda) = \frac{(1-\lambda)2y}{(k-1)x}$	$(y < x)$
		$K(y\|, x, \lambda) = \frac{(1-\lambda)2(k+1-y)}{(k-1)(k+1-x)}$	$(y > x)$

4.8.4 Some typical kernels

A number of typical kernels are given in Table 4.2. In Chapter 5 we also use lognormal kernels which in the d-dimensional case are defined as follows:

$$\left(\prod_{i=1}^{d} x_i \lambda \sigma_i \sqrt{2\pi}\right)^{-1} \exp\left\{-1/(2\lambda^2) \sum_{i=1}^{d} (y_i - x_i)^2/\sigma_i^2\right\}, \qquad (4.24)$$

where σ_i^2 is the sample variance of the observed values of x_i.

4.8.5 Kernel density estimation of a conditional kernel density function

When there is a covariate vector involved we then have to consider the modification to kernel density estimation as described in Section 4.8.2 to obtain an estimate of the conditional density function $p(y|x)$. To introduce the basic idea here let us suppose that x and y are both real numbers and consider a scattergram of the data set $D = \{(x_i, y_i) : i = 1, \ldots, n\}$. In terms of the conditional density function $p(y|x, \lambda)$ a kernel density function $K(y|x_i, \lambda)$ on Y asssociated with covariate x_i where x_i is close to x should contribute more reliably than a kernel $K(y|x_j, \lambda)$ where x_j is distant from x. This relative reliability may be made specific by the introduction of a weighting factor $w(x, x_i, \mu)$, which in some sense is larger the closer x_i is to x. Note that we have introduced the possibility that this weighting factor may depend on a weighting parameter μ and we also assume that $\sum_{i=1}^{n} w(x, x_i, \mu) = 1$. Such a weighted kernel density function would thus take the form

$$p(y|x, D, \lambda, \mu) = 1/n \sum_{i=1}^{n} K(y|y_i, \lambda) w(x, x_i, \mu).$$

One appropriate weighting factor which we shall use takes the form

$$1 - G\{d(x, x_i)/\mu\},$$

where G is a distribution function on R_+^1, d is a distance function and μ the weighting parameter for w.

The cross-validatory method of Section 4.8.2 can again be applied, selecting the values of λ and μ which maximize the pseudo-likelihood

$$L(\lambda, \mu|D) = \prod_{i=1}^{n} p(y_i|x_i, D_{-i}, \mu, \lambda),$$

where

$$p(y_i|x_i, D_{-i}, \lambda, \mu) = 1/(n-1) \sum_{j \neq i} K(y_i|y_j, \lambda) w(x_i, x_j, \mu).$$

Examples of the application of this kernel density estimation for conditional density functions will be found in Section 9.6.

4.9 Bibliographic notes

Details of the recently introduced methodology for compositional data analysis are available in Aitchison (1986); more recent expository papers are Aitchison (1997, 2001). The logistic-normal distribution was first developed in Aitchison and Shen (1980).

The resolution of the complete separation problem of binary regression is new to this monograph, as is the material on dealing with tree-structured types in statistical diagnosis.

The REML method of estimation of variance components was introduced by Patterson and Thompson (1971); Searle, Casella and McCulloch(1992) provide a detailed account of the topic. The package *nlme* was created by J.C. Pinheiro and D.M. Bates. The package is available free from

$$\text{http://nlme.stat.wisc.edu}$$

and for discussion and illustration see Pinheiro and Bates (2000).

For details of the now frequently used Gibbs sampling and MCMC approaches see Gelman et al. (1995) and Gilks, Richardson and Spiegelhalter (1996). The package *WinBUGS* was developed by Spiegelhalter et al. and is available free from

$$\text{http://www.mrc-bsu.cam.ac.uk/bugs/welcome.shtml;}$$

see Spiegelhalter et al. (2003) and Schollnik (2002) for illustrations and excellent discussion of the package.

The pioneer of biplot techniques in statistics was Gabriel (1971, 1981). The extension of this excellent graphical aid to compositional data is set out in Aitchison (1990) and Aitchison and Greenacre (2002).

There are now many approaches to non-parametric methods of kernel density estimation. For an overall view we suggest Silverman (1986), Wand and Jones (1995) and Bowman and Azzalini (1997); for more specific problems, see Aitchison and Aitken (1976), Aitchison and Lauder (1985), Titterington (1980) and Simonoff (1996).

4.10 Problems

Problem 4.1 On the assumption that the variability of D-part compositions in a selected set of cases follows a $L^D(\mu, \Sigma)$ distribution and that maximum likelihood estimates $\hat{\mu}, \hat{\Sigma}$ for μ, Σ have been computed show that the atypicality index of a referred patient R with composition z_R is given by

$$J\left[\frac{q_R}{\{q_R + (n-1)(1+h_R)\}} | \tfrac{1}{2}, \tfrac{1}{2}(n-d)\right],$$

where $q_R = \{\text{alr}(z_R) - \hat{\mu}\}\hat{\Sigma}^{-1}\{\text{alr}(z_R) - \hat{\mu}\}^T$, $h_R = 1/n$ and J is the incomplete beta function.

Problem 4.2 Three-part compositions (a, b, c) of skin tissue have been collected from 25 normal individuals and are recorded below. Display the data graphically in a triangular (ternary) diagram in S^2. If you are unfamiliar with triangular diagrams refer to the description in Chapter 11.

a	b	c	a	b	c
0.38	0.05	0.57	0.17	0.30	0.53
0.29	0.11	0.60	0.22	0.20	0.58
0.11	0.43	0.46	0.09	0.51	0.40
0.29	0.09	0.62	0.50	0.01	0.49
0.45	0.03	0.52	0.38	0.04	0.58
0.32	0.05	0.63	0.20	0.26	0.54
0.40	0.06	0.54	0.14	0.30	0.56
0.06	0.52	0.42	0.21	0.21	0.58
0.15	0.34	0.51	0.31	0.08	0.61
0.52	0.01	0.47	0.40	0.03	0.57
0.24	0.14	0.62	0.21	0.22	0.57
0.44	0.03	0.53	0.31	0.12	0.57
0.11	0.49	0.40			

Transform the data to logratio form and plot in R^2. Construct in R^2 a 95 per cent predictive region for a new logratio vector observation. Translate this region back to your ternary diagram.

Two new patients have been referred to the clinic with possibly abnormal skin tissue compositions (0.10, 0.50, 0,40) and (0.46, 0.03, 0.51). Are they within previous experience?

Problem 4.3 The data set below, recording the results of three diagnostic tests in standard units, has been recorded with the intention of developing a diagnostic system to differentiate between two types A and B of a recently identified syndrome. Application of standard binary logistic software has given a warning that there is no convergence and there are indications that in the estimation of parameters the estimates are growing very large. This suggests to you that this is a case of complete separation of the data for the two forms. You could verify this conjecture by finding a three dimensional hyperplane which separates the data sets. How would you find such a hyperplane?

After you have confirmed that there is complete separation the clinic involved in the study suggests that there is a further test (test 4) which may avoid this difficulty, with the following results for the 20 patients reported above.

Form A:	156	177	131	120	206	136	182	107	154	229
Form B:	110	175	148	159	140	65	154	307	220	139

You should check whether this additional test avoids the complete separation problem. Would you recommend that this extra test should be part of the differential diagnostic process?

Form	Test results		
	1	2	3
A	261	265	486
	297	290	866
	736	253	332
	269	69	266
	336	111	410
	323	111	241
	835	140	689
	419	94	492
	249	79	173
	245	100	222
B	271	215	218
	177	252	168
	177	410	197
	69	241	93
	165	174	296
	202	461	181
	112	321	63
	95	246	184
	137	300	263
	93	177	198

Problem 4.4 For readers with access to WinBUGS. For the data set of Problem 1.4 and the regression of final level on initial level and treatment follow the procedure detailed in Section 4.6 to estimate relevant parameters and for this simple situation compare your answers with a standard regression approach.

Problem 4.5 Review the software available to you and try to find a program for the singular value decomposition of multivariate data or even a biplot program. Apply the software so that you may construct a biplot for the female data of Problem 1.5. Construct an estimate of the covariance matrix and compare this with the estimates you obtain from the biplot.

For this biplot devise a method of plotting the male data of Problem 1.5. What conclusion do you draw from the relative positions of the female and male markers?

If in your biplot you have not considered the possibility of using a transformation, now repeat your analysis with the logarithms of the data. Comment on any differences that you observe.

Problem 4.6 The compositional biplot for the three part-compositional data set of Problem 4.2 should give an exact representation of the covariance structure and the relationship of the markers to the parts of the composition. Construct the appropriate biplot and verify the exact correspondence.

Plot the markers of the two new patients and consider what inferences you might draw from this graphical representation.

Problem 4.7 Suppose that the use of a kernel density method is being sought for the data set of Problem 4.3. Can you suggest any suitable kernels and how you might proceed to use these in the analysis of the three-part compositional data set?

Problem 4.8 Consider the special case of model (4.17),

$$y = X\phi^T + e,$$

where the e_i mutually independent $N(0, \sigma^2)$ random variables.

Show that the REML estimate of σ^2 is given by $rss/(n - p - 1)$ and that the maximised profile restricted loglikelihood is equal to

$$-0.5(n - p - 1)\{\log 2\pi + \log[rss/(n - p - 1)] + 1\} - 0.5 \log |X^T X|.$$

Derive expressions for the maximised profile restricted loglikelihood for the following special cases of (4.17): (i) $y_i = \mu + e_i$ and (ii) $y_i = \alpha + \beta x_i$.

CHAPTER 5

Experience

5.1 Introduction

In Chapters 1-4 we have repeatedly noted that the clinician, when dealing with a new patient, has often to draw heavily on previous experience. In this chapter we seek ways in which we may usefully quantify and summarize such experience. In particular, we try to find statistical counterparts to commonly voiced ideas such as 'normal range', 'within previous experience' and 'completely atypical'. We shall therefore be assuming that there exists some reliable and useful set of past observations or measurements. We leave to the next chapter any discussion of the problems that have to be considered in achieving this aim of a reliable and useful data set.

Statistically then our problem appears to be the following. We are given a set

$$D = \{(u_i, v_i) : i = 1, \ldots, n\}$$

of observations or measurements on n selected cases $S_1, \ldots, S_n$ with some information about how these data have been obtained. There is variability in these data and we have then to find some suitable and sensible probability mechanism which has plausibly given rise to this variability. We have in standard statistical language to go through some process of choosing and then fitting a statistical model to describe, for a generic case S, one or other of the conditional density functions $p_S(u|v), p_S(v|u)$. But our task does not finish there. The purpose in describing such past experience is to harness it to the investigation and management of a new referred patient R. How is the fitted statistical model to be adapted or developed for this use?

The nature of a typical observation (u, v) will vary from problem to problem. Sometimes we may be faced with an unconditional problem with, for example, no u present and the associated task of modelling the unconditional density function $p_S(v)$. Moreover the sample space of either u or v will also vary, with a real line, a d-dimensional real space, a d-dimensional simplex, a finite set of categories, or some product of these being possibilities. The problems of the remaining sections illustrate the variety of statistical problems that arise in attempts to describe such experience.

5.2 Single measurement variability

The simplest problems of describing experience involve a single continuous measurement v with no conditioning features. In clinical medicine a common practice based on a selected set $v_1, \ldots, v_n$ of measurements with sample mean m and sample variance s^2 is to quote, for example, a 95 per cent confidence interval $(m - 2s, m + 2s)$ as a normal range. In this section we use two contrasting clinical problems to provide some deeper insights into the nature of the statistical problems involved.

5.2.1 Plasma concentration of potassium

An autoanalyser is being introduced into routine use in a hospital for the analysis of standard blood plasma samples. Among the characteristics measured by the autoanalyser is the plasma concentration of K (potassium) recorded in meq/l. The question has been raised about the range of values of plasma K concentration as measured by the autoanalyser in normal, healthy persons and to this end plasma samples of 200 such individuals have been autoanalysed. The results are given in data set **potass**. Two new patients R_1 and R_2 have had blood samples taken and the autoanalyser has given associated plasma concentrations of 4.0 and 5.7 meq/l. What useful statements about these two patients can be made on the basis of the information available to us. In other words, how do these patients relate to past experience?

Histogram

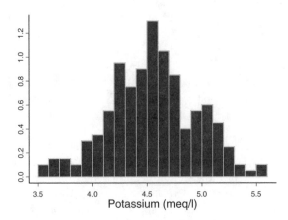

Figure 5.1 *Relative frequency histogram of plasma concentration of potassium in 200 normal, healthy subjects.*

Our first task is to obtain a clearer picture of the nature of the variability and with such extensive data this can be obtained from a histogram (Figure 5.1). The general form of this histogram suggests that we should be able to exploit a parametric model approach and its symmetry invites us to hope that the very tractable univariate normal statistical model $N^1(\mu, \sigma^2)$ will serve the purposes

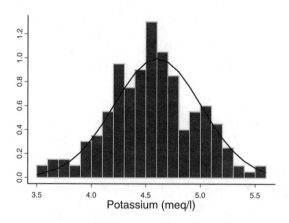

Figure 5.2 *Relative frequency histogram of plasma concentration of potassium in 200 normal, healthy subjects, with fitted normal density function.*

of the problem. The fitted normal model has $\hat{\mu} = 4.605$ and $\hat{\sigma} = 0.401$ meq/l. Figure 5.2 shows this fitted normal density function. We briefly indicate the use of techniques from Section 3.12 which provide support for this hope.

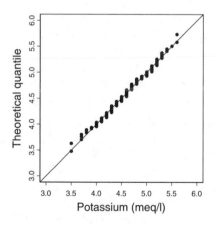

Figure 5.3 *A quantile-quantile plot of plasma concentration of potassium in 200 normal, healthy subjects, based on a theoretical normal probability model.*

Q-Q plot

Figure 5.3 shows the Q-Q plot for this data set. The straightness of the line encourages the view that the fitting of a univariate normal model is a reasonable approach to describing such variability, although we may note a tendency for the line not to pass through the centres of some of the groups. The Filliben correlation coefficient of 0.995 is extremely high and provides further support.

Box-Cox analysis

The profile likelihood curve is very flat with maximized value -693.3 occurring in the range $\lambda \in (1.2, 1.8)$, with the value at 1 only marginally different at -693.5. There is therefore no justification for consideration of a transformation to improve the validity of the normal model assumption.

Tests of normality

The Anderson-Darling, Cramer-von Mises and Watson tests can be performed in their marginal form. The computed values are $Q_A = 0.796$ for the Anderson-Darling statistic, marginally significant at the 5 per cent level, $Q_C = 0.142$ for the Cramer-von Mises statistic, significant at the 5 per cent level, and $Q_W = 0.143$ for the Watson statistic, just significant at the 2.5 per cent level. This apparent indication of some non-normality in these tests, at first sight disappointing, really arises because of the rounded nature of the observations, there being in effect only about one significant digit distinguishing them. We have found that the values of these test statistics can be substantially enlarged by extreme discretization of what are conceptually continuous measurements. For example, in the simulation of 200 observations from a $N^1(4.605, 0.1611)$ model, corresponding to the fitted model of this problem, the computed values of the three statistics were 0.412, 0.062, 0.053, all nonsignificant, whereas when the observations were rounded to one decimal place the corresponding computed test statistics were 0.926, 0.149, 0.140, all significant at the 2.5 per cent level. In such circumstances we see no difficulty in reconciling the apparent disparity between the previous analysis and the marginal test analysis and adopting a normal model.

The predictive distribution

In Section 3.10 we saw that inference based on the experience of a set of selected cases, here the 200 healthy persons, for the present referred patient is made through the predictive distribution defined in Property 3.10. Here we have $n = 200, \hat{\mu} = 4.605, \hat{\sigma}^2 = 0.1611$ and so the relevant Student distribution is $St^1\{199, 4.605, 0.1611(1 + 1/200)\}$. Because of the large number of selected cases this distribution is hardly distinguishable from the fitted normal distribution shown in Figure 5.2 and so we do not show a separate graph of its density function.

Atypicality indices

Although for such univariate measurements it may seem obvious if there are any outliers or influential observations in the selected set, we can follow the atypicality and influence diagnostic investigations set out in Sections 3.11-12 for the more general multivariate regression model. The atypicality indices of the selected cases computed on a leave-one-out basis range from 0.010 for $K = 4.1$, a value near the mean, to 0.995 for $K = 3.5$, the minimum recorded value. There are 13 cases in the ranges $K \leq 3.8$ and $K \geq 5.4$ with atypicality indices exceeding 0.95. These are also the cases with the highest Kullback-Liebler influence measures. In view of the number of selected cases these values do not seem exceptional and there seems to be no reason why we should consider their exclusion from the selected data set.

Assessment of the new cases

We assess the two new cases in terms of their atypicality indices. In terms of Property 3.11, with $c = d = 1, n = 200$, we have for case R_1

$$h_R = 1/200 = 0.005 \quad \text{and} \quad q_R = (4.0 - 4.605)^2/0.1611 = 2.27$$

and so an atypicality index 0.87, clearly within a reasonable range of experience. For R_2 we have $h_R = 0.005, q_R = 7.44$ with an atypicality index 0.993. These computations may seem unnecessary since for such a single continuous measurement we seem able to judge by simple comparison that R_1 is not untypical, whereas R_2, being above the observed range, is rather atypical of previous experience. This is indeed so but when we come to multivariate measurements such comparisons are problematic, particularly since it is extremely difficult to make allowances for correlated measurements in such judgements.

It must of course be realized that such analyses are built merely on the data presented and say nothing about the implications for the patient's condition and whether an attempt should be made to bring this aspect of the patient's condition nearer to the centre of the range. From a clinical point of view a plasma concentration of 5.7 meq/l with atypicality index 0.993 with no indication of other irregularities may not require any treatment. On the other hand a patient whose weight atypicality index is 0.993 may be strongly encouraged to diet.

Kernel density assessment

We can apply the techniques of Section 4.8 to obtain a kernel density assessment of the density function with the use of a normal kernel $K(v|v_i, \lambda)$. The maximized value -104.323 of the pseudo-likelihood function occurs at $\lambda = 0.356$. Figure 5.4 provides a graph of the resulting kernel density function. Recall from Section 4.8.4 that the bandwidth used is $\lambda\hat{\sigma} = 0.143$. We note that unlike the predictive density function there is a slight kink on the right hand side which accords with a similar feature in the histogram of Figure 5.1. Despite this the general results would be essentially the same as inference through the use of the normal parametric model. For example, the range of atypicality indices computed by the simulation technique of Section 4.8.3 is from 0.001 to 0.995 and those for the new patients with plasma potassium concentrations 4.0 and 5.7 meq/l are 0.862 and 0.993.

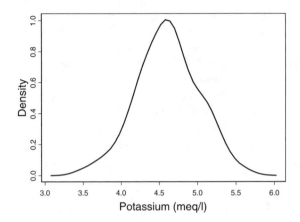

Figure 5.4 *Kernel estimate of the probability density function of plasma concentration of potassium in 200 normal, healthy subjects.*

5.2.2 Urinary excretion rate of pregnenetriol

Within data set `preg` there are 37 observations of urinary excretion rates (mg/24h) of pregnenetriol obtained from normal individuals. Uncritical use of an underlying normal model in this problem would lead to sample estimates $m = 0.832$ and $s^2 = 0.330$ for the mean and variance and consequently to $(-0.316, 1.98)$ as a two-standard-deviation normal range. The fact that such a range allows the possibility of negative excretion rates highlights the absurdity of such an approach. Any parametric modelling approach requires careful consideration of the nature of the variability.

Histogram

The histogram for this data set is shown in Figure 5.5 together with the obviously inappropriate predictive density function based on normal parametric modelling. The positive skewness of the histogram is evident, ruling out the possibility of normal modelling.

Q-Q plot

The curvature in the Q-Q plot of Figure 5.6 confirms the need for further investigation if some parametric modelling is to prove acceptable. The next step in such an investigation is to consider whether some form of transformation to normality is acceptable.

Box-Cox analysis

The profile likelihood has a maximum of -68.74 at $\lambda_1 = -0.25$ with values of -69.62 and -91.57 at $\lambda = 0$ and $\lambda = 1$, respectively. The test of the hypothesis that $\lambda = 1$ gives a computed test statistic value of 45.66 to be

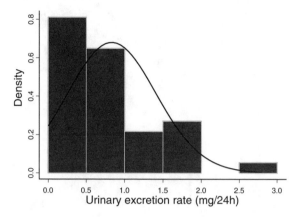

Figure 5.5 *Relative frequency histogram of excretion rates of pregnenetriol in 37 normal individuals, with superimposed fitted Student density function.*

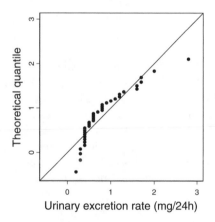

Figure 5.6 *Quantile-quantile plot of excretion rates of pregnenetriol in 37 normal individuals, based on a theoretical normal probability model.*

compared with percentiles of the $\chi^2(1)$ distribution and so we have no hesitation in deciding that a transformation is certainly necessary. Since there is a minor difference between the effects of using $\lambda = -0.25$ and $\lambda = 0$, associated with the logarithmic transformation, we choose the mathematically simpler logarithmic transformation. In effect we are making the assumption that a lognormal parametric model is appropriate. The improvement in the straightness of the Q-Q plot for the transformed data shown in Figure 5.7 is obvious and supports the appropriateness of this transformation.

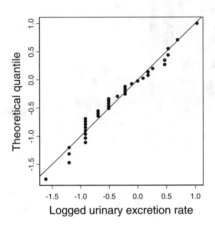

Figure 5.7 *Quantile-quantile plot of logged excretion rates of pregnenetriol in 37 normal individuals, based on a theoretical normal probability model.*

Tests of normality

For the untransformed data the computed values of the Anderson-Darling, Cramer-von Mises and Watson test statistics are $Q_A = 2.182$, $Q_C = 0.359$ and $Q_W = 0.312$, all of which are highly significant being well beyond the 1 per cent values. Although again there is some degree of discretization of this measurement it is clear that this in itself does not provide a reason for such high values of these test statistics. For the logarithmically transformed data the corresponding values of these test statistics are $Q_A = 0.600$, $Q_C = 0.092$ and $Q_W = 0.089$, none of which shows significant departure from normality.

The predictive distribution

The sample mean and variance of the transformed data are $m = 0.181$ and $s^2 = 0.391$ and the predictive distribution here takes the form of a logStudent distribution $\Lambda St^1(36, 0.181, 0.391(1 + 1/37))$. Figure 5.8 shows this predictive density function relative to the histogram.

Atypicality indices

Atypicality indices for the selected set based on the above predictive density function and on the leave-one-out method range from 0.031 for the case with pregnenetriol excretion rate 0.7 mg/24h to 0.980 for the case with pregnenetriol excretion rate 2.8 mg/24h, the largest recorded value. The cases with

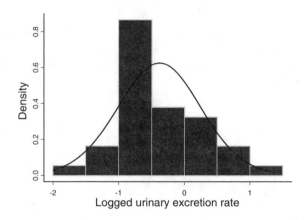

Figure 5.8 *Relative frequency histogram of logged excretion rates of pregnenetriol in 37 normal individuals, with fitted logStudent density function superimposed.*

the smallest and largest excretion rates are the only ones with atypicalities larger than 0.95.

Kernel density assessment

The pseudo-likelihood function has maximum value -36.713 which is attained at $\lambda = 0.550$. The atypicalities are mostly similar to those obtained via parametric analysis, especially in the tails of the distribution, but there are some discrepancies near the mode of the distribution due to the skewness in the kernel density estimate. The atypicalities were computed using simulation and they range from 0.039 to 0.985. The cases with the smallest and largest excretion rates have atypicalities larger than 0.95.

Comment

All the above forms of analysis may seem too elaborate for any univariate problem. It could be argued that it adds little to the sensible comparison of a new observation against the histogram. Two points can be made here. First we agree with this argument but point out that with modern computational aids there seems less tendency to trouble to draw histograms. Secondly while simple graphical comparison may be sufficient for univariate data, and possibly bivariate data, it is of little use in higher dimensional problems. Yet the univariate techniques carry over straightforwardly into higher dimensions.

5.3 Multiple measurement variability

5.3.1 Cortisol-cortisone variability in bilateral hyperplasia

As a simple illustrative example of describing experience of the variability of bivariate measurements of a group of selected cases we use the cortisol and cortisone measurements obtained from the 27 bilateral hyperplasia patients in the Cushing's syndrome data which have been extracted into data set `bilhyp`.

Scattergram

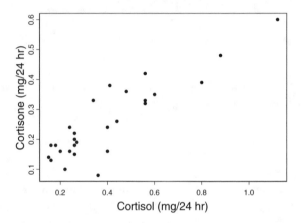

Figure 5.9 *Scattergram of the cortisol and cortisone concentrations in 27 patients with bilateral hyperplasia.*

Figure 5.9 provides the scattergram for the bivariate (cortisol, cortisone) concentrations of the 27 bilateral hyperplasia patients. Even at this simple graphical level we can see that the pattern is not symmetric about the mean vector, with indications of some positive skewness, raising some doubts as to any assumption of normality.

Q-Q plots

The Q-Q plots for the two concentrations are shown separately in Figure 5.10. The plots, particularly the cortisol plot, show a marked departure from the diagonal line.

Box-Cox analysis

The Box-Cox analysis applied separately to the two concentrations gives maximizing values $\lambda_1 = -0.338, \lambda_2 = 0.057$ with maximized univariate profile loglikelihoods of 7.93 and 21.03. If we compare these with the univariate profile loglikelihood values 0.85 and 18.05 at $\lambda_1 = 1$ and $\lambda_2 = 1$ we see that the values of the test statistic in (3.36) of 14.16 for cortisol and 5.96 for cortisone are

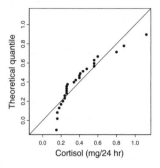 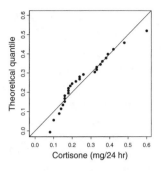

Figure 5.10 *Quantile-quantile plots of cortisol and cortisone concentrations in 27 patients with bilateral hyperplasia, based on a theoretical normal probability model.*

highly significant when compared against percentiles of the $\chi^2(1)$ distribution. We can use these as starting values for a bivariate Box-Cox analysis leading to the bivariate maximizing values $\lambda_1 = 0.187, \lambda_2 = 0.723$, substantially different from the univariate values, and with a maximized profile loglikelihood of 43.99. Comparison with the profile loglikelihood value 39.78 at $\lambda_1 = 1, \lambda_2 = 1$ gives a value of 8.42 for the test statistic in (3.36) which, when compared with percentiles of the $\chi^2(2)$ distribution, shows that there is a formal Box-Cox justification for a transformation. The profile loglikelihood surface is, however, relatively flat around the maximizing point with, for example, the values at $(0, 0), (0, 1), (0, 0.5)$ equal to 41.52, 43.06, 43.68, respectively, so that there is little to distinguish between the quality of a number of possible transformations.

Tests of normality

Table 5.1 *Values of the modified test statistics for the bilateral hyperplasia data*

Test	Variable(s)	Anderson-Darling	Cramer-von Mises	Watson
Marginal				
	Cortisol	1.397	0.204	0.173
	Cortisone	0.813	0.132	0.119
Bivariate angle				
	Cortisol-Cortisone	0.444	0.065	0.062
Radius		0.504	0.087	0.059

Table 5.1 shows the values of the marginal, bivariate angle and radius Anderson-Darling, Cramer-von Mises and Watson test statistics. All three

marginal tests for cortisol show substantial departure from normality at the 1 per cent significance level. There is similar evidence of departure from normality in the marginal tests for cortisone at the 5 per cent level of significance. This supports our earlier visual assessment of the Q-Q plots. None of the bivariate angle nor radius tests suggests any significant departure from bivariate normality.

Conclusion

How can we assess all this evidence regarding the normality or otherwise of the bivariate concentration vector? The scattergram, Q-Q plots, univariate Box-Cox analyses and marginal tests of normality all suggest that some transformation is indicated. The bivariate Box-Cox analysis also suggests that a transformation is necessary and the flatness of the profile loglikelihood surface assures us that a range of transformations is certainly feasible. Both the univariate and bivariate Box-Cox analysis suggest that a logarithmic transformation for cortisol is appropriate and, with the flatness of the profile loglikelihood surface in mind, it seems sensible to consider whether a logarithmic transformation of both concentrations is supportable. Applied to the logged data none of the battery of normality tests shows any significant departure from normality. Moreover the Q-Q plots for the transformed data, shown in Figure 5.11, are admirably diagonal.

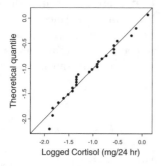 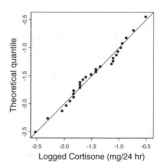

Figure 5.11 *Quantile-quantile plots of logged cortisol and cortisone measurents in 27 patients with bilateral hyperplasia, based on a theoretical normal probability model.*

The predictive distributions

In view of the above conclusion we shall work, in our parametric analysis, on the assumption that the bivariate concentrations are distributed lognormally as $\Lambda^2(\mu, \Sigma)$. The sample estimates are

$$\hat{\mu} = [\ -1.067 \quad -1.473 \ ], \qquad \hat{\Sigma} = \begin{bmatrix} 0.2948 & 0.2108 \\ 0.2108 & 0.2438 \end{bmatrix}.$$

The predictive distribution appropriate to new patients is then of logStudent form

$$\Lambda St^2 \left[k, \hat{\mu}, \{1 + 1/n\}\hat{\Sigma} \right],$$

where $k = 26$, $n = 27$.

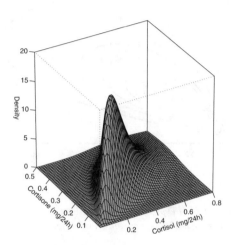

Figure 5.12 *Predictive logStudent density surface of cortisol and cortisone concentrations in patients with bilateral hyperplasia.*

In Figure 5.12 we provide on the untransformed concentration space a mesh diagram of the surface of this predictive density function. Comparison with the scattergram of Figure 5.9 shows a reasonable correspondence with the nature of the variability of the data. We can report here that had we decided not to transform the data and assumed a bivariate normal model we would have found, as in the case of the pregnenetriol data of Section 4.2, that the predictive distribution would have allowed the possibility of negative values of the concentrations. This indeed is a compelling reason for considering logarithmic transformations when faced with essentially positive measurements.

Atypicality indices of selected cases

The atypicality indices of the selected cases computed on the basis of the predictive distribution and on the leave-one-out principle range from 0.092 to 0.9998, the only index exceeding 0.95 being 0.9998 for selected case 13, the case with the smallest cortisone concentration. Within a group of 27 we may expect one case to have atypicality index above 0.95 and there is no clinical evidence to regard this case as special.

Regions of experience

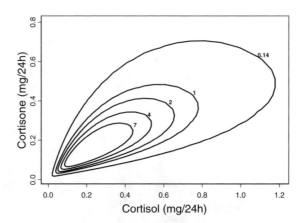

Figure 5.13 *Contour plot of the predictive logStudent density surface of cortisol and cortisone concentrations in patients with bilateral hyperplasia.*

With such bivariate data we can use isoprobability contours of the probability density surface (loci of points with the same probability density) to define what could be termed a region of experience. Figure 5.13 shows a set of such contours at heights 7, 4, 2, 1, and 0.14 for the concentration measurements. More specifically we could define a region of actual experience as the region within the contour associated with the most atypical selected case. This is provided by the outermost contour of Figure 5.13. An alternative to the use of isoprobability contours is to define a region in terms of atypicality contours. For example, a *region of 95 per cent experience* would have its boundary as the locus of points whose atypicality indices are 0.95. A claim for such a region is that we may expect 95 per cent of future cases to have bivariate measurements within this region. For a predictive distribution of the form $\Lambda St^d\{k, \hat{\mu}, (1 + n^{-1})\hat{\Sigma}\}$ we can find the equation of such a boundary. First we determine the value of $t \equiv t_{95}$ satisfying

$$J\left\{t \mid \tfrac{1}{2}d, \tfrac{1}{2}(n - d)\right\} = 0.95.$$

Then, any bivariate vector u whose corresponding Mahalanobis distance

$$q = (\log u - \hat{\mu})\hat{\Sigma}^{-1}(\log u - \hat{\mu})^T$$

satisfies $q/\{q + (n^2 - 1)/n\} = t_{95}$ is on the boundary of the region of 95 per cent experience. Thus the equation of the boundary is

$$(\log u - \hat{\mu})\hat{\Sigma}^{-1}(\log u - \hat{\mu})^T = \frac{(n^2 - 1)}{n}\frac{t_{95}}{1 - t_{95}}.$$

Figure 5.14 shows the region of 95 per cent experience for the bilateral hyperplasia group.

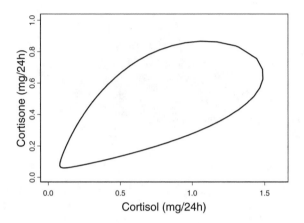

Figure 5.14 *95% region of experience of cortisol and cortisone concentrations in patients with bilateral hyperplasia.*

Kernel density assessment

Assessment of the density function by the non-parametric kernel method is straightforward. Being aware of the inappropriateness of the normal kernel in the pregnenetriol study of Section 4.2 we adopt the lognormal kernel defined in (4.24) with $d = 2$ to ensure that no negative measurements are possible with our method of assessment. The pseudo-loglikelihood maximization method then leads to estimate $\lambda = 0.465$ of the smoothing parameter for the density estimate. Figure 5.15 provides a mesh diagram of this kernel assessment of the density function. Using the corresponding kernel assessments we can obtain by the mesh method of Section 4.8.3 kernel atypicalities for the selected cases. The main disagreements between the predictive and kernel assignments of atypicality indices are that the kernel method assigns an atypicality index of only 0.605 for case 13 and indicates one different possible outlier in case 5, the case with the largest values of both concentrations, with an atypicality index of 1.00. These discrepancies are clearly caused by the differences already identified.

Assessment of referred patients

As an illustration of the assessment of new patients we consider the 7 selected cases of adenoma, A1–A7, in data set **cush**. We can compute atypicality

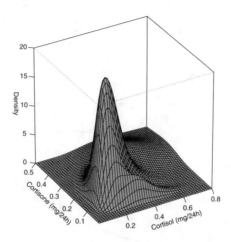

Figure 5.15 *Plot of bivariate kernel density estimate based on the bilateral hyperplasia data.*

indices with respect to the bilateral hyperplasia group on the basis of our parametric or non-parametric analyses above. These are shown in Table 5.2. It is clear that, while there is some variation in the indices of the cases showing no appreciable atypicality, both assessments are identifying the most atypical cases, namely A1 and A7.

Table 5.2 *Atypicality indices for 7 adenoma patients computed using parametric and kernel methods*

Method	Patient						
	A1	A2	A3	A4	A5	A6	A7
Parametric	0.98	0.67	0.28	0.82	0.28	0.85	0.99
Kernel	0.99	0.63	0.53	0.74	0.54	0.80	0.99

5.3.2 Coagulation measurements in genetic counselling in haemophilia

In order to use the coagulation measurements of data set `haemo` for genetic counselling in haemophilia we have clearly to investigate the possibility of describing the nature of the variability of the bivariate vectors of measurements in both the carrier and non-carrier selected groups.

Scattergram

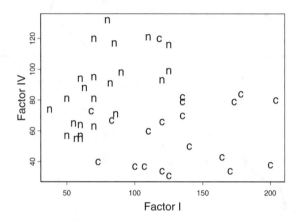

Figure 5.16 *Scattergram of coagulation measurements recorded on 20 carriers (c) and 23 non-carriers (n) of haemophilia.*

Figure 5.16 provides the scattergram for the bivariate coagulation measurements of the 20 carriers and 23 non-carriers in the selected set. It is clear that these measurements provide some separation of the two types and our purpose here is to attempt to quantify this separation by obtaining appropriate predictive distributions to describe the differences in this experience.

Q-Q plots

The Q-Q plots for the two coagulation measurements of the carriers and the non-carriers are shown in Figure 5.17. The plot showing some departure from the diagonal line is that for the first coagulation measurement of the non-carriers, but the departure does not appear to be particularly strong.

Box-Cox analysis

For the 20 carriers, Box-Cox analysis applied separately to the two coagulation measurements gives maximizing values $\lambda_{11} = 0.582, \lambda_{12} = -0.042$. Using these as starting values for a bivariate Box-Cox analysis we obtain the bivariate maximizing values $\lambda_{11} = 0.585, \lambda_{12} = -0.036$ with a maximized profile loglikelihood of -190.72. Since the profile loglikelihood value is -192.24 at $\lambda_{11} = 1, \lambda_{12} = 1$, comparison of the value 3.04 of the test statistic in (3.36) with percentiles of the $\chi^2(2)$ distribution shows that there is no Box-Cox justification for a transformation. Indeed the profile loglikelihood surface is very flat around the maximizing value with, for example, the value -191.07 at $\lambda_{11} = 0, \lambda_{12} = 0$. A similar analysis of the 23 non-carriers gives, for the two

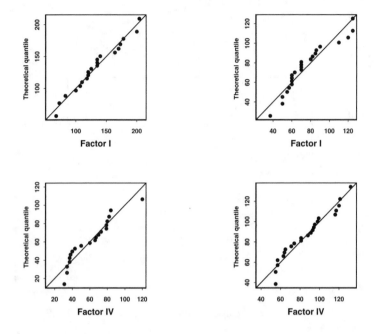

Figure 5.17 *Quantile-quantile plots of the coagulation measurements for 20 carriers and 23 non-carriers of haemophilia.* **Top left.** *Factor I measurement for carriers.* **Top right.** *Factor I measurement for non-carriers.* **Bottom left.** *Factor IV measurement for carriers.* **Bottom right.** *Factor IV measurement for non-carriers.*

univariate analyses, $\lambda_{21} = -0.244, \lambda_{22} = 0.115$, and for the bivariate analysis $\lambda_{21} = -0.151, \lambda_{22} = 0.155$ with a maximized profile loglikelihood of -202.97. The value of the profile likelihood function is -205.85 at $\lambda_{21} = 1, \lambda_{22} = 1$ and -203.03 at $\lambda_{12} = 0, \lambda_{22} = 0$. Since the value of the test statistic in (3.36) comparing the maximized value and the value at $\lambda_{21} = 1, \lambda_{22} = 1$ is 5.76, comparison with percentiles of the $\chi^2(2)$ distribution shows that there is again no Box-Cox justification for the use of a transformation.

Tests of normality

Table 5.3 shows the values of the marginal, bivariate angle and radius Anderson-Darling, Cramer-von Mises and Watson test statistics separately for the carrier and non-carrier cases. Comparing the results with the critical values in Table 3.2 we see that the only tests showing significant departure from normality are the marginal tests for the first coagulation measurements in the non-carrier cases. This accords with the experience in the Q-Q plots above.

Table 5.3 *Values of the modified test statistics for the haemophilia data*

Test	Variable(s)	Anderson- Darling	Cramer- von Mises	Watson
Carriers				
Marginal				
	Factor I	0.310	0.048	0.048
	Factor IV	0.774	0.099	0.099
Bivariate angle				
	Factor I-Factor IV	0.223	0.005	0.019
Radius		0.352	0.044	0.036
Non-carriers				
Marginal				
	Factor I	0.999	0.145	0.131
	Factor IV	0.505	0.059	0.059
Bivariate angle				
	Factor I-Factor IV	0.471	0.044	0.039
Radius		0.438	0.059	0.045

Conclusion

Any slight evidence for use of a transformation here appears to be confined to the first measurement of the non-carrier group, with a logarithmic transformation the obvious choice. Such a transformation would involve specification of different parametric models for the carrier and non-carrier groups. While there is no theoretical reason for resisting such an asymmetrical approach there may be some awkwardness in clinical practice in such asymmetry. Moreover the obvious flatness of the profile loglikelihood surfaces and the maximizing values $(0.585, -0.036)$ for carriers and $(-0.151, 0.155)$ for non-carriers suggest that a sensible compromise solution may be to use a logarithmic transformation of all measurements. From the viewpoint of normality assumptions the effects of this decision are that the Q-Q plots for the transformed data are slightly more diagonal in appearance and only the marginal tests of normality for the second coagulation measurement of the carriers, with Anderson-Darling, Cramer-von Mises, Watson test statistic values of 0.830, 0.129, 0.132, are just significant at the 5 per cent significance level.

The predictive distributions

In view of the above conclusion we shall work, in our parametric analysis, on the assumption that the bivariate coagulation measurements are distributed lognormally as $\Lambda^2(\mu_1, \Sigma_1)$ and $\Lambda^2(\mu_2, \Sigma_2)$, respectively, in the carrier and non-carrier groups. The sample estimates are

$$\hat{\mu}_1 = [\ 4.85 \quad 4.02\ ], \qquad \hat{\mu}_2 = [\ 4.28 \quad 4.42\ ],$$

$$\hat{\Sigma}_1 = \begin{bmatrix} 0.0952 & 0.0077 \\ 0.0077 & 0.1566 \end{bmatrix}, \qquad \hat{\Sigma}_2 = \begin{bmatrix} 0.0989 & 0.0530 \\ 0.0530 & 0.0774 \end{bmatrix}.$$

The predictive distributions appropriate to new patients are then of logStudent form

$$\Lambda St^2 \left\{ k_i, \hat{\mu}_i, (1 + 1/n_i)\hat{\Sigma}_i \right\} \qquad (i = 1, 2),$$

where $k_1 = 19, k_2 = 22, n_1 = 20, n_2 = 23$. In Figure 5.18 we provide a mesh diagram of the surfaces of the two probability density functions. It can be seen that these reflect the separation and roughly elliptical shape of the groups in the scattergram of Figure 5.16.

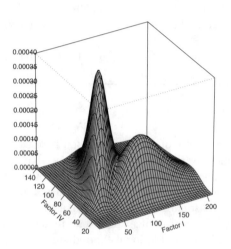

Figure 5.18 *Probability density surfaces of the coagulation measurements for the carriers and non-carriers of haemophilia.*

Atypicality indices of selected cases

The atypicality indices of the selected cases computed on the leave-one-out principle range from 0.085 to 0.926 for the carrier group and from 0.005 to 0.955 for the non-carrier group, so that there is no need here to consider whether any of these cases should be regarded as outliers.

Regions of experience

As for the bilateral hyperplasia concentrations discussed above we can provide a region of 95 per cent experience for the bivariate coagulation measure-

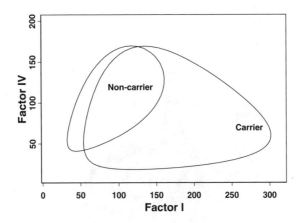

Figure 5.19 *95% regions of experience of the coagulation measurements for carriers and non-carriers of haemophilia.*

ments. These are shown separately for the carrier and non-carrier groups in Figure 5.19.

Kernel density assessment

Assessment of the density functions by the non-parametric kernel method is straightforward. Since the bivariate measurements are all well above zero the use of a spherical bivariate normal kernel does not carry the danger of introducing the possibility of negative measurements as in the case of the pregnenetriol study in Section 5.2. Equally a lognormal kernel is available; see (4.24) with $d = 2$. We prefer the lognormal approach because of its conformity with the decision to use lognormal parametric modelling. The pseudo-loglikelihood maximization method then leads to estimates $\lambda_1 = 0.660, \lambda_2 = 0.543$ of the smoothing parameters for the carrier and non-carrier groups. Figure 5.20 shows the mesh surfaces of the two assessed kernel density functions for the carriers and non-carriers, which are in broad agreement with the parametric picture of Figure 5.18. Using these kernel assessments we can obtain by the mesh method kernel atypicalities for the selected cases. These are in rough agreement with the atypicalities found by lognormal parametric modelling, ranging from 0.004 to 0.840 for carriers and from 0.001 to 0.788 for non-carriers. Within the framework of this kernel density approach there is again no evidence of outliers within the selected groups.

Assessment of the referred patients

For the 15 new patients of data set newhaem we can compute atypicality indices with respect to the carrier and the non-carrier groups on the basis of our parametric or non-parametric analyses above. Since we shall require

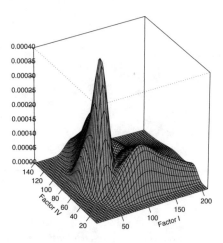

Figure 5.20 *Kernel density surfaces of the coagulation measurements for the carriers and non-carriers of haemophilia.*

the ratio of the carrier to non-carrier densities in Chapter 8 we provide those 'odds' in Table 5.4 together with the atypicalities. We shall reserve further comments on these new cases until we consider the role of the assessments in the setting of genetic counselling.

5.3.3 Experience of adenoma in Conn's syndrome

In our analyses so far we have had the advantage of graphical aids such as histograms, scattergrams and mesh surface diagrams, allowed by the low dimensions of the measurement vectors. We have seen that, relative to these lower-dimensional data sets, concepts such as data transformation, predictive and kernel density assessments and atypicality indices reflect what we can see visually about our measurement experience. When we are faced with higher-dimensional measurement vectors the same forms of analysis apply but we have less recourse to graphical methods associated with the full measurement vector. As an illustration of the problems of quantifying experience of the variability of higher-dimensional measurements we investigate the possibility of describing the adenoma experience in the selected group A1–A20 in data set **conn**. We use abbreviated labels: N (sodium), K (potassium), C (carbon dioxide), R (renin), A (aldosterone), S (systolic BP) and D (diastolic BP).

Table 5.4 *Atypicalities of 15 new patients with respect to the carrier and non-carrier groups, computed using the parametric and kernel methods. The 'odds' in favour of the carrier group are also given*

	Atypicalities				Odds Ratio
	Carriers		Non-Carriers		
	Parametric	Kernel	Parametric	Kernel	
N1	0.77	0.71	0.69	0.56	0.40
N2	0.99	1.00	1.00	1.00	5.62
N3	0.97	0.97	0.47	0.48	0.02
N4	0.26	0.32	0.86	0.91	3.60
N5	0.64	0.65	0.83	0.76	1.24
N6	0.91	0.94	0.93	0.97	0.68
N7	0.78	0.69	0.95	0.93	2.68
N8	0.73	0.61	0.85	0.74	1.06
N9	0.99	1.00	0.96	0.98	0.01
N10	0.31	0.45	0.96	0.96	11.23
N11	0.87	0.87	0.64	0.62	0.17
N12	0.18	0.32	0.94	0.96	10.46
N13	0.41	0.33	1.00	1.00	7543.99
N14	0.37	0.05	0.94	0.87	7.58
N15	0.65	0.73	0.33	0.50	0.27

Q-Q plots

Only two of the seven Q-Q plots, those for N and A in Figure 5.21, show any appreciable departure from the diagonal line. The main feature of the N plot is the gap between the eighth and ninth points, due to the gap between 141.0 and 143.0 in the recorded N values. Clinically there is no reason for such a gap since values within the range (141.0,143.0) are common in the new patients, and we are clearly experiencing an effect of the small sample available. We shall see the effects of this feature in our further analysis.

Box-Cox analysis

Use of Box-Cox analysis as a sledge-hammer approach to decisions on transformation is here fraught with difficulties. For example, a univariate Box-Cox analysis of the N concentrations leads to a maximizing value $\lambda_N = 18.2$ with maximized profile loglikelihood -47.62, whereas the profile loglikelihood values at $\lambda_N = 1$ and $\lambda_N = 0$ are -47.28 and -47.36, hardly differing from the maximized value. In view of our comment above about the unusual nature of the gap in the N values it would certainly seem non-sensical to attempt to raise the N concentrations to the power 18 in order to obtain a marginal improvement in the normality of the sample. The unusual nature of the N concentrations renders attempts to subject the full seven-dimensional mea-

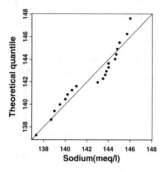
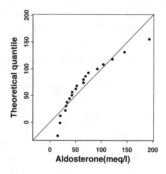

Figure 5.21 *Quantile-quantile plots of the concentrations of sodium (left) and aldos-terone (right) in blood plasma for 20 patients with an adenoma, based on a theoretical normal probability model.*

surement vector to a multivariate Box-Cox analysis impossible because of resulting ill-conditioning and near-singularity of matrices. Multivariate Box-Cox analysis applied to the six-dimensional vector (K,C,R,A,S,D) results in a maximizing vector $\lambda = [0.45, 0.46, 1.26, -0.21, -0.028, -1.20]$ with maximized profile loglikelihood -342.66, compared with values -350.68 and -347.70 at $\lambda = [1, 1, 1, 1, 1, 1]$ and $\lambda = [0, 0, 0, 0, 0, 0]$. When twice the differences from the maximized profile loglikelihood value are compared against percentiles of the $\chi^2(7)$ distribution there is nothing to distinguish between the last two vectors of transformations, while the first two show a significant difference. Before we decide on a course of action we report the results of the battery of tests of normality.

Tests of normality

For the seven-dimensional vector here there are altogether 21 marginal tests, 63 bivariate angle tests and 3 radius tests. Of these, only the three marginal tests for N and A show significant departure from normality, all at the 5 per cent significance level, corroborating our view of the corresponding Q-Q plots. The values of the Anderson-Darling, Cramer-von Mises, Watson test statistics are 0.879, 0.153, 0.151 for N and 0.984, 0.148, 0.126 for A.

Conclusion

The results of the Q-Q plots and the tests of normality suggest that we should first concentrate on the N and A concentrations. We have already concluded that the sample of N concentrations is unusual and that a wide range of Box-Cox transformations seem equally plausible. For the A concentrations the value $\lambda_A = -0.21$ suggests that a logarithmic transformation may be appropriate. When this is applied the Q-Q plot is beautifully diagonal and the Anderson-Darling, Cramer-von Mises and Watson marginal test statistics re-

duce to the non-significant values 0.126, 0.015, 0.015. We can also report that
the associated bivariate angle and radius test statistics all remain insignificant.

Let us now examine the R concentrations. The Box-Cox analysis with
$\lambda_R = 1.26$ suggests that there is no need to transform the R concentrations.
Since some of the R concentrations, such as 0.7 for A3 and 0.9 for A15, are low
we have to consider whether an assumption of normal variability might lead
to the possibility of negative concentrations as in the case of the pregnenetriol
study considered above. The estimated mean and standard deviation of the R
concentrations are 3.35 and 1.29 and so the estimated probability of a negative
concentration on the basis of a normality assumption is $\Phi(-\mu_R/\sigma_R) = 0.0047$,
probably too large for comfort. In order to avoid this possibility of allowing
negative concentrations for R we therefore advocate the use of a logarithmic
transformation. We have thus reached a position of advocating logarithmic
transformations for R and A, with knowledge that such a transformation for
N is also a possibility. The further fact that there is no significant difference
between the six-dimensional maximized profile loglikelihood -342.66 and the
value -347.70 associated with an overall logarithmic transformation of all
concentrations suggests that we should follow through the consequences of
applying a logarithmic transformation to all seven concentrations. With such
a transformation the only tests of normality suggesting significant departure
from normality are those for the R concentration, with Anderson-Darling,
Cramer-von Mises, Watson test statistics 1.50, 0.223, 0.186, all significant at
the 1 per cent significance level. Since in this case the logarithmic transformation has been introduced to ensure positivity of concentration we prefer to
persist with the transformation at the expense of some marginal departure
from normality.

Biplot

We now investigate the possibility of providing a graphical view of this
adenoma experience in terms of a biplot; see Section 4.7 for the theoretical
detail. We naturally use logarithmically transformed concentrations and since
the variances of the logged concentrations vary between 0.00035 for R and
0.471 for A we shall also use the standardization technique of Section 4.7.
Figure 5.22 provides this biplot, which captures a proportion 0.57 of the total variability. We can immediately see how the rays reflect the correlation
structure of the data if we examine the main correlations (> 0.4) between the
logged concentrations emphasised in the following array:

$$
\begin{bmatrix}
 & K & C & R & A & S & D \\
N & -0.088 & \mathbf{0.407} & -0.112 & 0.102 & 0.072 & -0.059 \\
K & & -\mathbf{0.620} & -0.060 & -\mathbf{0.418} & -0.259 & -0.080 \\
C & & & 0.135 & \mathbf{0.529} & 0.388 & 0.086 \\
R & & & & 0.041 & 0.280 & 0.052 \\
S & & & & & & \mathbf{0.701}
\end{bmatrix}.
$$

Recall that for this type of biplot a correlation between two measurements,
such as N and R, is represented by the cosine of the angle NOR, and that

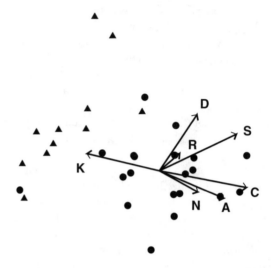

Figure 5.22 *Biplot of the logged concentrations of sodium, potassium, carbon diox-ide, renin and aldosterone in blood plasma together with systolic and diastolic blood pressures in 20 patients with an adenoma (circles) and 11 patients with bilateral hyperplasia (triangles).*

because this two-dimensional plot accounts for only 57 per cent of the total variation in the data the representation is very approximate here. Note that the positive correlation of 0.701 between S and D is reflected in the acuteness of the angle between the rays OS and OD. Similarly the negative correlation of −0.620 between K and C corresponds to the obtuseness of the angle between OK and OC. Acute angles between ON and OC and between OA and OC correspond, respectively, to the positive correlations 0.407 and 0.529 between the associated logged concentrations, and obtuse angle KOA corresponds to the negative correlation −0.418 between K and A. Indeed it can be verified that for this data set the signs of all the correlations correspond to the acuteness or obtuseness of all the associated angles.

In addition to the case markers for the adenoma cases we have plotted the case markers for the bilateral hyperplasia cases B1–B11. It is clear that there is some separation of the two groups which is encouraging from the point of view of differential diagnosis, the main aim of the analyses of this data set. Before we discuss the interpretation of the case markers we note that there is complete overlap of the projections of the adenoma and bilateral hyperplasia case markers on the S and D rays so that we can anticipate that, considered individually, these have no diagnostic value in differential diagnosis in Conn's syndrome, a view substantiated later in Chapter 8. We therefore reduce the complexity of the diagram by providing in Figure 5.23 the biplot for the five-dimensional concentration vector (N, K, C, R, A). This biplot retains a proportion 0.66 of the total variability. It is again easy to check that the angles between rays are in good accord with the correlation structure of the concentrations.

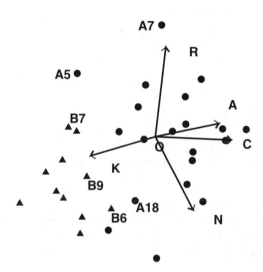

Figure 5.23 *Biplot of the logged concentrations of sodium, potassium, carbon dioxide, renin and aldosterone in blood plasma in 20 patients with an adenoma (circles) and 11 patients with bilateral hyperplasia (triangles).*

Recall that the biplot through its case markers and rays gives an approximate representation of the complete data set in the sense that projections of case marker vectors on a ray indicate the extent to which that standardized concentration exceeds or falls short of the average for the data set. For example, we can see that A7 is substantially above average in R; indeed it is the adenoma case with the largest R. Case A5, with its large negative projection on OC, is well below average in C; it is in fact the adenoma case with the smallest C value. From the relative positions of the adenoma and the bilateral hyperplasia cases we might anticipate from the biplot that, for example, a case of Conn's syndrome with large K and small R may be more likely to be of bilateral hyperplasia than of adenoma type. Equally, small C or A may also indicate bilateral hyperplasia. In Chapter 8 we shall be in a position to test such conjectures. The advantage of the biplot is that it provides a graphical representation of the complete data set which may prove useful in explaining in a consultative context the outcome of some sophisticated statistical analysis.

The predictive distribution

On the assumption that the concentration vector (N, K, C, R, A) is lognormally distributed as $\Lambda^5(\mu, \Sigma)$ we can obtain the predictive distribution, appropriate to inference of any referred patient, as of logStudent form,

$$\Lambda St^5(k, \hat{\mu}, (1 + 1/n)\hat{\Sigma}),$$

where $k = 19$, $n = 20$, and

$$\hat{\mu} = \begin{bmatrix} 4.96 & 1.20 & 3.38 & 1.10 & 3.96 \end{bmatrix},$$

$$\hat{\Sigma} = 10 \times \begin{bmatrix} 0.0035 & -0.0028 & 0.0073 & -0.0113 & 0.0131 \\ -0.0028 & 0.2974 & -0.1026 & -0.0562 & -0.4943 \\ 0.0073 & -0.1026 & 0.0920 & 0.0706 & 0.3480 \\ -0.0113 & -0.0562 & 0.0706 & 2.9621 & 0.1540 \\ 0.0131 & -0.4943 & 0.3480 & 0.1540 & 4.7056 \end{bmatrix}.$$

Atypicality indices of selected cases

The atypicality indices of the selected adenoma cases A1–A20 can be readily evaluated by the leave-one-out method. These range from 0.095 for A19 to 0.984 for A3, the case with the smallest R concentration of 0.7, and 0.974 for A16, the case with the largest A concentration of 192.7. There is nothing here clinically to suggest that we should regard any of these cases as outliers.

Kernel density assessment

Assessment of the density functions by the non-parametric kernel method is again straightforward. We use a lognormal kernel for all the reasons put forward in our discussion of transformations; see (4.24) with $d = 5$. The maximization based on the pseudo-loglikelihood method then leads to an estimate $\lambda = 0.847$ of the smoothing parameter. The kernel density assessments associated with the 20 selected cases A1–A20 are then

$$10^{-5} \times \begin{bmatrix} 0.116 & 0.654 & 0.098 & 0.766 & 0.044 & 0.740 & 0.117 & 0.780 & 0.541 & 0.104 \\ 0.305 & 0.655 & 0.674 & 0.301 & 0.118 & 0.014 & 0.293 & 0.184 & 0.626 & 0.368 \end{bmatrix}.$$

Because of the higher dimensionality the mesh method of computing kernel atypicality indices is not practicable. We can, however, identify the most atypical cases judged on the basis of low kernel densities as A16 and A3, in agreement with the parametric findings above.

Assessment of the bilateral hyperplasia cases

We have already seen in the biplot some ways in which the bilateral hyperplasia cases differ from the adenoma cases. We can also calculate their atypicality indices with respect to the adenoma group. The two largest atypicality indices are 0.906 for B4, the case with the overall smallest values of C and A, and 0.829 for B1. The fact that these atypicality indices are not extreme is in agreement with the overlap of the two groups in the biplot and suggests that there will be a degree of uncertainty in the differential diagnosis of Conn's syndrome.

We can also obtain the kernel density assessments for these cases with respect to the adenoma kernel density above. For B1–B11 these are

$$10^{-5} \times [\, 0.108 \; 0.131 \; 0.812 \; 0.136 \; 0.221 \; 0.329 \; 0.271 \; 0.257 \; 0.996 \; 0.167 \; 0.031 \,].$$

The most atypical on the basis of lowest kernel density is B11, the bilateral hyperplasia case with the highest K and A concentrations. Note, however, that its kernel density 0.031×10^{-5} is larger than that of A16 and so, on this kernel assessment, less atypical than A16.

5.4 Conditional variability

Often a clinical measurement of interest may depend on other known characteristics or features of the patient and so in any attempt to define normal ranges or regions it is important to take such features into account in attempting to describe experience. A simple example is the now well known fact that the range of blood pressure in healthy individuals rises with age; see, for example, Pickering (1968, chapter 28). We now turn our attention to this type of problem in two particular situations.

5.4.1 Anti-diuretic hormone variability in healthy persons

The problem of describing experience in the measurement of anti-diuretic hormone (ADH) has been outlined in Section 1.6. The statistical problem is to try to determine the extent, if any, to which ADH is dependent on gender (G) and urine osmolarity (UO).

Scattergram

The scattergram of ADH against urine osmolarity measurement is shown in Figure 5.24. We take as a starting point in modelling a tentative maximal normal linear model with interaction between gender and osmolarity:

$$\text{ADH} = \alpha_G + \beta_G \text{UO} + \text{error} \quad (G = M, F).$$

Box-Cox analysis

With this maximal model we apply a Box-Cox transformation to the response ADH and find that the maximizing $\lambda = -0.12$ with maximized profile loglikelihood -355.3 compared with the value -373.1 at $\lambda = 1$. The value 35.6 of the test statistic in (3.36) in comparison with percentiles of the $\chi^2(1)$

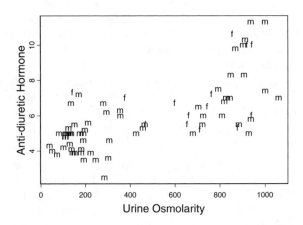

Figure 5.24 *Scattergram of anti-diuretic hormone measurement and urine osmolarity in 61 healthy male patients (m) and 14 healthy female patients (f).*

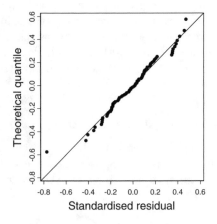

Figure 5.25 *Quantile-quantile plot of standardised residuals obtained from a simple linear regression of logged anti-diuretic hormone measurement on logged urine osmolarity and gender in 75 healthy patients.*

distribution is highly significant (P < 0.001) and, since the value at $\lambda = 0$ of -355.6 is hardly different from the maximum -355.6, we opt for a logarithmic transformation. It seems sensible then to consider taking log UO as covariate to produce effectively a multiplicative model

$$E(\log \text{ADH} \mid G, \text{UO}) = \alpha_G + \beta_G \log \text{UO} \quad (G = M, F), \quad (5.1)$$

with independent $N(0, \sigma^2)$ errors. This model is now taken to be the maximal model. Re-application of Box-Cox analysis, that is consideration of a Box-Cox power transformation to log ADH, yields a maximizing power λ close to 0, confirming the reasonableness of using the logarithm of ADH as the response variable.

Tests of normality

We can investigate the assumption of normality of the error term in the maximal model of (5.1) by the three marginal tests. The computed values of the Anderson-Darling, Cramer-von Mises and Watson test statistics are 0.393, 0.043 and 0.044, all attesting to reasonable normality of error, and this is confirmed by the diagonal nature of the corresponding Q-Q plot of Figure 5.25.

Lattice of hypotheses

Table 5.5 *Hypothesis-testing for the ADH data*

Level	Model	Hypothesis tested	Residual s.s. (d.f)	F	P
4	$\alpha_G + \beta_G \log \text{UO}$		4.00 (71)		
3a	$\alpha_G + \beta \log \text{UO}$	$\beta_M = \beta_F$	4.07 (72)	1.40	0.24
3b	$\alpha + \beta_G \log \text{UO}$	$\alpha_M = \alpha_F$	4.08 (72)	1.58	0.21
2a	α_G	$\beta_M = \beta_F = 0$	6.34 (73)	20.86	10^{-7}
2b	$\alpha + \beta \log \text{UO}$	$\alpha_M = \alpha_F$ $\beta_M = \beta_F$	4.12 (73)	1.12	0.33
1	α	$\alpha_M = \alpha_F$ $\beta_M = \beta_F = 0$	6.92 (74)	17.34	10^{-8}

Having established a maximal model we now turn our attention to questioning whether ADH does depend on gender and urine osmolarity UO. The lattice for testing such dependence is shown in Figure 5.26. Following the testing strategy of Section 3.10 we proceed up the lattice only as far as level 2, where

$$E(\log \text{ADH} \mid G, \text{UO}) = \alpha + \beta \log \text{UO}$$

is acceptable as a working model. In other words, there is no need to introduce the complexity of different regressions for males and females. A summary of

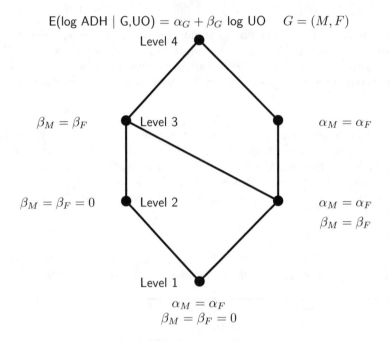

Figure 5.26 *Lattice of hypotheses for the ADH Study.*

the test statistics and p-values is given in Table 5.5. In this case the tests are exact and standard F-tests have been used.

Predictive distribution

Our parametric working model is that ADH follows a lognormal distribution $\Lambda^1(\alpha + \beta \log \mathrm{UO}, \sigma^2)$. With estimates

$$\hat{\alpha} = 0.462, \qquad \hat{\beta} = 0.220, \qquad \hat{\sigma}^2 = 0.0565$$

and $k = 73, n = 75$, so that $(1 + 1/n)\hat{\sigma}^2 = 0.0572$, the appropriate predictive distribution for application to a new referred patient is of logStudent form

$$\Lambda St^1 \left(73, 0.462 + 0.220 \log \mathrm{UO}, 0.0572\right).$$

Atypicality indices of the selected cases

On the basis of the predictive distribution and on the leave-one-out principle we can compute the atypicality indices of the 75 selected cases. These range from 0.002 to 0.999; case S48, with the smallest ADH value, has an atypicality of 0.999 and case S14, with the largest ADH value, has an atypicality of 0.950. There appears to be nothing exceptional clinically about S14 and S48 and in a sample of size 75 we might expect a few cases with atypicality indices exceeding 0.95.

Kullback-Liebler influence

Another way of testing the concordance of the data and model is through the Kullback-Liebler divergence measure of influence as described in Section 3.12.5. The Kullback-Liebler measures range from $< 10^{-4}$ to 0.0043, 0.0046, 0.0073, 0.0077 for S14, S7, S41, S48, respectively. We have already discussed S14 and S48. S7 has the largest ADH value, equally with S14, and S41 has the smallest value of UO. Examination of standardized residuals identifies only one case, S48, outside the range $(-3, 3)$. Overall there seem to be no grounds for excluding any of the selected cases as outliers.

Assessment of new cases

We are now in a position to assess the new patients N1–N6 in data set **newadh** by their atypicality indices as computed with the above predictive distribution.

Patient	N1	N2	N3	N4	N5	N6
Atypicality	0.137	0.821	0.987	0.987	0.048	0.931

These atypicalities give the clinician an indication of which cases may be abnormal in their ADH measurements. For example, patient N3 has clearly an abnormally high ADH relative to his low value of UO, whereas patient N4 has an abnormally low ADH relative to her low UO.

5.4.2 Calcium content of bones

A new method of measurement of the calcium contents CH and CF of the heel and the forearm is under study and the extent to which the variability depends on the following factors and other characteristics of the individual is of interest:

G:	Gender
A:	Age
H:	Height
W:	Weight
SA:	Surface area
MF:	Strength of forearm
ML:	Strength of leg
DC:	Diameter of os calcis
AC:	Area of os calcis
DR:	Diameter of radius and ulna

The objective is to use this experience to determine whether a new patient can be regarded as having normal calcium contents CH and CF, conditional on any of these other characteristics which may be found to affect calcium measurements. An aspect of this problem is the fact that some features, such as G, A, H and W, are easy to record whereas the others are more trouble-some. To some extent then an aim is to find out which, if any, of the more troublesome measurements are necessary to obtain a satisfactory conditional model to describe variability in the bivariate measurement (CH, CF). Suppose that we start our analysis on the basis of a maximal model of normal linear regression form, as in Definition 3.8, with the response vector y the bivariate calcium vector (CH, CF) and the covariate vector x of the form [1, G, A, H, W, SA, MF, ML, DC, AC, DR], where 1 is a 'dummy variable' and $G = -1$ for males and $G = +1$ for females.

Box-Cox analysis

Starting with univariate analysis we find maximizing values $\lambda_{CF} = 0.810$, $\lambda_{CH} = 1.02$ with corresponding profile loglikelihood values $-407.7, -357.62$. The fact that these are almost identical with the values at $\lambda_{CF} = 1, \lambda_{CH} = 1$ suggests that no transformation will be necessary. Starting with the univariate maximizing values we find that a bivariate Box-Cox analysis gives a maximizing vector $(\lambda_{CF}, \lambda_{CH}) = (0.750, 1.021)$ with corresponding profile loglikelihood -762.1, hardly different from the value -763.4 at $(\lambda_{CF}, \lambda_{CH}) = (1, 1)$. On formal Box-Cox analysis therefore there is no need for any transformation.

Q-Q plots

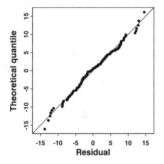 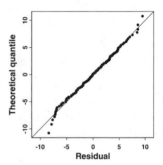

Figure 5.27 *Quantile-quantile plots of residuals obtained from fitting the maximal model: CH response (left) and CF response (right).*

The Q-Q plots associated with this maximal model are shown in Figure 5.27. Both are satisfactorily diagonal.

Tests of normality

By comparing the results in Table 5.6 with the critical values contained in Table 3.2 we see that the test statistics for all marginal, bivariate angle and radius tests of normality of residuals are well below significance levels, confirming the conclusions from the above Box-Cox analysis and the Q-Q plots.

Lattice of hypotheses

In the following analysis we take an additive model as being the maximal model, thus ignoring the possibility that gender might significantly interact

Table 5.6 *Values of the modified test statistics for the calcium data*

Test	Variable(s)	Anderson-Darling	Cramer-von Mises	Watson
Marginal				
	CH residual	0.417	0.071	0.069
	CF residual	0.170	0.015	0.015
Bivariate angle				
	CH-CF residuals	0.213	0.018	0.018
Radius		0.997	0.118	0.049

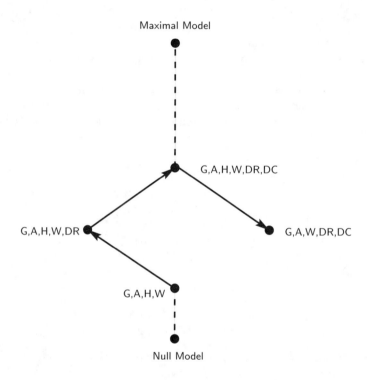

Figure 5.28 *Lattice of hypotheses for the calcium data.*

with at least one of the covariates; we leave this issue to be considered as an end-of-chapter problem. Since the covariate vector here is ten-dimensional the full lattice of hypotheses has 1024 nodes. We have, however, a convenient starting node for our investigation of this lattice since we can explore to what extent the easily recorded covariates (G, A, H, W) are necessary or sufficient to provide a satisfactory description of experience. Figure 5.28 gives details at some of the nodes explored. First, testing the (G, A, H, W) hypothesis within the maximal model gives a significance probability $< 10^{-7}$. We must therefore consider the various ways of supplementing (G, A, H, W). At the next higher level the introduction of one of SA, MF, ML, DC, AC, DR leads to significance probabilities $< 10^{-4}$ except for DR which gives a significance probability 0.0075. We then explore at the next higher level which covariate it may be necessary to add to (G, A, H, W, DR). At this level the introduction of one of SA, MF, ML, DC, AC leads to significance probabilities 0.0048, 0.0041, 0.0055, 0.41, 0.065, respectively. Thus starting with (G, A, H, W) we have arrived at (G, A, H, W, DC, DR) as a reasonable working model, but we must obviously now ask the question whether some of G, A, H, W may not be necessary. Now starting with (G, A, H, W , DC, DR) and moving to the next lower level in the lattice by deleting one of G, A, H, W we obtain significance probabilities of $< 10^{-5}$, $< 10^{-10}$, 0.14, 0.028. We can thus exclude H from our consideration and arrive at a working model involving (G, A, W, DC, DR). Denoting [CH CF] by y and [1 G A W DC DR] by x we are now interested in using the normal linear model $y = xB + \text{error}$ in our assessment of new patients.

Note that our investigation of the assumption of normality above was in relation to the residuals in the maximal model. We confirm here that within the working model there is also no significant evidence against the normality assumption.

Predictive distribution

The estimates of B and Σ are

$$\hat{B} = \begin{bmatrix} -4.219 & 10.374 \\ -3.768 & -3.700 \\ -0.315 & -0.239 \\ 0.146 & 0.040 \\ 0.764 & 0.112 \\ 0.356 & 0.724 \end{bmatrix}$$

and

$$\hat{\Sigma} = \begin{bmatrix} 42.16 & 5.80 \\ 5.80 & 17.49 \end{bmatrix}.$$

The conditional predictive distribution associated with a new referred patient R with covariate vector x_R is then

$$St^2 \left[k, x_R \hat{B}, (1 + h_R)\hat{\Sigma} \right]$$

where $k = 121$ and h_R is the 'hat' value for the new patient as defined in Property 3.10. We note here the direction of the effects, as anticipated by the clinicians involved, with calcium content on average higher for males than females, decreasing with age, increasing with weight, diameter of os calcis and diameter of radius and ulna.

Atypicality indices of the selected cases

The above predictive distribution allows us to compute the atypicality indices of the 127 selected cases on the leave-one-out principle. There are just two cases S103 and S11 with atypicality indices 0.964 and 0.959 exceeding 0.95. While S103 has the smallest W and a low DC value neither of the two cases appears exceptional clinically, and there is no reason to consider their exclusion from the past experience data set.

Kullback-Liebler influence

The largest Kullback-Liebler influence measure is 0.106 associated with S118, well above the next largest 0.047 of S27, all other selected cases having values less than 0.040. Again there appears to be nothing exceptional clinically in the apparently influential S118.

Assessment of new cases

With the predictive assessment we can readily compute the atypicality indices of the four new patients N1–N4 from data set **newbones**.

Patient	N1	N2	N3	N4
Atypicality	0.997	0.685	0.798	0.938

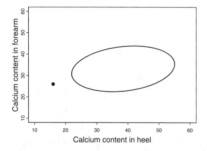 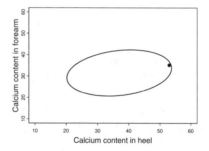

Figure 5.29 *95% regions of previous experience for referred patients N1 (left) and N4 (right), with the points indicating their actual calcium contents.*

Of these clearly N1 and possibly N4 require further investigation. For conditional descriptions it is possible to produce a region of previous experience for any specific covariate vector x along lines similar to the argument of Section 5.3.1, with $k = 121, b = x\hat{B}, c = (1 + h)\hat{\Sigma}$; note however that the raw data are used here and the calculations are based on Property 3.4. The 95 per cent regions of previous experience corresponding to the covariate vectors of N1 and N4 are shown in Figure 5.29, with the positions of the patients' (CH, CF) also shown. Given their respective conditioning features, N1 is clearly deficient in both his calcium contents whereas N4 appears to be rather high in the calcium content of her heel.

A multiplicative model: an alternative approach

While the above analysis is no doubt adequate as a practical tool for the assessment of new patients it is inevitably an artefact. If we reflect on the nature of the 'predictor' we see that it contains a feature which is in part an additive linear combination of weight and diameters. This seems unlikely in terms of 'natural laws'; a more natural a priori expectation is that calcium content is in some way proportional to some powers of these measurements. We can thus consider the adoption of a maximal 'multiplicative' model which incorporates this possibility, and the simplest starting point is to use logarithmically transformed variables throughout, apart from G, and then to investigate a normal linear regression model with these transformed data. We can report here that testing with the lattice of hypotheses leads to a working model of the form

$$[\log CH \quad \log CF] = [\ 1 \quad G \quad \log A \quad \log W \quad \log DR\ ]B + \text{error},$$

with B and Σ estimated by

$$\hat{B} = \begin{bmatrix} 1.740 & 1.347 \\ -0.165 & -0.134 \\ -0.428 & -0.371 \\ 0.419 & 0.066 \\ 0.458 & 0.905 \end{bmatrix}$$

and

$$\hat{\Sigma} = \begin{bmatrix} 0.05321 & 0.01454 \\ 0.01454 & 0.03318 \end{bmatrix}.$$

Note that with this multiplicative model there is one less covariate, namely DC, involved in the working model. In practical terms this means that there is one less of the awkward measurements to be made. In terms of the predictive distribution arising from this multiplicative approach new patient N1 has a large atypicality index 0.999, with the others N2, N3, N4 having atypicality indices 0.659, 0.829, 0.748, respectively. In our view this multiplicative model is still very much an artefact. Moreover, the three marginal tests associated with the CH residual all give significant departure from normality at the one per cent significance level, and there are six atypicality indices above 0.95 compared with only two for the additive model. In view of all these disadvantages we prefer the above additive approach.

5.5 Compositional variability

The data recorded on patients in clinical medicine are sometimes compositional in nature, that is where what are recorded are the proportions in which parts of some whole occur. In this section we consider how to describe variability in such data in relation to two specific problems.

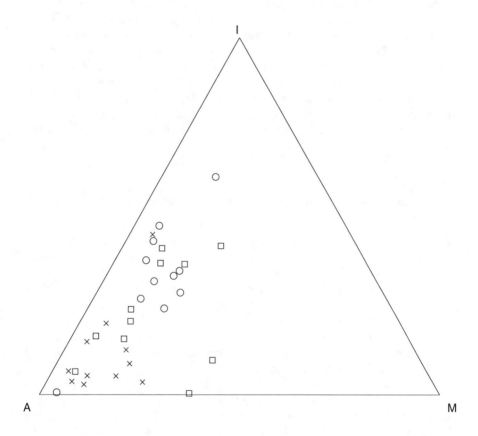

Figure 5.30 *Ternary diagram for plots of three-part cell compositions (I, A, M) for normal persons (×), patients with Crohn's disease (□) and patients with ulcerative colitis (○).*

5.5.1 Ulcerative colitis and Crohn's disease

In an attempt to find some means of differential diagnosis between ulcerative colitis and Crohn's disease specimens of gut from 22 patients, 11 with known ulcerative colitis and 11 with known Crohn's disease, were examined and the cells from these specimens classified into three categories I, A and M. In addition these cells were also counted in the gut of 11 normal persons. Since the amount of gut varies it is the relative numbers or the proportions of these cells that are of interest in exploring the possibility of their use in diagnosis. Data set **crohn** shows the proportions of (I, A, M) cells in the 33 cases. Since each case provides a three-part composition we can obtain a graphical view of the variability by plotting each composition as a point in a ternary diagram as described in Section 4.2; see Figure 5.30. It is clear from the degree of overlap in the ternary diagram that, while there may be some degree of discrimination between normal and ulcerative colitis and between normal and Crohn's disease, there is no possibility that such compositions can distinguish between ulcerative colitis and Crohn's disease. These views are readily confirmed by testing of relative hypotheses after a logratio transformation as indicated in Section 4.2. Tests of equality of bivariate mean logratios are significant for a normal, ulcerative colitis comparison (P<0.05) and for a normal, Crohn's disease comparison (P<0.05) but there is no significant difference between ulcerative colitis and Crohn's disease (P = 0.48). Since the primary aim of the study was to find some form of differential diagnosis between ulcerative colitis and Crohn's disease, there seems little point in continuing this line of enquiry.

5.5.2 Comparison of steroid metabolite concentrations in normal adults and children

We recall here the problem of differential diagnosis in Cushing's syndrome outlined in Section 1.10. In a previous attempt at diagnosis it was found that a three-year old child was wrongly diagnosed as highly likely to have the adenoma form when in fact the correct diagnosis was adrenal carcinoma. This misdiagnosis is not surprising when we appreciate that the Cushing syndrome patients in data set cush have ages ranging from 16 to 67 years. Since children obviously excrete less per 24 hours than adults there is no reason to suppose that a diagnostic system based on adult amounts of various excreted steroid metabolites should be in any way applicable to children. Data set cushkids records concentrations (mg/24 hrs) of 14 steroid metabolites of 30 normal children; recall that data set cush introduced in Section 1.10 records the same steroid metabolite concentrations of 37 normal adults. In considering the general question of modelling the variability of these adults and children we must have in mind the following question. Is it possible that a satisfactory differential system can be built on the compositional aspect of the data rather than the actual amounts? If this is so can such a system be applied to children?

In order for such a procedure to be feasible we require to investigate the hypothesis that the compositional variability of steroid metabolites in children is the same as that in adults. At the same time we may investigate a related hypothesis that compositional variability in either group is independent of total metabolite excretion. In our modelling let x_A denote the composition formed from the steroid metabolite vector of a typical adult and t_A the associated total of the steroid metabolites. Let (x_C, t_C) be the corresponding composition and total for a typical child. A convenient way to model the joint density function $p(x,t)$ of the adult (composition, total) vector (x_A, t_A) is in the marginal, conditional form $p(t_A)p(x_A|t_A)$, where, for our adult data sets, we can take $p(t_A)$ to be of lognormal form $\Lambda^1(\mu_A, \sigma_A^2)$ and $p(x_A|t_A)$ of logistic-normal form $L^1(\alpha_A + \beta_A t_A, \tau_A^2)$. Modelling for the children's data is similar with subscript C replacing subscript A. We note that the parametric form adopted for the variability of the total steroid metabolite is of no immediate interest since our questions relate specifically to the conditional distribution. Tests of the hypotheses $\beta_A = 0$ and $\beta_C = 0$ of no dependence of composition on total are readily carried out and result in significance probabilities P $=0.009$ and P $=0.029$. Thus we have to conclude that there is a dependence of composition on total both in adults and in children and we have to conclude that there is no great hope that a differential diagnostic system devised for adults is likely to be adaptable to children.

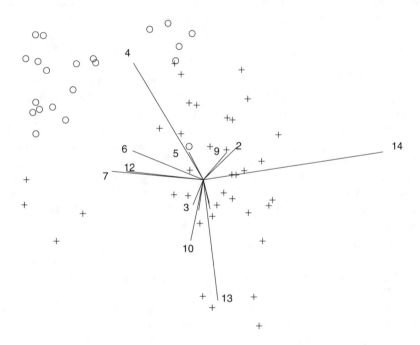

Figure 5.31 *Compositional biplot for steroid metabolites in adults (+), with the relative positions of children (o).*

We note also that if we had made a direct comparison of the compositions formed from the adults and the children we would, for example, have found a highly significant difference in their means. This is all very obvious if we construct a compositional biplot for adults and also show on the biplot the compositional markers for the children, as in Figure 5.31. Note how the children are fairly well separated from the adults, having, for example, low proportions of metabolites 13 (pregnanetriol) and 14 (pregnenetriol) compared with adults.

5.6 Multivariate binary data

So far we have considered the description of variability of data vectors whose components are continuous or compositional. Other forms are possible and as an example of the nature of such forms we tackle the problem of describing the variability in experience in the problem of diagnosing Keratoconjunctivitis sicca.

5.6.1 Describing experience in Keratoconjunctivitis sicca

The reliable diagnosis of Keratoconjunctivitis sicca (KCS) in patients with rheumatoid arthritis by an opthalmic specialist is not always available at a rheumatic clinic. In such circumstances the question arises as to whether it is possible to use non-specialists and ten binary features (presence or absence of certain symptoms) of patients to differentiate between cases of KCS and non-KCS.

Data set kcs shows these binary features in 77 rheumatoid arthritis patients, A1–A40 with KCS and B1–B37 with no KCS. This data set was obtained by an opthalmic specialist first screening a group of rheumatoid arthritis patients for KCS. Once the members A1–A40 of this KCS group had been identified a group B1–B37 of similar size of patients with no KCS was taken as controls. Selection of these cases has thus been made on the basis of disease type u (1 for KCS, 2 for non-KCS) with subsequent recording of the 10-dimensional multivariate binary feature vector v. In terms of our study here we wish to seek a method of describing the variability in the ten-dimensional binary vectors separately for each of the two groups.

Multivariate binary kernel density estimation

As we have earlier stated in Section 4.8 there are difficulties in the construction of satisfactory parametric forms for modelling multivariate binary data. We therefore consider the non-parametric approach of kernel density estimation. Let y be a typical D-dimensional binary vector and $x_1, \ldots, x_D$ be the binary vectors of the n selected subjects of one of the groups. Then we consider a kernel of form

$$K(y|x, \lambda) = \lambda^{d(x,y)}(1 - \lambda)^{D-d(x,y)},$$

where $0 \leq \lambda < 1$ and $d(x,y)$ is the number of coincidences between the components of x and y. As in Section 4.8 the smoothing parameter λ is selected on the criterion of maximizing the pseudo-likelihood

$$\frac{1}{n}\prod_{i=1}^{n}\sum_{j \neq i} K(x_j|x_i, \lambda)$$

with respect to λ. For the two groups the maximizing smoothing parameters are $\lambda_1 = 0.980$ and $\lambda_2 = 0.844$ with maximized pseudo-loglikelihoods -94.04 and -249.09.

Atypicality assessments

For the ten-dimensional binary vector here the discrete sample space consists of 1024 ($= 2^{10}$) distinct points and there is no difficulty in computing the kernel density

$$p(y|D) = \frac{1}{n} \sum_{i=1}^{n} K(y|x_i, \lambda)$$

for each $y \in \{0,1\}^{10}$. These densities can then be arranged in descending order; then the cumulative sums computed from this ordered set provide the atypicalities of the associated vectors. For the 40 subjects with KCS the atypicalities, computed using the mesh method, range from 0.05 to 0.97, with only three subjects having a value above 0.9. Only one subject has an atypicality of more than 0.95 but there are no clinical grounds for not including them in the analysis.

5.7 Bibliographic notes

The statistical analyses in this chapter are on the whole direct applications of the methodology set out in Chapters 3 and 4 and so we draw attention only to a few aspects of the analysis. The Box-Cox transformation analysis first appeared in Box and Cox (1964); see also Aitkin et al. (1989) for its application to general linear modelling. As pointed out in Chapter 3 the multivariate tests of normality are based on Stephens (1982) with a concise set of tables available in Aitchison (1986). Much of the description of clinical experience depends on the use of a predictive distribution as described in detail in Aitchison and Dunsmore (1975), where there is also a full discussion of atypicality indices as a tool for assessing where individual patients lie in relation to previous experience. The assessment of conditional variability is highly dependent on the use of lattice testing and the reader is referred to Chapter 3 for details and references. For analyses involving compositional data again refer to Aitchison (1986). The problem of describing experience of Keratoconjunctivitis sicca in rheumatoid arthritis patients is considered in Anderson et al. (1972) and the use of the multivariate binary kernel method first appeared in Aitchison and Aitken (1976).

5.8 Problems

Problem 5.1 A clinic is attempting to set up a means of describing normal experience of a newly discovered enzyme and has made determinations of the enzyme concentration in 150 normal individuals. The results in standard units are given below.

207	243	237	247	228	156	198	200	186	219
257	219	247	259	209	253	194	205	209	226
306	223	261	227	252	210	236	236	195	256
226	331	157	193	227	253	185	196	227	241
249	225	166	198	227	259	179	243	209	257
221	211	195	219	203	178	322	216	228	198
289	328	230	192	250	183	190	270	282	271
210	216	183	240	246	255	235	287	227	212
227	184	225	308	147	172	221	170	207	155
222	255	249	236	228	268	291	199	267	211
226	266	242	207	211	194	191	277	165	274
183	238	208	211	246	296	250	204	253	295
237	225	209	260	269	212	207	212	232	208
281	204	249	217	198	246	216	225	254	262
214	214	327	261	230	214	216	256	237	210

As consultant you are asked to investigate this possibility and to suggest a means of ascribing atypicality indices to new patients. You are further asked to demonstrate your method on patients whose recorded enzyme concentrations are 150, 280, 350.

Problem 5.2 A clinic consults you on the possible use of the concentrations (meq/l) of two hormones a and b in the detection of patients who may have an overactive excreting gland. The clinic has determined the hormone levels in 45 individuals known to have normal excretion and the hormone levels are recorded in Table 5.7.

Since the clinic may decide to use only one of the hormone levels to detect patients with overactive glands you are asked to consider each hormone separately in your analysis of this experience and report to the clinic. You decide also to consider how you would use both hormone levels as a means of detecting irregular glandular behaviour.

How would you assign atypicality indices to two patients who have levels (20.7, 25.6) and (30.4, 25.9), respectively, on hormones (a, b)?

Problem 5.3 Two indicators of a certain blood disease have been recorded in 24 patients and the clinic has asked you to provide a means of detecting whether new patients suspected of having the disease are within this previous experience. The clinic is particularly interested in having some easy graphical means of putting any screening method into operation. The data are shown in Table 5.8.

Table 5.7 *Data for Problem 5.2*

Hormone		Hormone		Hormone	
a	b	a	b	a	b
6.5	11.1	2.7	20.4	11.7	24.3
7.8	11.7	9.2	15.8	7.6	11.9
5.3	12.9	6.8	12.9	19.6	28.7
4.8	8.6	10.0	8.4	2.5	11.1
6.2	11.1	10.8	8.8	3.8	13.1
3.5	11.8	7.0	19.1	4.6	17.2
8.6	7.7	9.1	18.6	29.3	11.4
7.9	17.3	6.0	9.4	9.7	9.8
7.2	7.3	6.0	16.6	5.6	20.4
1.8	9.0	5.8	13.3	7.5	8.3
5.3	7.1	4.0	10.5	6.1	16.6
8.7	18.1	8.6	8.5	13.7	9.9
9.3	9.1	16.1	13.7	7.5	16.2
8.3	5.2	5.1	4.9	12.4	16.8
7.2	16.6	5.4	5.7	11.5	8.5

Table 5.8 *Data for Problem 5.3*

Indicator 1	Indicator 2	Indicator 1	Indicator 2
20.8	6.1	9.3	8.3
3.5	15.5	10.4	8.5
47.7	10.9	1.9	18.4
17.8	5.1	29.4	5.2
16.5	7.2	5.1	12.7
16.5	6.8	30.9	5.2
8.6	7.5	7.6	11.2
9.4	10.2	12.3	8.4
6.1	10.3	5.3	10.8
7.6	10.7	22.9	5.4
19.7	6.9	8.4	10.5
9.7	10.0	7.9	11.2

What conclusions would you draw about two new patients with indicators (15.0, 10.5) and (5.0, 9.5)?

Problem 5.4 There is a need to describe experience in the levels of two hormones, A and B, in normal individuals so that it may be possible to screen persons suspected of being susceptible to a hormone deficiency condition. The

hormone levels (in standard units) of 30 normal persons have been determined
and recorded as below.

You are asked to describe this normal experience and, if possible, to devise
a graphical method whereby persons outside this normal experience may be
easily detected.

In particular, how would you report on the normality or otherwise of two
new patients, the first with (A, B) levels (2.1, 6.9) and the second with
(A, B) levels (3.9, 5.0)?

Hormone levels		Hormone levels		Hormone levels	
A	B	A	B	A	B
3.71	4.74	1.35	11.40	9.27	1.64
6.72	4.24	1.67	7.38	10.63	1.62
1.91	6.33	7.00	2.34	8.63	2.62
1.23	7.82	1.42	4.62	1.11	9.59
4.81	3.46	2.03	6.03	2.33	4.33
2.79	3.81	1.90	7.24	2.36	7.96
1.59	11.64	8.54	1.49	3.37	4.75
2.55	6.44	2.87	3.22	1.81	6.61
0.65	9.86	1.26	7.83	1.36	9.42
5.85	2.00	1.22	6.28	1.98	4.99

Problem 5.5 A problem in defining normal experience has arisen in a new
blood screening situation which isolates a certain constituent of blood plasma.
It is now possible to determine the proportions of the three parts a, b, c of
this constituent. For twenty-five normal individuals this composition has been
determined in the hope that it will provide some indication of the nature of
variability within normal individuals. The compositional data are given below.

a	b	c	a	b	c
0.21	0.11	0.68	0.15	0.08	0.77
0.19	0.21	0.60	0.25	0.29	0.46
0.26	0.22	0.52	0.20	0.43	0.37
0.14	0.15	0.71	0.16	0.24	0.60
0.19	0.16	0.65	0.05	0.12	0.83
0.16	0.13	0.71	0.20	0.26	0.54
0.19	0.22	0.59	0.23	0.59	0.18
0.31	0.45	0.24	0.32	0.27	0.41
0.11	0.32	0.57	0.08	0.04	0.88
0.09	0.05	0.86	0.20	0.18	0.62
0.28	0.17	0.55	0.12	0.22	0.66
0.11	0.18	0.71	0.11	0.07	0.82
0.21	0.17	0.62			

You are asked to report on the possibility of describing normal experience and in particular whether you can provide a simple graphical means of determining whether a new individual is within normal experience.

Three new patients have been referred to the clinic and the proportions of a, b, c have been determined. You are asked to make some statement about how these patients relate to normal experience.

a	b	c
0.21	0.35	0.44
0.35	0.11	0.54
0.14	0.43	0.43

Problem 5.6 Re-read Section 5.3.3 and apply the analyses described there to obtain an appropriate description of the experience in the hyperplasia group of Cushing's syndrome, restricting your analysis to the first seven concentrations. In your analysis consider how you can compare this experience with that of the adenoma group.

Problem 5.7 In a study of lethargic patients the responses of ten men and ten women to different doses of a stimulus are given in the following table. You have been asked to investigate fully the extent to which response depends on the stimulus and gender.

Stimulus	Response	Gender
1	3.74	M
2	3.94	M
3	4.11	M
4	5.52	M
5	4.96	M
6	9.54	M
7	8.09	M
8	11.70	M
9	10.40	M
10	12.31	M
1	0.02	F
2	2.45	F
3	6.77	F
4	5.34	F
5	8.57	F
6	8.56	F
7	10.30	F
8	9.88	F
9	11.39	F
10	16.18	F

If you are asked to predict the response of a new male patient to a stimulus of 8.5 units, how would you respond? In what way, if any, would your response differ if the new patient had been female?

Problem 5.8 Refer to Problem 1.3. It has been suggested that the blood compositions of Form A patients are dependent on the three symptoms, whereas the blood compositions of form B patients are not dependent on the three symptoms. Investigate this conjecture.

Problem 5.9 A study has been carried out to see if the composition of four constituents a, b, c, d in tissue obtained at biopsy is in any way dependent on the size (mg) of the specimen analysed. The study so far has investigated 16 patients with the results recorded below. You have been asked to investigate the situation and to recommend whether or not more patients should be investigated.

Percentages of constituents				Size
a	b	c	d	mg
29	9	22	40	44
35	15	19	31	16
33	8	25	34	40
25	10	30	35	123
21	10	15	54	35
22	12	18	48	32
27	11	19	43	68
27	13	18	43	27
29	12	17	42	11
28	12	21	39	18
43	7	23	26	46
36	9	17	38	14
29	11	20	40	72
21	15	19	46	32
28	10	25	37	30
34	12	15	39	36

Problem 5.10 Consider the use of the symptom data of Problem 1.3 for purposes of differential diagnosis of forms A and B. Do you consider the multivariate kernel approach of Section 5.6 adequate for this purpose?

Problem 5.11 In a study of obesity in a certain group of 40 men a clinic has been assigning indices of obesity, breathlessness and unfitness, all measured on the scale of 0 to 1, and is now wondering to what extent these indices relate to height (cm), girth (cm), weight (kg) and a diet index, also measured on a scale of 0 to 1. The data are given in Table 5.9. You are asked to produce a full report on the clinic's question.

Problem 5.12 Review Section 5.4.2 and investigate the possibility that gender interacts with the covariates.

Problem 5.13 Review and prepare a report on Problem 1.5.

Table 5.9 *Data for Problem 5.11*

Obesity	Breath-lessness	Unfitness	Height (cm)	Girth (cm)	Weight (kg)	Diet index
0.35	0.59	0.74	169	111	76	0.68
0.54	0.79	0.75	149	93	64	0.64
0.57	0.77	0.75	162	126	78	0.67
0.62	0.84	0.97	145	125	77	0.89
0.28	0.78	0.59	155	107	63	0.58
0.48	0.80	0.99	158	117	70	0.96
0.33	0.64	0.91	150	101	60	0.82
0.63	0.69	0.35	164	117	81	0.42
0.44	0.74	0.53	153	110	69	0.53
0.87	0.86	0.47	163	156	100	0.47
0.80	0.67	0.78	172	116	105	0.61
0.66	0.71	0.55	171	116	81	0.56
0.82	0.70	0.61	163	122	85	0.66
0.77	0.77	0.87	184	138	103	0.87
0.61	0.79	0.94	153	130	89	0.71
0.72	0.77	0.65	163	127	90	0.59
0.78	0.79	0.72	156	125	89	0.61
0.70	0.76	0.71	167	129	87	0.72
0.36	0.71	0.70	158	108	65	0.70
0.23	0.61	0.71	179	106	66	0.63
0.72	0.84	0.64	161	144	106	0.55
0.18	0.64	0.63	184	93	64	0.63
0.78	0.80	0.96	172	147	110	0.82
0.26	0.64	0.99	171	105	65	0.93
0.22	0.49	0.36	159	90	61	0.46
0.85	0.85	0.75	166	153	108	0.73
0.72	0.78	0.82	164	131	89	0.70
0.25	0.58	0.84	147	91	56	0.77
0.53	0.73	0.79	171	124	83	0.66
0.63	0.77	0.95	170	133	90	0.89
0.58	0.74	0.68	168	115	85	0.60
0.67	0.74	0.99	165	123	88	0.87
0.54	0.67	0.95	168	114	89	0.80
0.76	0.75	0.94	171	123	91	0.91
0.34	0.69	0.79	169	112	76	0.68
0.62	0.82	0.84	154	136	76	0.77
0.16	0.61	0.94	164	92	54	0.85
0.51	0.71	0.91	167	111	75	0.84
0.84	0.77	0.67	168	130	98	0.64
0.59	0.71	0.93	168	115	86	0.78

CHAPTER 6

Observation and Measurement

6.1 Introduction

In our analysis of experience in the preceding chapter we proceeded on the assumption that the observations and measurements constituting the data were worth using. In this chapter we take a more critical look at the problems of observing and measuring. Clinical medicine abounds with difficult problems of measurement such as the conformity of measurements made by different clinicians under similar working conditions, the identification of sources of variability, the transferability of data from one clinic to another, the comparison of different methods of measurement, the development of measurement strategies to eliminate or at least to counter any sources of irreproducibility and the consensus problems between different observers for both continuous and categorical data. Since all of these problems involve variability and uncertainty the statistician has often an important role to play in assessing the merits of a method of observing or measuring, in advising on how the method may be improved and in quantifying the effects of any remaining imprecision.

First we identify the various components of observational problems by considering a number of simple examples. We then examine particular problems when more than one observer is involved. This kind of problem is clearly a fundamental one. If two clinicians investigating the same patient make different observations the whole question of communicability of information is raised. Observer error studies are now a popular form of such investigation.

6.2 The components of an observational problem

Consider the following everyday clinical observational problem. A clinician examining a patient decides that it would be sensible to measure the patient's blood pressure. His standard equipment for this purpose is a sphygmometer or a non-mercury equivalent. A rubber cuff connected to a mercury manometer or a non-mercury equivalent is placed round the seated patient's upper arm and inflated until the column of mercury is seen to be above the blood pressure expected. The clinician then places his stethoscope on the patient's lower arm and gradually releases the pressure in the cuff. At a certain stage in this releasing process the clinician will hear characteristic sounds (Korytuk sounds) which indicate that the pressure in the cuff is now equal to the patient's systolic blood pressure, that is the pressure at the pumping stroke of the heart. He then reads off this pressure (in mm Hg) on the mercury column. He then proceeds to release further the air in the cuff until further characteristic sounds are heard. His reading this time is the patient's diastolic blood pressure, at the refilling stroke of the heart. These two readings, systolic and diastolic blood pressures, are recorded as an indication of the patient's circulatory condition.

We can now begin to identify the different components of any observational situation with reference to this example. First a clinician may be involved in recording blood pressures for a whole series of his patients. It is therefore convenient to have a suitable name for the series of entities measured, and we refer to such an entity as a *case*. We use this impersonal word since the case may refer not to a person but to a petri dish with bacterial colonies which a technician has the task of counting or to a blood sample of origin unknown to the steroid chemist who has to analyse it. For each case there is some defined characteristic or *feature* which it is of interest to observe or measure. In the present example the feature is systolic blood pressure or diastolic blood pressure. Instead of considering these two one-dimensional features separately we can refer to the two-dimensional feature blood pressure with components systolic blood pressure and diastolic blood pressure. To observe or measure a defined feature we need a technique or *method* of observing or measuring. In the illustrative example the method is described as the sphygmometric method, and the feature is measured by this method in terms of the effect of blood pressure on the height of the mercury column. There are other methods of recording blood pressures, e.g. by a direct catheter insertion method or a Rose-box method, and interest may centre on the compatibility or the relative effectiveness of such methods. The clinician plays an important role as *observer* in this measurement process and it is clearly important in modern medicine that there should be no subjective component in the measurement. It is highly desirable that the measurement should be substantially the same as would be obtained by any other clinician or qualified observer.

There is another important component of our illustrative example which we must not overlook, namely the *conditions*, whether temporal, psychological, environmental or material, under which the measurement is made. Normally the method should spell out as precisely as possible the controlled conditions under which the measurement process should be conducted and the observer should try to ensure that the conditions are strictly adhered to. In the sphygmometric method we carefully specified that the patient was to be seated. But what if he or she has had to rush to the consulting room in order to arrive in time, or is bubbling over with indignation at being kept waiting for half an hour, or has recently taken a sedative to reduce apprehension of the consultation. Do such variable conditions have an effect on the measurement? Or should reclining rather than sitting be a recommended condition to ensure greater consistency? Clearly in any observational problem the *conditions* component may play an important role.

When called upon to analyse any observational problem concerning some feature the statistician is well advised as a very first step to identify the components: case, method, observer, conditions.

Earlier in this section we begged an important question of measurement by talking about a defined feature. For some features such as number of fingers or age verified by birth certificate there may be no serious problem here but for others such as the extent of mobility of a recently broken arm or skin thickness there are clearly problems of definition. For the apparently simple feature such as blood pressure there are serious problems. If a person's blood pressure is continually monitored over 24 hours very large fluctuations will occur depending apparently not only on the person's physical activity but also on his or her mental activity or stress or psychological state. If there is such a dynamic feature temporal variability in what sense is it sensible or meaningful to attempt to search for a single measurement? Is it perhaps necessary to take a series of measurements spaced through time or even a continuous record to characterise the feature we envisage when we talk about blood pressure? The statistician may well have a role to play resolving such questions. The basic criterion of good observation or measurement is reproducibility. It is as well to realise that as an operational criterion the concept of reproducibility is related to the working circumstances under which we wish the observed or measured feature to be meaningfully communicable. If for the feature of plasma concentration of aldosterone a hospital will ensure that all its measurements are made by one method (double isotope) under identical conditions (specimen collection, storage) then the only practical concern is, that for a given case, method and conditions, the measurements made by different observers (steroid laboratory technicians) should be substantially the same. If such were the case we would say that there is (observer|case, method, conditions) reproducibility. In this terminology the components of observation to the left of the vertical bar are those which can vary in working circumstances and those components to the right are those factors which we are satisfied are held constant under measurement circumstances.

Once the kind of reproducibility of importance is specified we can begin to consider the kind of *design* required for a measurement study to investigate the extent of the reproducibility. In the present case we would want either all the observers (if few in number) or a random selection of such observers to make replicate determinations on aliquots of a random selection of cases or blood samples. Since any valid method is going to be applied to many cases it is only sensible to investigate measurement over a representative subset of cases. We would insist on *replicates* for two reasons. First to allow the investigation of whether there is any interaction between observers and cases. If we find that there is observer variability then for any satisfactory measurement of this plasma concentration we must clearly insist on the one observer carrying out all determinations unless we can find subtler ways of overcoming this irreproducibility. Even with a single observer we may not be out of the woods since we have to consider (replicate|case, method, observer, conditions) reproducibility, in other words how variable are replicate determinations made on the same case with the same method by the same observer under the same conditions.

Again if two clinics, one using a double isotope method under constant conditions and the other a radioimmunoassay method under constant conditions and both clinics using more than one observer, are obliged to produce compatible results we would require to investigate (method, observer|case, conditions) reproducibility. For a satisfactory design for such a reproducibility investigation we should ideally have enough aliquots from each blood sample (case) to allocate at least two to each (method, observer) combination.

It is surely now clear that there is a great variety of reproducibility problems and that the design and analysis of the observational experiment must be dictated by the circumstances of the practical situation. In particular areas of study specialist words for reproducibility have been coined such as precision, sensitivity, selectivity, repeatability. It is, however, sensible for the statistician to model carefully any new situation in terms of the concepts just presented. These concepts will be amply demonstrated and developed in the practical applications in the remainder of this chapter.

It will be convenient to use a consistent subscript notation throughout to identify the various components, and we use the subscript i for cases and j for observers.

We summarise the main problems of observational experiments in terms of the following questions which may usually be usefully posed.

 (i) Identify case, feature, method, observer, conditions, replicate.

 (ii) Does the method of measurement adequately represent the feature of interest? Is the method of measurement feasible on grounds of cost, ethics, etc?

(iii) Under what operational circumstances should observations be reproducible?

(iv) Can we design an observational experiment to test for this reproducibility?

 (v) If so, can we analyse the experiment to test for the reproducibility?

(vi) If there is irreproducibility is it of practical consequence in terms of clinical vs. statistical significance and, if so, can we identify the sources of the irreproducibility?

(vii) If irreproducibility is of practical importance and we cannot control the factors responsible are there any devices of measurement by which we can overcome its effect?

The role of sources of variation in maximal parametric modelling

We have outlined the possible sources of variation that can affect an observed value. We now consider how these sources affect our approach to (a) model fitting then (b) building up our experience.

We take the approach that in this situation our experimental data set D constitutes observations made under different combinations of the conditions. The probability model describing D is based on the probability model $p(v|u, \delta)$ describing the observed v for true u under the given experimental conditions, where δ is the parameter in the maximal probability model $p(v|u, \delta)$. The aim of the exercise is to analyse D to see to what extent we can reduce or relate our maximal model to a working theoretical model $p(v|D)$ for a new case, estimated from D and indeed how the appropriate form of the probability model fitted to D dictates how we build up future experience in a fashion that appropriately reflects the sources of variation in the observations in D.

6.3 An observer error study of a diagnostic ratio

In the examination of heart X-rays radiologists regard the ratio of the transverse diameter of the heart to the transverse diameter of the thorax as a useful diagnostic index. Traditionally the magnitude of this diagnostic ratio is judged visually without any direct measurement being recorded. The question now being posed is whether this ratio could be quantified in the sense that its computation from measurements made by one radiologist would be conformable with that from measurements made by another radiologist. Only in such circumstances would such a quantitative index be reliably objective.

To investigate the feasibility of this index as a worthwhile recordable measurement an observer error study had been carried out as part of a larger scale assessment of the measurability of heart X-rays.

Five consultant radiologists were each presented with 65 heart X-rays on a standard displaying screen in randomised order and asked, by actual measurement with a ruler, to record certain lengths and angles whose definitions all had agreed. Table 6.1 shows the six basic measurements recorded in data set dratio.

Table 6.1 *Definition of the heart X-ray measurements*

v_1 :	Heart size: midline to right heart border at widest part.
v_2 :	Heart size: midline to left heart border at widest part.
v_3 :	Transverse diameter of thorax at widest part.
v_4 :	Aortic knuckle: midline to right aortic margin.
v_5 :	Aortic knuckle: midline to left aortic margin.
v_6 :	Cardiac shadow area, by planimetry.

For the moment we shall confine our attention to the diagnostic ratio which is defined as $(v_1 + v_2)/v_3$. For two of the radiologists 15 of the heart X-rays were presented once again in a randomised order without the radiologist's knowledge that these were repeats. These data are recorded in data set dratio2.

Our first task in the analysis of this problem is to identify its components in the terminology of the preceding paragraph and these are given in Table 6.2. Since we are concerned only with the one simple method of measurement and fairly constant measurement conditions we concentrate on the problem of case

Table 6.2 *Components in the diagnostic ratio study*

Case:	heart X-ray
Feature:	diagnostic ratio
Observer:	radiologist
Method:	visual study and measurement with a ruler
Conditions:	visual inspection conditions, such as lighting

reproducibility over observers. We adopt the notation

$$v_{ijr} \quad (i = 1, \ldots, 15; \; j = 1, 2; \; r = 1, 2)$$

to denote the rth replicate measurement of the diagnostic ratio of the jth radiologist on the ith heart X-ray. Our aim then is to model the variability in the v_{ijr} and to investigate the extent to which this depends on case and observer. Since in this application the cases and the observers are simply representative of the wider population of cases and observers we adopt a random effects approach in our modelling. The fact that there is replication allows us to consider the possibility of case-observer interaction in the variability. Our model then sets

$$v_{ijr} = \mu + a_i + b_j + (ab)_{ij} + e_{ijr}$$

where the a_i, b_j and $(ab)_{ij}$ are the random effects due to case, observer and case×observer interaction and all are independently distributed as $N(0, \sigma_a^2)$, $N(0, \sigma_b^2)$ and $N(0, \sigma_{ab}^2)$, respectively, and the error terms e_{ijr} are distributed, again independently, as $N(0, \sigma_e^2)$. Our first aim is to apply a maximum likelihood procedure to the testing of the lattice of hypotheses concerning σ_a^2, σ_b^2 and σ_{ab}^2. To achieve this we have to obtain the parameters of the normal distribution of the 60-dimensional vector

$$v = \begin{bmatrix} v_{1,11} & v_{1,12} & v_{1,21} & v_{1,22} & v_{2,11} & v_{2,12} & v_{2,21} & v_{2,22} & \cdots & v_{15,22} \end{bmatrix}.$$

We may rewrite the model as the following linear mixed-effects model for v, denoting by c a column-vector all of whose entries are unity.

$$v = \mu c + Z_1 r_1^T + Z_2 r_2^T + Z_3 r_3^T + e, \tag{6.1}$$

where

$$\begin{aligned} r_1 &= [a_1, a_2, \ldots, a_{15}], \\ r_2 &= [b_1, b_2], \\ r_3 &= [(ab)_{1,1}, (ab)_{1,2}, \ldots, (ab)_{15,1}, (ab)_{15,2}] \end{aligned}$$

and

$$Z_1^T = \begin{bmatrix} 1111 & 0000 & \cdots & 0000 \\ 0000 & 1111 & \cdots & 0000 \\ \vdots & \vdots & \ddots & \vdots \\ 0000 & 0000 & \cdots & 1111 \end{bmatrix},$$

$$Z_2^T = \begin{bmatrix} 11 & 00 & 11 & 00 & \cdots & 11 & 00 \\ 00 & 11 & 00 & 11 & \cdots & 00 & 11 \end{bmatrix},$$

$$Z_3^T = \begin{bmatrix} 11 & 00 & \cdots & 00 \\ 00 & 11 & \cdots & 00 \\ \vdots & \vdots & \ddots & \vdots \\ 00 & 00 & \cdots & 11 \end{bmatrix}$$

and so the distribution of v, and hence the likelihood,

$$L\left(\mu, \sigma_a^2, \sigma_b^2, \sigma_{ab}^2, \sigma_e^2 | v\right)$$

is determined.

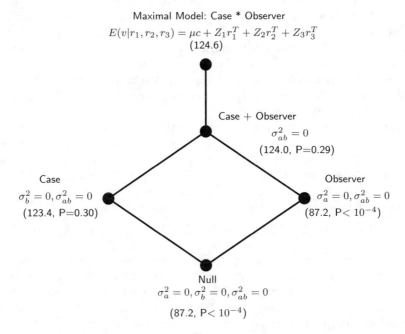

Figure 6.1 *Lattice of hypotheses for the diagnostic ratio study. At each node the value of the REML loglikelihood is shown, together with the P-value associated with the approximate test of the stated hypothesis within the maximal model.*

The variance components were estimated using the method of restricted maximum likelihood (REML) under the maximal model, and the hypotheses of the lattice of Figure 6.1 were tested using the *nlme* software package. For the maximal model the REML estimates are

$$\hat{\mu} = 0.450, \quad \hat{\sigma}_a^2 = 2.58 \times 10^{-3}, \quad \hat{\sigma}_b^2 = 2.86 \times 10^{-5},$$

$$\hat{\sigma}_{ab}^2 = 9.04 \times 10^{-5}, \quad \hat{\sigma}_e^2 = 2.97 \times 10^{-4},$$

with maximized REML loglikelihood 124.6. The results obtained using standard lattice testing from lower to higher levels and given in Figure 6.1 lead to a working model associated with a case only effect:

$$v_{ijr} = \mu + a_i + e_{ijr},$$

with REML estimates

$$\hat{\mu} = 0.450, \quad \hat{\sigma}_a^2 = 2.60 \times 10^{-3}, \quad \hat{\sigma}_e^2 = 3.76 \times 10^{-4}.$$

The P-values reported in Figure 6.1 are based on asymptotic likelihood ratio tests. However, due to the fact that in each case the hypothesis lies on the boundary of the parameter space, the P-values need to be viewed with some caution. Normally, in order to compute more exact P-values, one would conduct Monte Carlo versions of the tests, but in this case the results are so clear that these are omitted. We note that while the observer error is not deemed statistically significant its magnitude relative to the case error can be estimated from the maximal model as $\hat{\sigma}_b/\hat{\sigma}_e = 0.09$. It is up to the clinician to decide whether this is clinically significant. We may also obtain from the *nlme* output confidence intervals for σ_a and σ_e and they are $(0.0348, 0.0749)$ and $(0.0158, 0.0238)$, respectively.

It is important to distinguish between two different uses to which the working model may be put. First suppose that heart X-rays of the study are from normal, healthy persons and we wish to provide some indication of the normal range of diagnostic indices. Then the appropriate distribution on which to base the variability of a diagnostic index v is $\phi(v|\mu, \sigma_a^2 + \sigma_e^2)$ or some predictive equivalent, and so an appropriate 95 per cent normal range would be

$$\left\{ \hat{\mu} - 2\sqrt{(\hat{\sigma}_a^2 + \hat{\sigma}_e^2)}, \hat{\mu} + 2\sqrt{(\hat{\sigma}_a^2 + \hat{\sigma}_e^2)} \right\} = (0.341, 0.556).$$

Suppose, however, that we are assessing a new case and an observer has recorded v for the diagnostic ratio, and we wish to make some statement about the true diagnostic ratio u. Here we are not interested in the variability between cases and any inference about imprecision must be based on the appropriate distribution, namely $\phi(v|u, \sigma_e^2)$. Thus as an approximate 95 per cent interval for β we could take $(v - 2\hat{\sigma}_e, v + 2\hat{\sigma}_e)$ so that for an observed diagnostic ratio of 0.490 we would obtain an interval $(0.451, 0.529)$.

In our maximum likelihood analysis for arriving at a normal range and at a measure of imprecision for a new case we used an estimative method. We now provide a Bayesian analysis which uses the predictive method and which also avoids the possibility of negative components of variance.

For the normal range problem the working model for predicting the variability of a new case with a possibly new observer is $\phi(v|\mu, \sigma_a^2 + \sigma_e^2)$ for one replicate v. The predictive form for this model can be estimated simultaneously with the variance components to give highest posterior density estimates. We also compute a 95 per cent prediction interval for a future observation and, given an observed diagnostic ratio of 0.49, a 95% inverse prediction interval for the corresponding true diagnostic ratio u. This analysis was performed using the WinBUGS package with the following model.

$$
\begin{aligned}
v_{ijr} &\sim \mathrm{N}(\mu_i, \sigma_e^2), \\
\mu_i &\sim \mathrm{N}(\mu, \sigma_a^2), \\
v_1 &\sim \mathrm{N}(\mu, \sigma_a^2 + \sigma_e^2), \\
v_2 &\sim \mathrm{N}(u, \sigma_e^2).
\end{aligned}
$$

Note that the model for the v_{ijr} has been expressed using hierarchical recentering so as to avoid problems due to lack of identifiability. The term v_1 denotes a future observed diagnostic ratio, while v_2 and u denote, respectively, an observed and the corresponding true diagnostic ratio. The following independent non-informative priors were also used.

$$
\begin{aligned}
\mu &\sim \mathrm{N}(0, 10^6), \\
u &\sim \mathrm{N}(0, 10^6), \\
\sigma_a &\sim \mathrm{U}(0, 100), \\
\sigma_e &\sim \mathrm{U}(0, 100).
\end{aligned}
$$

In WinBUGS, three parallel chains were run. The results from a burn-in of 5,000 samples were discarded. The chains were run for a further 5,000 samples and the output was used to check the equilibrium of the process. Examination of autocorrelation plots and trace plots suggested that the chains were mixing well and were in equilibrium and this was supported by the Brooks-Gelman-Rubin convergence statistics. A further 5,000 samples were generated from the three chains and the results are given in Table 6.3.

Table 6.3 *WinBUGS output for the observer error study of diagnostic ratio*

Node	Mean	SD	MC error	2.5%	Median	97.5%
v_1	0.4499	0.0636	5.276E-4	0.3250	0.4501	0.5755
v_2	0.4899	0.0199	1.450E-4	0.4510	0.4900	0.5290
μ	0.4501	0.0151	1.317E-4	0.4190	0.4502	0.4796
σ_a	0.0564	0.0126	1.362E-4	0.0378	0.0545	0.0872
σ_e	0.0199	0.0022	2.432E-5	0.0162	0.0197	0.0247

From the 2.5% and 97.5% columns we may find highest posterior intervals for σ_a and σ_e and the predictive intervals for v_1 and v_2 and the true diagnostic ratio, which are in reasonable agreement with the REML results. We note that the Bayesian intervals for v_1 and u are slightly wider than their estimative counterparts, as we would expect because the uncertainties in the parameter estimates are being accounted for in the modelling.

6.4 An observer error study of multivariate heart measurements

In a larger study of heart X-ray measurements five consultant radiologists recorded the six measurements $v_1, \ldots, v_6$ of Table 6.1 for each of 65 cases presented in randomized order, different for each radiologist. The complete set of 325 six-dimensional vectors of measurements is given in data set `dratio`.

If v_{ij} denotes the vector of measurements of the ith heart X-ray by the jth radiologist then the simple fixed effects multivariate model

$$v_{ij} = \mu + \alpha_i + \beta_j + e_{ij}$$

will allow us to investigate the possibility of a radiologist effect. Note that there is no replication within an observer in this study so that there is no possibility of investigating case×observer interactions. For the sake of simplicity we use fixed effects rather than random effects. This, of course, means that the results are applicable only to the cases and observers included in this experiment and that generalisation to other cases and observers is strictly not possible on statistical grounds. The relevant lattice of hypotheses is shown in Figure 6.2. The appropriate tests used here are discussed in Section 3.10 and depend on the values of the determinants of the sums-of-squares and cross-products residual matrices which are also shown in logged form in Figure 6.2. All hypotheses are rejected so that we require to use the maximal model with case effects, as we would expect, and observer effects.

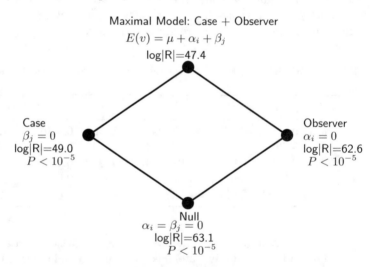

Figure 6.2 *Lattice of hypotheses for multivariate heart measurements. At each node the value of the logged residual determinant is shown, together with the P-value associated with the approximate test of the stated hypothesis within the maximal model.*

In view of the finding in Section 6.3 that there was no statistically significant observer error in diagnostic ratio assessments it is of interest to ask whether, despite significant error differences in this larger study, the diagnostic ratio may retain this stable between-observer property. By taking a random-effects approach and performing a similar linear mixed-effects analysis to that discussed in Section 6.3 we display the results of lattice-testing in Figure 6.3. Since there is no replication there is no possibility of investigating case×observer interaction. Box-Cox analysis and Q-Q plotting suggest that no transformation is required. The inference is the same as for the previous study in that there is significant variability among the cases but no significant observer variability. The 95% confidence intervals for σ_α and σ_e are (0.047, 0.067) and (0.012, 0.014) respectively.

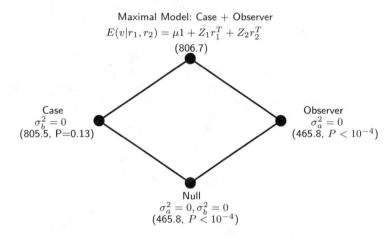

Figure 6.3 *Lattice of hypotheses for the second diagnostic ratio study. At each node the value of the REML loglikelihood is shown, together with the P-value associated with the approximate test of the stated hypothesis within the maximal model.*

6.5 An observer error study of cell counts

The objectives of this study are to determine whether 'observer error', either in the form of an observer being unable to reproduce stable relative counts of labelled to unlabelled cells or in the form of variability across selected areas of tissue, is important and to provide an idea of the degree of precision attaching to the counting process for a future patient. In the pilot study considered here only one observer A is involved, making one count on a first area of tissue and two (replicate) counts on a second area of tissue for each of ten cases. For the purposes of our statistical analysis it is convenient to imagine three 'observers', defined in the following way:

Observer 1 is A with his only count on area 1.
Observer 2 is A with his first count on area 2.
Observer 3 is A with his second count on area 2.

Note also that since only one person is involved in the counting process there is no possibility of assessing the variability that there may be between different persons assigned the counting process. Data set `cells` provides information on the numbers L, U of labelled and unlabelled cells counted within each area.

Since each pair (L, U) is essentially determining the composition of the area we use the natural logratio transformation $v = \log(L/U)$ in order to investigate sources of variability. We again consider a linear mixed model approach that is similar to that used in Section 6.3. Let v_{ij} denote the logratio count recorded for case i $(i = 1, 2, \ldots, 10)$ by 'observer' j $(j = 1, 2, 3)$. As a first step in our analysis we may therefore imagine the maximum possible explanation in the variation of the v_{ij} in terms of the model

$$v_{ij} = \mu + a_i + b_j + e_{ij},$$

where μ is a general mean, the a_i are mutually independent $N(0, \sigma_a^2)$ random effects, the b_j are mutually independent $N(0, \sigma_b^2)$ random effects and the ϵ_{ij} are independent $N(0, \sigma_e^2)$ random errors. Therefore σ_a^2 and σ_b^2 are components of variability due respectively to cases and observers.

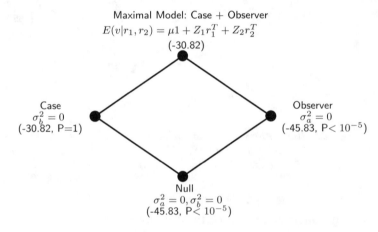

Figure 6.4 *Lattice of hypotheses for cell count study. At each node the value of the REML loglikelihood is shown, together with the P-value associated with the approximate test of the stated hypothesis within the maximal model.*

Hypotheses of interest can then be posed within this model in terms of these variance components. The hypothesis $\sigma_a^2 = 0$ means that there is no variation in logratio count from case to case, whereas the hypothesis $\sigma_b^2 = 0$ indicates that there is no variability among observers. Figure 6.4 shows the complete lattice of hypotheses together with the associated tests. Standard lattice testing results in the acceptance of the 'inter-case variability' hypothesis as our working model. There is no statistically significant variability among observers in addition to case-to-case variation. The 95% confidence intervals for σ_a and σ_e are $(0.66, 1.73)$ and $(0.30, 0.56)$ respectively.

Having reported this finding to the observer we added the following comments. All the above is concerned with statistical significance. Let us put to you another view of observer error studies which is more concerned with clinical significance.

The objective of an observer error study is surely to determine the extent to which variability within an observer (for example, you on replicated counts) or between observers (this cannot be assessed in your study) is clinically significant. Suppose that your true observer count proportion $p_T = L/(L+U)$ and in log-ratio form $v_T = \log\{p_T/(1-p_T)\}$. In terms of our modelling above the logratio

$$v = \log \frac{p}{1-p}$$

varies for a given case about a mean v_T normally with standard deviation σ. You can imagine σ to make allowance for all the various kinds of observer error (replication and area) you are prone to, together with any other unexplained error. In other words, we are supposing that the only differences lies in cases but that counting is prone to imprecision. From the *nlme* output a safe estimate $\hat{\sigma}$ of σ would then be $\hat{\sigma} = 0.411$. Then we could place a 95 per cent confidence interval (making allowance for observer and other error) on v_T as approximately

$$v_{\text{obs}} - 2 \times 0.411 < v_T < v_{\text{obs}} + 2 \times 0.411$$

leading to a corresponding confidence interval for p_T:

$$\frac{\exp(v_{\text{obs}} - 0.822)}{1 + \exp(v_{\text{obs}} - 0.822)} < p_T < \frac{\exp(v_{\text{obs}} + 0.822)}{1 + \exp(v_{\text{obs}} + 0.822)}.$$

Thus if the observed proportion of L to $L+U$ is $p_{\text{obs}} = 0.1$ (10 per cent) then $v_{\text{obs}} = \log(0.1/0.9) = -2.197$ so that the confidence interval for the true proportion p_T is

$$0.047 < p_T < 0.202.$$

Thus if, for example, the treatment of the new case depends on this proportion being below, say, 0.15 a single count leading to an observed proportion 0.1 would leave doubts about whether to treat, or not.

6.6 A comparison of large and small X-rays for diagnosis

An interesting problem of observer error was introduced in Section 1.7. The storage of standard X-rays is becoming an increasingly pressing problem and various alternatives have been suggested. The current investigation concerns the possibility of replacing the large film by a small one prepared from it. Should a diagnostic assessment of the patient be required later when the large film has been destroyed will the small film be adequate for this purpose? To obtain a fair assessment of the relative effectiveness of the two sizes we clearly require to study the diagnostic performance of radiologists presented with large and small films for the same set of patients, whose diagnosis is known from other investigations.

In the study large and corresponding small X-rays of 90 patients, suffering from a variety of conditions, were used. Each of three consultant radiologists was presented with the sequence of 90 large films in random order and asked to reach a diagnosis for each. They were then asked later to reach diagnoses based on the 90 small films presented again in a random order different from the order for the large films. Since the correct diagnosis was known for each of the 90 cases the diagnosis reached by the radiologist for a particular film could be recorded simply as correct (C) or wrong (W). Data set xrays presents these results.

Since the diagnosis is known for each case we can conveniently consider the observation v as a binary response with $v = 1$ denoting a correct, and $v = 0$ a wrong, diagnosis. For case i $(i = 1, \ldots, 90)$ let v_{ijk} be the response of observer j $(j = 1, 2, 3)$ with the kth size of X-ray film ($k = 1$ for large, $k = 2$ for small). A now standard way of modelling the response probabilities is

$$\Pr(v_{ijk} = 1 | \text{case } i, \text{observer } j, \text{size } k) = \frac{\exp(\mu + \alpha_i + \beta_j + \gamma_k)}{1 + \exp(\mu + \alpha_i + \beta_j + \gamma_k)},$$

$$\Pr(v_{ijk} = 0 | \text{case } i, \text{observer } j, \text{size } k) = \frac{1}{1 + \exp(\mu + \alpha_i + \beta_j + \gamma_k)}.$$

Since there is no replication in this study there is no possibility of investigating any interactions and we have not introduced any interaction terms in the linear predictor $\mu + \alpha_i + \beta_j + \gamma_k$.

The parameter dimension 96 here is high and although it is feasible to proceed to a formal maximization of the full likelihood based on the v_{ijk} data there is an elegant way of avoiding the embarrassment of the large number of parameters. While it has been convenient in our initial modelling to introduce the parameters α_i $(i = 1, \ldots, 90)$ to remind ourselves that cases may differ in difficulty these α_i are essentially nuisance parameters and of no immediate interest. We virtually know that the α_i will differ and we need concentrate only on $\beta_1, \beta_2, \beta_3$ and γ_1, γ_2. This can be achieved by conditional density functions or probabilities, which do not depend on the nuisance parameters and from which a 'partial likelihood' may be formed and used to investigate relevant hypotheses. To simplify our exposition of this partial likelihood method we confine attention first to the radiologists' performance with the large X-rays.

Analysis of the large X-ray study

In our modelling of performance with the large X-rays we may drop the subscript k and let v_{ij} denote the response (correct or wrong) on the ith case by the jth observer and adopt the full model with

$$\Pr(v_{ij} = 1 | \text{case } i, \text{observer } j) = \frac{\exp(\mu + \alpha_i + \beta_j)}{1 + \exp(\mu + \alpha_i + \beta_j)},$$

$$\Pr(v_{ij} = 0 | \text{case } i, \text{observer } j) = \frac{1}{1 + \exp(\mu + \alpha_i + \beta_j)}.$$

For each case we can list in Table 6.4 eight possible triplets of responses

Table 6.4 *Large X-rays: response probabilities*

Observers			Probability
1	2	3	
C	C	C	$\delta_{i1}\delta_{i2}\delta_{i3}/\Delta_i$
W	C	C	$\delta_{i2}\delta_{i3}/\Delta_i$
C	W	C	$\delta_{i1}\delta_{i3}/\Delta_i$
C	C	W	$\delta_{i1}\delta_{i2}/\Delta_i$
W	W	C	δ_{i3}/Δ_i
W	C	W	δ_{i2}/Δ_i
C	W	W	δ_{i1}/Δ_i
W	W	W	$1/\Delta_i$

together with the associated probabilities given by the full model, with the notation

$$\delta_{ij} = \exp(\mu + \alpha_i + \beta_j), \quad \Delta_i = \prod_{j=1}^{3}(\delta_{ij} + 1).$$

We have grouped the response triplets according to the total number of wrong diagnoses as it is on the basis of conditioning of these totals that we can eliminate the nuisance parameters. For example, given that exactly one diagnosis is wrong the conditional probability that it is observer 1 who has the wrong diagnosis (that is, that the triplet recorded is (1 0 0)) is

$$\frac{\delta_{i2}\delta_{i3}/\Delta_i}{\delta_{i2}\delta_{i3}/\Delta_i + \delta_{i1}\delta_{i3}/\Delta_i + \delta_{i1}\delta_{i2}/\Delta_i}$$

$$= \frac{\exp(\beta_2 + \beta_3)}{\exp(\beta_2 + \beta_3) + \exp(\beta_1 + \beta_3) + \exp(\beta_1 + \beta_2)}$$

which does not depend on the nuisance parameters. The complete set of these conditional probabilities is listed in Table 6.5. In this table

$$\Delta_1 = e^{\beta_2+\beta_3} + e^{\beta_1+\beta_3} + e^{\beta_1+\beta_2}, \quad \Delta_2 = \sum_{i=1}^{3} e^{\beta_i}.$$

Each of the recorded response triplets contributes its appropriate conditional probability to the partial likelihood, which is simply the product of all these conditional probabilities. Note that the triplets (0, 0, 0) and (1, 1, 1) make no contribution to the partial likelihood. This is intuitively obvious since any case for which all three radiologists get the diagnosis correct (or wrong) provides no possible clue as to the relative accuracies of the radiologists.

The parametrization of the model as specified is conveniently symmetric in $\beta_1, \beta_2, \beta_3$ but these parameters are technically not identifiable. For example, $\beta_1 + \kappa, \beta_2 + \kappa, \beta_3 + \kappa$ yield the same conditional probabilities and therefore

Table 6.5 *Large X-rays: partial likelihood formulae*

| Observers | | | Contribution to |
1	2	3	Partial Likelihood
W	C	C	$e^{\beta_2+\beta_3}/\Delta_1$
C	W	C	$e^{\beta_1+\beta_3}/\Delta_1$
C	C	W	$e^{\beta_1+\beta_2}/\Delta_1$
W	W	C	e^{β_3}/Δ_2
W	C	W	e^{β_2}/Δ_2
C	W	W	e^{β_1}/Δ_2

the same partial likelihood as $\beta_1, \beta_2, \beta_3$. This is easily remedied for computational purposes by the introduction of a simple constraint such as $\beta_1 = 0$ or $\beta_1 + \beta_2 + \beta_3 = 0$ and working effectively with two parameters β_2, β_3. The hypothesis H of no observer error can then be expressed as $\beta_2 = \beta_3 = 0$ and this can be tested readily within the maximal model M with general β_2, β_3. The maximized loglikelihoods are $l_M = -26.86, l_H = -28.56$. Since the generalized likelihood ratio test at the 5 per cent level rejects the hypothesis of no observer differences if $2(l_M - l_H) > 5.99$, the 95 percentile of the $\chi^2(2)$ distribution, and since here $2(l_M - l_H) = 3.4$, there is clearly in this study no significant evidence of any radiologist effect. It should be pointed out, however, that although there are 90 cases in the study only 25 of these contribute to the partial likelihood so that the effective sample size is 25.

Comparison of large and small X-rays

Returning to the main problem of whether there is any difference in the use of large and small X-rays we have the unconditional probabilities associated with the v_{ijk}.

$$\Pr(v_{ijk} = 1|\text{case } i, \text{observer } j, \text{size } k) = \frac{\exp(\mu + \alpha_i + \beta_j + \gamma_k)}{1 + \exp(\mu + \alpha_i + \beta_j + \gamma_k)},$$

$$\Pr(v_{ijk} = 0|\text{case } i, \text{observer } j, \text{size } k) = \frac{1}{1 + \exp(\mu + \alpha_i + \beta_j + \gamma_k)}.$$

Again we can rid ourselves of the nuisance parameters α_i by constructing for each sextuplet of responses a partial likelihood based on conditional probabilities given the total number of wrong diagnoses recorded. This process is obviously more complicated than that for the large X-ray study and we shall illustrate the contributions to the partial likelihood by a few examples. Consider the sextuplet of responses ordered as follows:

Observer 1		Observer 2		Observer 3	
Large	Small	Large	Small	Large	Small

Table 6.6 *Probabilities of response configurations with two wrong diagnoses*

Observer 1		Observer 2		Observer 3		Probability
Large	Small	Large	Small	Large	Small	
W	W	C	C	C	C	$\delta_{i21}\delta_{i22}\delta_{i31}\delta_{i32}/\Delta_i$
W	C	W	C	C	C	$\delta_{i12}\delta_{i22}\delta_{i31}\delta_{i32}/\Delta_i$
W	C	C	W	C	C	$\delta_{i12}\delta_{i21}\delta_{i31}\delta_{i32}/\Delta_i$
W	C	C	C	W	C	$\delta_{i12}\delta_{i21}\delta_{i22}\delta_{i32}/\Delta_i$
W	C	C	C	C	W	$\delta_{i12}\delta_{i21}\delta_{i22}\delta_{i31}/\Delta_i$
C	W	W	C	C	C	$\delta_{i11}\delta_{i22}\delta_{i31}\delta_{i32}/\Delta_i$
C	W	C	W	C	C	$\delta_{i11}\delta_{i21}\delta_{i31}\delta_{i32}/\Delta_i$
C	W	C	C	W	C	$\delta_{i11}\delta_{i21}\delta_{i31}\delta_{i32}/\Delta_i$
C	W	C	C	C	W	$\delta_{i11}\delta_{i21}\delta_{i22}\delta_{i31}/\Delta_i$
C	C	W	W	C	C	$\delta_{i11}\delta_{i12}\delta_{i31}\delta_{i32}/\Delta_i$
C	C	W	C	W	C	$\delta_{i11}\delta_{i12}\delta_{i22}\delta_{i32}/\Delta_i$
C	C	W	C	C	W	$\delta_{i11}\delta_{i12}\delta_{i22}\delta_{i31}/\Delta_i$
C	C	C	W	W	C	$\delta_{i11}\delta_{i12}\delta_{i21}\delta_{i32}/\Delta_i$
C	C	C	W	C	W	$\delta_{i11}\delta_{i12}\delta_{i21}\delta_{i31}/\Delta_i$
C	C	C	C	W	W	$\delta_{i11}\delta_{i12}\delta_{i21}\delta_{i22}/\Delta_i$

Table 6.6 lists all the response sextuplets for which exactly two responses are wrong together with the conditional probabilities. The notation used sets

$$\delta_{ijk} = \exp(\mu + \alpha_i + \beta_j + \gamma_k),$$

$$\Delta_i = \prod_{j=1}^{3}\prod_{k=1}^{2}\{1 + \exp(\mu + \alpha_i + \beta_j + \gamma_k)\}.$$

Each conditional probability is obtained from the corresponding unconditional probability by dividing by the sum of the fifteen unconditional probabilities. The probabilities are given in Table 6.6 and we now discuss the form of the exponents of some of them. Thus for response pattern WW CC CC the exponent contains $-2\beta_1$. This pattern provides no direct information on the relative merits of large and small X-rays so that γ_1 and γ_2 are missing from the exponent, whereas it indicates for that case the inferiority of observer 1 relative to observers 2 and 3 with the $-2\beta_1$ feature. Similarly for response pattern CW CC CW the exponent contains $-\beta_1 - \beta_3 + \gamma_1 - \gamma_2$ and this indicates support for large against small with $\gamma_1 - \gamma_2$ in the exponent and also indicates that observers 1 and 3 are inferior in this case with a subsequent $-\beta_1 - \beta_3$ in the exponent.

It should now be obvious how conditional probabilities can be constructed for other sextuplets and how the partial likelihood can be constructed as a product of all the conditional probabilities associated with recorded sextu-

Table 6.7 *Comparison of models for X-ray data*

Model	Dimension	Loglikelihood
Observer + Size	4	-107.4
Observer	3	-107.5
Size	2	-107.6
Null	1	-109.4

plets. We note again that the all correct sextuplet (CC CC CC) and the all wrong sextuplet (WW WW WW) make no contribution to the partial likelihood since neither gives information with respect to differences in observer or size.

Again the non-identifiability of the parameters caused by the symmetric development can be easily removed by setting $\beta_1 = 0$ and working with the parameters β_2, β_3 and $\gamma = \gamma_1 - \gamma_2$. The relevant maximized loglikelihoods and the parameter dimensions are given in Table 6.7. Clearly, no significant observer or size effects are detected.

6.7 Bacteria counts

We now reconsider the data on hospital bacterial counts which were first discussed in Section 1.8 and displayed in Table 1.4. We denote the count on the ith plate from the jth observer by v_{ij} and take as maximal model the following Poisson regression model with hierarchical random-effects:

$$M_2: \quad v_{ij} \sim Po(\mu_{ij})$$

with

$$\log \mu_{ij} = \mu + a_i + b_{ij},$$

where the a_i and the b_{ij} are mutually independent with $a_i \sim N(0, \sigma_1^2)$ and $b_{ij} \sim N(0, \sigma_2^2)$ and μ is a fixed effect. In this model the parameter σ_1^2 represents the variability in bacterial count from plate to plate while σ_2^2 is the variability in count among observers within plates. We also consider two special cases of model M_2: in model M_1 σ_2^2 is zero and so only plate-to-plate count variability is allowed for and in model M_0 the mean count is taken to be a fixed constant and both σ_1^2 and σ_2^2 are zero. All three models were fitted and parameter estimates and model deviance computed using WinBUGS. The parameters μ, σ_1 and σ_2 were assumed to be a priori independent with 'non-informative' priors

$$\mu \sim N(0, 10^4) \qquad \sigma_1 \sim U(0, 100) \qquad \sigma_2 \sim U(0, 100).$$

In the case of model M_2 three parallel chains were run from dispersed initial values for the parameters. The results of the first 5,000 iterations were discarded as burn-in and the chains run for a further 5,000 iterations during which convergence was monitored. Examination of trace and autocorrelation plots showed that the chains were stationary and that the chain for σ_1 indicated the presence of a fair degree of autocorrelation. The BGR convergence statistics were checked and showed no cause for alarm. Due to the autocorrelation in the σ_1 chain the chains were each run for a further 10,000 iterations, giving 30,000 in all. As the Monte Carlo error was sufficiently small relative to the standard deviation of σ_1, in particular, estimates were based on the results of these 30,000 iterations. As the models M_1 and M_0 are simpler than M_2 the diagnostics were checked using the trace and autocorrelation plots of a single chain and convergence was faster. The results for all three models are shown in Table 6.8.

Table 6.8 *Bacterial count models, interval estimates and deviances*

Model	95% HPD Intervals			Deviance
	α	σ_1	σ_2	
M_2	(3.8, 5.0)	(1.01, 1.98)	(0.040, 0.096)	40.7
M_1	(3.8, 5.0)	(1.01, 1.98)	—	80.2
M_0	(5.1, 5.2)	—	—	13,400.0

Clearly models M_1 and M_2 are strongly preferred to model M_0 on the basis of mean posterior deviance. The drop in deviance from model M_1 to model M_2 is also large and this suggests that we should adopt the maximal model M_2. This means that there is significant observer variability within plates in addition to the (much larger) variability from plate to plate.

6.8 Bibliographic notes

The objective of this chapter has been to give an overall view of how observer error studies in a variety of forms can be used to ensure that the data used to describe experience are reliable and reproducible. There is a wide literature on such observer error studies and since most of it involves standard types of analysis such as analysis of variance with fixed, random or mixed effects we need not pick out any particular reference text; see, however, Dunn (1989). What we do wish to emphasise is again the good sense of constructing at the outset of such analyses a lattice of all the relevant hypotheses rather than use so-called ANOVA (analysis-of-variance tables) and MANOVA (multivariate analysis of variance tables), which, in our view, are little more than computational devices. In a way this chapter emphasises the good sense of spending time modelling the situation presented. Good examples of this are the cell-count problem of Section 6.5 and the comparison of large and small X-rays of Section 6.6. In the first it is important to realise the compositional nature of the data and model accordingly. In the second the fact that some of the data provide no information on the relative merits of large and small X-rays can be easily overlooked. For example, we can report that when such a data set is presented to mature statistical students in a practical class there is a tendency to amalgamate the data into an uninformative contingency table and apply an inappropriate chi-squared test. The analyses presented in Section 6.6 are based on the concept of partial likelihood; see Cox (1975).

6.9 Problems

Problem 6.1 The determination of granule densities on microscopic slides has been causing problems and so a series of observer error studies has been conducted. The three studies are described in the tables below. You are asked to report on the nature of the variability and to make recommendations on future practice.

Replicate determinations of granule densities in five fields by two observers.

Observer		Field			
	1	2	3	4	5
1	1.98	1.22	1.16	1.27	0.98
	1.87	1.40	1.11	1.35	0.90
	1.86	1.20	1.21	1.46	0.99
2	2.68	1.65	1.14	1.57	0.79
	2.66	1.57	1.23	1.65	0.93
	2.68	1.68	1.14	1.45	0.75

Replicate determinations of granule densities in ten fields by a single observer.

				Field					
1	2	3	4	5	6	7	8	9	10
2.05	1.96	1.75	3.10	2.70	1.20	6.90	4.90	6.60	6.30
2.08	1.73	1.72	3.60	2.62	1.42	6.90	4.20	6.68	6.54
2.02	1.87	1.84	3.75	2.80	1.42	6.50	4.71	6.88	6.60
2.05	2.05	1.10	3.84	2.97	1.48	6.30	4.32	6.07	6.50
1.98	2.02	1.60	3.85	2.89	1.37	6.93	4.61	6.80	6.15
1.97	2.06	1.38	3.75	3.00	1.38	6.62	4.51	6.45	6.70
1.85	1.89	1.67	3.95	3.10	1.42	6.21	4.57	6.56	6.18
2.14	1.82	1.50		3.07	1.44	6.50	4.25	6.25	6.45
2.19	1.88	1.76			1.24	6.55	4.67	6.64	6.37
2.28	1.50	1.74			1.46	6.80	4.48	6.40	6.50

Determinations made by a single observer of granule densities in unstained (U) and stained (S) sections from ten different fields.

					Field					
	1	2	3	4	5	6	7	8	9	10
U	1.18	1.70	0.84	3.39	3.10	4.96	2.13	1.70	2.50	0.96
S	1.33	2.20	1.02	3.48	5.60	5.06	3.18	1.73	2.67	1.80

Problem 6.2 New safety measurements in a hypertension clinic have meant the replacement of the standard column-of-mercury meter by another cuff-meter. Also there is a proposal that an innovative automatic recorder of blood pressure should be introduced. A pilot investigation into the reproducibility of blood pressure reading has been conducted. Three clinicians in the course of their routine work have used the cuff-meter on 20 different patients, 60 patients in all, and their readings on these patients have been simultaneously recorded by the automatic method, unseen by the clinicians. The results for systolic blood pressures (mg Hg) are given below.

		Clinician			
C1		C2		C3	
auto	cuff	auto	cuff	auto	cuff
172	171	210	215	190	188
201	203	212	219	192	187
181	183	191	198	173	168
173	177	201	208	195	189
168	167	185	190	207	202
184	182	192	195	230	222
205	207	193	198	197	194
167	166	214	219	226	220
193	193	203	210	188	186
195	196	195	202	170	170
188	189	188	198	181	178
214	215	190	196	184	180
207	210	173	178	207	204
250	253	209	215	170	164
171	169	217	222	193	189
198	199	176	182	174	171
210	209	227	234	143	140
184	182	186	192	200	194
205	205	198	206	179	173
227	227	202	205	217	212

You are asked to investigate the reliability of the use of the cuff-meter relative to the automatic recorder.

Do you consider this investigation as satisfactory? If not, what design improvements would you recommend?

Problem 6.3 A new analytical technique for determining the percentages of four parts (a, b, c, d) of the enzyme content of blood plasma is under consideration. Three biochemists have trained in the new technique and have been invited to analyse aliquots of 15 specimens with the results recorded below.

Biochemist											
B1 Percentages				B2 Percentages				B3 Percentages			
a	b	c	d	a	b	c	d	a	b	c	d
23	10	49	18	25	10	49	16	23	11	49	17
25	14	48	13	25	15	48	12	24	15	49	12
18	13	50	19	18	13	51	18	17	14	50	19
24	13	47	16	26	13	46	15	25	12	47	16
28	11	47	14	28	12	47	13	25	13	48	14
25	10	48	17	24	11	49	16	24	11	48	17
26	9	46	19	28	9	45	18	27	9	45	19
27	9	48	16	27	9	50	14	28	9	47	16
29	10	45	16	30	10	45	15	28	10	46	16
33	12	43	12	33	12	45	10	33	12	44	11
35	14	40	11	36	14	40	10	33	14	42	11
28	13	45	14	28	14	46	12	27	14	46	13
21	10	46	23	22	10	47	21	21	10	46	23
25	14	47	14	25	15	48	12	23	14	49	14
22	14	46	18	22	14	49	15	21	14	48	17

Investigate the new technique from the viewpoint of reliability.

Problem 6.4 Review and prepare a report on Problem 1.1.

Problem 6.5 In diagnosing a certain type of kidney dysfunction the clinical problem is to decide which of the two kidneys, right or left, is the cause of the problem. A new radiological technique has been suggested and to investigate its effectiveness three radiologists have used the technique on 20 patients and made decisions left (L) or right (R) for each case. The correct answer is available after substantial further investigation. The results recorded below give the correct side and the sides chosen by the three radiologists.

Correct	Radiologists		
answer	R1	R2	R3
L	L	L	L
R	R	L	R
R	R	R	L
R	R	L	R
L	L	L	L
R	R	R	R
R	L	R	R
L	L	L	L
R	R	R	R
L	L	R	L
R	R	R	R
R	R	L	R
L	L	L	L
L	L	L	R
R	R	R	R
R	R	R	R
L	L	R	L
L	L	L	L
R	R	R	L
R	L	R	R

You are asked to consider whether the new technique is reliable.

CHAPTER 7

Indirect Measurement: Assay and Calibration

7.1 Introduction

When the statistical analysis described in Chapter 6 indicates that a direct method of measurement cannot produce valid or reproducible observations, due to too great variability in the conditions or materials involved in measurement, we have then to study methods of indirect measurement. Assays of many biochemical substances are of this type. Similar types of problem arise if different methods of measurement are used in different clinics or if there is a proposal to replace an established method by some cheaper or more efficient alternative method.

We consider the appropriate applied statistical techniques for investigating the reliability of the indirect measurement and its usefulness for predicting the direct measurement. This can be achieved through the statistical technique of calibration, leading to the calibrative density function. The complexity of the calibration problem depends on the underlying functional relationship between the direct and indirect measurements and the sources of variability affecting the indirect measurement method. We look first of all at situations where a linear relationship can be assumed, and investigate the problems posed by the sources of variability met in practice. We also consider how non-linear relationships can be handled in a tractable form. For both linear and non-linear situations we present approximations as well as full Bayesian analysis and illustrate their use.

Following the stability arguments of Chapter 2, the general calibration problem is concerned with assessing the calibrative density function $p(u|v, D)$ for the unknown direct measurement u, given the observation v associated with the referred case and the data set $D = \{(u_i, v_i) : i = 1, \ldots, n\}$ of selected cases observed under the identical experimental conditions. A parametric model $p(v|u, \theta)$ is assumed for the distribution of v given both u and a vector of unknown parameters θ. These parameters belong to a parameter set Θ and they are involved in the functional relationship between the indirect and direct measurements and also the relevant sources of variability. Based on a prior distribution $p(\theta)$ on θ and the data D, the posterior distribution $p(\theta|D)$ of θ given the data D is formed. We also assume a prior distribution $p(u|D)$ for u; this may depend on the observed u_i contained in D, in the case of a natural calibration experiment, or simply be a function $p(u)$ of u. The predictive density function for a future value v given the corresponding u and the data

D is then obtained as

$$p(v|u, D) = \int_{\Theta} p(v|u, \theta)p(\theta|D)d\theta.$$

The calibrative density of u given v and D is then given by

$$p(u|v, D) = \frac{p(v|u, D)p(u|D)}{\int_U p(v|u, D)p(u|D)du},$$

or as

$$p(u|v, D) = \frac{p(v|u, D)p(u)}{\int_U p(v|u, D)p(u)du},$$

if a separate prior assessment $p(u)$ is available. The complexity, tractability and subsequent realism of $p(u|v, D)$ will depend on a functional relationship between u and v and the diversity of sources of experimental variation.

We look first at situations where a linear relationship can be assumed and investigate the problems posed by the sources of variability met in practice; we then consider the non-linear case.

7.1.1 Simple linear calibration

The data set $D = \{(u_i, v_i) : i = 1, \ldots, n\}$ consists of independent pairs of measurements sampled in the conditional form $p(v|u)$ or the joint form $p(u, v)$ such that

$$E(v_i|u_i) = \alpha + \beta u_i + e_i, \tag{7.1}$$

where $\theta = (\alpha, \beta, \sigma^2)$ and the e_i are mutually independent $N(0, \sigma^2)$ random variables. We denote a future pair of values of the measurements by (u, v) and assume that $p(v|u, D)$ is $N(\alpha + \beta u, \sigma^2)$. We now describe briefly two approximate methods for the computation of a calibrative interval for u together with a fully Bayesian analysis in which all parameter uncertainties are taken into account. Of these methods the Bayesian approach is generally the preferred option.

Estimative approach

Ignoring the uncertainty in the estimation of the parameter θ we may take $p(v|u, D)$ to be $N(\hat{\alpha} + \hat{\beta}u, \hat{\sigma}^2)$, where $\hat{\alpha}$ and $\hat{\beta}$ are the maximum likelihood estimates of α and β and $\hat{\sigma}^2$ is given by $rss/(n-2)$, where rss denotes the residual sum of squares associated with the simple linear regression model. It follows that

$$\frac{v - \hat{\alpha} - \hat{\beta}u}{\hat{\sigma}} \sim N(0, 1)$$

and that a $100c\%$ confidence interval for u is given by

$$\frac{v - \hat{\alpha}}{\hat{\beta}} \pm N(0, 1; (1 + c)/2)\frac{\hat{\sigma}}{\hat{\beta}},$$

where $N(0, 1; p)$ denotes the pth quantile of the $N(0, 1)$ distribution.

Classical approach

In the classical approach, a calibrative interval for u is based on the pivotal function result

$$\frac{(v - \hat{\alpha} - \hat{\beta}u)^2}{\hat{\sigma}^2(1 + 1/n + (u - \bar{u})^2/S_{uu})} \sim F(1, n - 2),$$

where $\bar{u} = 1/n \sum_{i=1}^{n} u_i$ and $S_{uu} = \sum_{i=1}^{n}(u_i - \bar{u})^2$. A $100c\%$ confidence set for u is then given by

$$\frac{(v - \hat{\alpha} - \hat{\beta}u)^2}{\hat{\sigma}^2(1 + 1/n + (u - \bar{u})^2/S_{uu})} \leq F(1, n - 2; c),$$

where $F(a, b; c)$ denotes the cth quantile of the $F(a, b)$ distribution. Equating both sides of this inequality one obtains a quadratic equation which may be solved for the unknown u. In the usual case, where the slope parameter β is significantly non-zero, this procedure provides a finite calibrative interval for u.

Predictive approach

In the following approach based on the predictive density $p(v|u, D)$ a fully Bayesian analysis is employed to take full account of the uncertainty in the parameter θ. Assuming a vague prior distribution on θ it may be shown that the predictive distribution $p(v|u, D)$ is

$$St^1 \left[n - 2, \hat{\alpha} + \hat{\beta}u, (1 + 1/n + (u - \bar{u})^2/S_{uu})\hat{\sigma}^2 \right].$$

In a natural calibration experiment the prior distribution $p(u|D)$ takes the form

$$St^1 \left[n - 1, \bar{u}, (1 + 1/n)\frac{S_{uu}}{(n - 1)} \right].$$

The calibrative density function is then obtained by Bayes's formula as

$$p(u|v, D) = \frac{p(v|u, D)p(u|D)}{\int_U p(v|t, D)p(t|D)dt}.$$

Computation of the calibrative interval requires the use of numerical integration techniques, but as an alternative we use Gibbs sampling via the package WinBUGS. The methods defined here are illustrated using the aldosterone data in Section 7.2.

7.1.2 Non-linear calibration

In cases where the relationship between the indirect and direct measurement methods does not have the linear form of (7.1) we resort to non-linear regression modelling based on the model

$$E(v_i|u_i) = g(u_i; \theta) + e_i, \tag{7.2}$$

where g is a smooth, monotonic function and the e_i are mutually independent $N(0, \sigma^2)$ random variables. We again consider two approximate methods together with the fully Bayesian approach.

Estimative approach

By replacing the parameter θ by its maximum likelihood estimate $\hat{\theta}$ we may write down the pivotal function

$$\frac{v - g(u; \hat{\theta})}{\hat{\sigma}} \sim N(0, 1).$$

In cases where feasible solutions exist, we may then obtain a 100c% calibrative interval for u by solving the equations

$$g(u; \hat{\theta}) = v - \hat{\sigma} N(0, 1; (1 + c)/2),$$
$$g(u; \hat{\theta}) = v + \hat{\sigma} N(0, 1; (1 + c)/2),$$

where $N(0, 1; p)$ denotes the pth percentile of the $N(0, 1)$ distribution.

Asymptotic approach

Solving for u the equation $v = g(u; \theta)$ expresses u as a parametric function $h(v; \theta)$ of θ, where h is the inverse of the function g. An approximate 100c% calibration interval for u may then be obtained using the standard asymptotic theory of maximum likelihood as

$$h(v; \hat{\theta}) \pm N(0, 1; (1 + c)/2) \sqrt{d^T C d},$$

where d is the gradient vector of the function h, with respect to the components of θ, evaluated at $\hat{\theta}$ and C is the estimated covariance matrix of $\hat{\theta}$.

Predictive approach

Exact distributional results are not available in the non-linear case and so there is even more need for numerical methods. We will use Gibbs sampling via the WinBUGS package in order to compute calibration intervals using a fully Bayesian method. The methods for computation of calibrative intervals in the non-linear case are illustrated in Sections 7.5 and 7.6.

7.2 Calibration of methods for aldosterone

It is the intention of a steroid laboratory to change its method of determining the plasma concentration of aldosterone from a double isotope method to a radioimmunoassay method. The reasons for this intention are diminished cost, increased speed and smaller blood sample required. The problem is that the double isotope method has been used to make determinations which have formed the basis of a satisfactory differential diagnostic method. If a changeover to the new radioimmunoassay method is to be made then it is clearly necessary to compare these two methods for compatibility, and if differences are established we must find a means of determining equivalent double isotope measurements.

To investigate this problem two aliquots of each of 72 blood samples, selected to give a spread over the range of anticipated values, are used, one aliquot being assigned to the double isotope method and the other aliquot to the radioimmunoassay method. The results are shown in data set `aldo`.

Previous work has established reasonable (observer, conditions, method) reproducibility so that our entire attention can now be devoted to dealing with (method | case) reproducibility, where we drop the irrelevant factors of observer and conditions. We must clearly treat the problem as one of calibration with the variable u denoting double isotope determination and v radioimmunoassay determination.

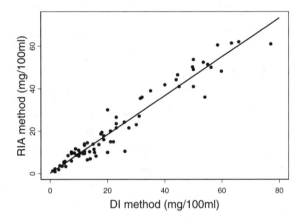

Figure 7.1 *Concentrations of aldosterone in blood plasma, determined by the radioimmunoassay (RIA) and double isotope (DI) methods.*

As a first step in this calibrative application we verify which marginal and conditional probability functions are stable and estimable from D. The sampling is in fact joint since each blood sample is split into two aliquots. Thus $p(u,v)$ is the basic sampling form represented in the data. Figure 7.1 shows the scattergram of the $(u,v) = (DI, RIA)$ data. The plot suggests that it might be reasonable to assume a linear relationship between RIA and DI, although there is clear evidence of heterogeneity especially for small values of DI. It would be worth adopting a weighted analysis and considering transformations but we leave such considerations as an end-of-chapter problem. In the practical context it is the higher values of DI and RIA that are of most direct interest, although we apply the methods also for a small value of RIA to indicate how the method breaks down with the current model.

The joint nature of the sampling gives us the choice of direct modelling of the conditional form $p(u|v)$ or indirect modelling through $p(u|v) \propto p(v|u)p(u)$, the more 'standard' calibration problem in most calibrative data sets. We can conveniently use this application to illustrate the standard problem. With (u_i, v_i) denoting the double isotope (DI) and radioimmunoassay (RIA) concentrations of the ith blood sample we are here dealing with the standard normal linear model defined in (7.1). The standard estimates of α, β (with estimated standard errors) and σ^2 are

$$\hat{\alpha} = 0.1539 \ (0.8699), \quad \hat{\beta} = 0.9148 \ (0.0286), \quad \hat{\sigma}^2 = 20.75,$$

with $\bar{u} = 23.95$ and $S_{uu} = 25398.46$.

Table 7.1 *At three given aldosterone concentrations determined by the radioimmunoassay (RIA) method, point estimates and 95% interval estimates of the corresponding aldosterone concentrations which would be obtained using the double isotope method are given, based on the Estimative, Classical and Predictive approaches*

RIA	Estimative		Classical		Predictive	
50	54.5	(44.7, 64.3)	54.6	(44.4, 64.8)	54.6	(44.4, 65.0)
25	27.2	(17.4, 36.9)	27.2	(17.2, 37.2)	27.2	(17.0, 37.3)
6	6.4	(−3.4, 16.2)	6.3	(−3.8, 16.4)	6.3	(−3.9, 16.4)

The methods described in Section 7.1.1 were applied for three values of RIA and the results are provided in Table 7.1. In the Bayesian analysis, the model assumptions given in Section 7.1.1 were adopted, the DI data were mean-centred and the prior distributions on α, β, σ and u were taken to be independent with

$$\alpha \sim N(0, 10^6), \quad \beta \sim N(0, 10^6), \quad \sigma \sim U(0, 100), \quad u \sim N(0, 10^6).$$

In WinBUGS initial values of the variables were generated randomly from the prior distributions and three parallel chains were run. The results from a burn-in of 1,000 samples were discarded. The chains were run for a further 4,000 samples and the output was used to check the equilibrium of the process. Autocorrelations plots and trace plots suggested that the chains were mixing well and were in equilibrium and this was confirmed by considering the Brooks-Gelman-Rubin convergence statistics. A further 5,000 samples were generated from each chain and they were used to produce 95% highest posterior density intervals for the unknown DI concentrations. The posterior mean of the samples is taken as the point estimate. The posterior densities are symmetric in this case.

The three methods produce very similar point and interval estimates of the unknown DI concentration in all three cases. The last interval at RIA=6 is obviously unrealistic, as the DI concentration is a positive quantity. As already indicated this interval is included only for the purpose of illustration.

7.3 Glucose calibration

The glucose calibration problem concerns the use of a reflectance meter in the diagnosis of neonatal hypoglycaemia. The standard measurement of glucose concentration here is the biochemical oxidase method. The new method of assessing glucose concentration is the reflectance meter method. Data set `gluc` gives replicated reflectance meter readings for a set of individuals, whose biochemical measurement was also determined. We denote by u_i the biochemical oxidase measurement and by v_{ij} $(j = 1, \ldots, n_i)$ the n_i reflectance meter measurements of the ith individual $(i = 1, \ldots, 52)$. We note that in data set `gluc` n_i is either 2 or 3. The data are shown in Figure 7.2.

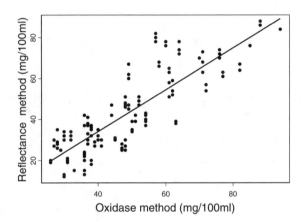

Figure 7.2 *Concentrations of glucose obtained using the reflectance meter and biochemical oxidase methods, with two or three replicate measurements on each sample.*

The plot exhibits a lot of variation but a linear relationship captures the main upward trend in the data. Note that there are two components of variation in the reflectance meter readings due to the variability among replicate readings within individuals and also the variability from individual to individual. One way to account for these sources in the modelling would be to take, in the model of (7.1), the random error for the ith individual to be the sum of two independent terms with respective variances σ_I^2 and σ_B^2. Then the variance of the random errors is the sum $\sigma_I^2 + \sigma_B^2$ and these variances appear as a sum in the modelling. Hence, as far as calibration is concerned, there is no advantage in splitting the error variation into these separate terms. Therefore, we adopt a simple linear regression model and assume that

$$v_{ij} = \alpha + \beta u_i + e_{ij},$$

where the e_{ij} are mutually independent $N(0, \sigma^2)$ random variables.

The consultative question of interest is:

Given r replicate measurements $v = (v_1, v_2, \ldots, v_r)$ of the glucose concentration made using the reflectance meter method, how accurately can we predict u the corresponding concentration that would have been obtained using the biochemical oxidase method?

In order to produce calibrative intervals for u we require to make the following changes to the formulae given in Section 7.1.1, with $\bar{v} = 1/r \sum_{i=1}^{r} v_i$ denoting the average of the replicate readings.

Estimative approach

The 100c% calibrative interval for u is based on the following pivotal function result

$$\frac{\bar{v} - \hat{\alpha} - \hat{\beta}u}{\hat{\sigma}/\sqrt{r}} \sim N(0, 1),$$

and is given by

$$\frac{\bar{v} - \hat{\alpha}}{\hat{\beta}} \pm N(0, 1; (1 + c)/2) \frac{\hat{\sigma}}{\sqrt{r}\hat{\beta}}.$$

Classical approach

The 100c% calibrative interval for u is based on the pivotal function

$$\frac{(\bar{v} - \hat{\alpha} - \hat{\beta}u)^2}{\hat{\sigma}^2(1/r + 1/n + (u - \bar{u})^2/S_{uu})} \sim F(1, n - 2),$$

and is defined by the set of values of u which satisfy the inequality

$$\frac{(\bar{v} - \hat{\alpha} - \hat{\beta}u)^2}{\hat{\sigma}^2(1/r + 1/n + (u - \bar{u})^2/S_{uu})} \leq F(1, n - 2; c).$$

Predictive approach

The predictive distribution $p(v|u, D)$ is

$$St^1 \left[n - 2, \hat{\alpha} + \hat{\beta}u, (1/r + 1/n + (u - \bar{u})^2/S_{uu})\hat{\sigma}^2 \right].$$

The methods described in Section 7.1.1 were applied for varying numbers of replicates and the results are provided in Table 7.2.

In the Bayesian analysis, the model assumptions given in Section 7.1.1 were adopted, the oxidase data were mean-centred and the prior distributions on α, β, σ and u were taken to be independent with

$$\alpha \sim N(0, 10^6), \quad \beta \sim N(0, 10^6), \quad \sigma \sim U(0, 100), \quad u \sim N(0, 10^6).$$

In WinBUGS, the initial values for the variables were generated randomly from the prior distributions and three parallel chains were run. The results from a burn-in of 1,000 samples were discarded. The chains were runs for a further 4,000 samples and the output was used to check the equilibrium of the process. Autocorrelations plots and trace plots suggested that the chains were mixing well and were in equilibrium and this was confirmed by considering the Brooks-Gelman-Rubin convergence statistics. A further 10,000 samples were

Table 7.2 *The glucose concentrations, as determined by the reflectance meter method, are given in two sets of data with varying numbers of replicates. Point estimates and 95% interval estimates of the corresponding glucose concentrations which would be obtained using the biochemical oxidase method are given, based on the Estimative, Classical and Predictive approaches*

v	Estimative		Classical		Predictive	
30	36.0	(17.8, 54.3)	35.9	(17.4, 54.5)	35.8	(15.9, 55.5)
30,32	37.0	(24.1, 49.9)	36.9	(23.8, 50.1)	36.8	(22.5, 51.2)
30,32,33	37.7	(27.1, 48.2)	37.6	(26.8, 48.4)	37.5	(25.7, 49.1)
60	65.4	(47.1, 83.6)	65.5	(46.9, 84.0)	65.5	(45.5, 85.9)
60,62	65.9	(53.0, 78.8)	66.0	(52.8, 79.2)	66.0	(51.7, 80.2)
60,62,63	67.0	(56.5, 77.5)	67.1	(56.3, 78.0)	67.2	(55.4, 79.3)

generated from the three chains and they were used to produce 95% highest posterior density intervals for the unknown glucose concentration that would have been obtained using the biochemical oxidase method. The posterior mean of the samples is taken as the point estimate. The posterior densities are symmetric in this case.

The point and interval estimates are very similar in each case for all three methods, with the Bayesian intervals being wider. The intervals are reflecting a good deal of uncertainty in the estimate of glucose concentration which would be obtained using the biochemical oxidase method. The use of replicates results in a real gain in precision; in going from a single measurement to three replicate measurements the width of the interval is generally reduced by about 41%. Even then the glucose concentration has an estimated error of $\pm$ 10.5 mg/100ml.

7.4 Calibration of foetal age by crown rump length

This application concerns the measurements in data set `foetal`. In this data set crown rump length of the foetus in 194 pregnant women was recorded along with the maturity in days of the foetus established to within three days. The measurements were in some instances replicated over time as summarized in the following table

r	1	2	3	4	5	6	7	8
n_r	146	13	11	6	8	5	1	4

where r denotes the number of replicates over time and n_r is the number of women with r replicates. The data are shown in Figures 7.3 and 7.4.

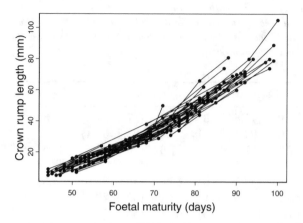

Figure 7.3 *Plot of crown rump length against foetal maturity for the women who were measured on more than one occasion, with a line connecting the data from each foetus.*

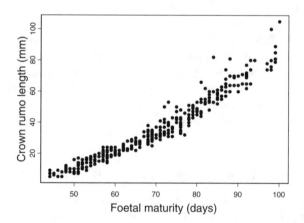

Figure 7.4 *Plot of crown rump length against foetal maturity for the women who were measured on only one occasion.*

The plots show a reasonably clear relationship between crown rump length and foetal maturity but it appears to be non-linear. The plots suggest that the square root of crown rump length is used as the response and this is supported by Box-Cox analysis. The individual subject line plots of Figure 7.3 suggest that we consider a model which can take into account the possibility of random between-subject variation in the intercepts and slopes of the individual plots.

For purposes of exposition of the calibrative method the imprecision in maturity is ignored at this stage, but it will be dealt with later in Section 7.7. The consultative questions here can be identified as follows.

Given the crown rump length v of a referred pregnant woman with foetus of unknown maturity u how can we use the past experience in data set foetal *to obtain the calibrative distribution $p(u|v, D)$? How accurate is this as a predictor of maturity? If we take replicate measurements $v = (v_1, \ldots, v_r)$ over fixed known time intervals how much more accurate is our predictor of maturity?*

We assume that the square roots of the crown-rump length measurements v_{ij} are linearly dependent on maturity u_{ij} and adopt the linear mixed-effects model

$$v_{ij} = \alpha + \beta u_{ij} + a_i + b_i u_{ij} + e_{ij} \quad (j = 1, \ldots, n_i; \ i = 1, \ldots, 194) \quad (7.3)$$

as the maximal model, where the random variables a_i, b_i and e_{ij} are mutually independent with $a_i \sim N(0, \sigma_a^2), b_i \sim N(0, \sigma_b^2)$ and $e_{ij} \sim N(0, \sigma_e^2)$. In this model the parameters α and β denote the fixed-effect population level intercept and slope terms while the a_i and the b_i denote, respectively, random intercept and slope effects. The model may be written more compactly in the vector-matrix form

$$v = X\phi^T + Z_1 r_1^T + Z_2 r_2^T + e, \quad (7.4)$$

where

$$\phi = [\alpha, \beta]$$
$$r_1 = [a_1, a_2, \ldots, a_{194}]$$
$$r_2 = [b_1, b_2, \ldots, b_{194}]$$

and

$$X^T = \begin{bmatrix} 1_N \\ u \end{bmatrix},$$

$$Z_1 = \text{diag}\{1_{n_1}, 1_{n_2}, \ldots, 1_{n_{194}}\},$$

$$Z_2 = \text{diag}\{u_1, u_2, \ldots, u_{194}\},$$

where $u_i = \{u_{i1}, \ldots, u_{in_i}\}(i = 1, 2, \ldots, 194)$, $u = \{u_1, u_2, \ldots, u_{194}\}$, $N = \sum_{i=1}^{i=194} n_i$ and 1_n denotes a $n \times 1$ column vector containing 1s. This maximal model was fitted using the package *nlme* and the results are shown in Table 7.3.

The intervals for the fixed effect parameters α and β do not contain zero and so each of these terms is required in the model in addition to the others. The interval for σ_a is fairly wide, indicating that it has not been estimated very precisely, whereas the intervals for the other two standard deviations are fairly precise. The size of σ_b might initially suggest that the random slope variation is not important but recall that the size of this term is dependent on the scale of the covariate. In order to test whether either of the two variance components are required in the model we consider the lattice of hypotheses shown in Figure 7.5. We find that the random intercept variation is not required in the

Table 7.3 *Point and interval estimates of the parameters of the model (7.3)*

Parameter	Estimate	95% Interval
α	-2.827	$(-2.991, -2.662)$
β	0.122	$(0.120, 0.125)$
σ_a	0.114	$(0.0237, 0.553)$
σ_b	0.00318	$(0.00208, 0.00486)$
σ_e	0.238	$(0.212, 0.268)$

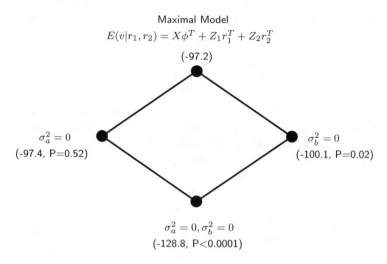

Maximal Model
$$E(v|r_1, r_2) = X\phi^T + Z_1 r_1^T + Z_2 r_2^T$$

(-97.2)

$\sigma_a^2 = 0$
(-97.4, P=0.52)

$\sigma_b^2 = 0$
(-100.1, P=0.02)

$\sigma_a^2 = 0, \sigma_b^2 = 0$
(-128.8, P<0.0001)

Figure 7.5 *Lattice of hypotheses for the crown rump length study. At each node the value of the REML loglikelihood is shown, together with the P-value associated with the approximate test of the stated hypothesis within the maximal model.*

model and that the random slope variation is required. Hence we take as our working model

$$v = X\phi^T + Z_2 r_2^T + e, \tag{7.5}$$

in which the individual linear relationships for the women are assumed to have the same fixed intercept but randomly-varying slopes. The parameter estimates obtained with this model are given in Table 7.4. These results are very similar to the estimates obtained using the maximal model.

We proceed to answer the consultative question posed above. Given the complexity of this model we consider only a full Bayesian analysis in the package WinBUGS. We consider an individual referred woman whose foetus has a crown rump length measurement of 35mm at an unknown maturity of u_1 days. In addition we have a sequence of crown rump length measure-

Table 7.4 *Point and interval estimates of the parameters of the model (7.5)*

Parameter	Estimate	95% Interval
α	-2.823	$(-2.986, -2.660)$
β	0.122	$(0.120, 0.125)$
σ_b	0.00353	$(0.00294, 0.00425)$
σ_e	0.240	$(0.215, 0.269)$

ments of 28, 35 and 48mm from this woman, taken at 7-day intervals, with corresponding unknown maturity values of $u_2 - 7$, u_2 and $u_2 + 7$ days.

In the Bayesian analysis, the prior distributions on β, σ, σ_b, u_1 and u_2 were taken to be independent with

$$\beta \sim N(0, 10^6), \sigma \sim U(0, 10), \sigma_b \sim U(0, 10), u_1 \sim N(0, 10^6), u_2 \sim N(0, 10^6).$$

The initial values of the variables were generated randomly from the prior distributions and three parallel chains were run. The results from a burn-in of 1,000 samples were discarded. The chains were run for a further 4,000 samples and the output was used to check the equilibrium of the process. Autocorrelations plots and trace plots suggested that the chains were mixing well and were in equilibrium and this was confirmed by considering the Brooks-Gelman-Rubin convergence statistics. A further 10,000 samples were generated from the three chains and they were used to produce 95% highest posterior density intervals for the unknown maturity. The posterior distributions are fairly symmetric. In the case where there is a single CRL measurement of 35mm the estimate of the maturity of the foetus is 71.3 days, with 95% highest posterior density interval (65.8, 76.9). In the case where the sequence of three CRL measurements is available the estimate of maturity is 72.1 days with 95% highest posterior density interval (68.9, 75.2). Hence the effect of using a sequence of three CRL measurements rather than a single measurement is to reduce the length of the calibrative interval from 11.1 days to 6.3 days, a reduction of 43% and thus a useful gain in precision.

7.5 Radioimmumoassay of angiotensin II

Data were collected in a designed calibration experiment in which the concentration of angiotensin II u_i in the ith vial was recorded together with the percentage bound v_i, as described in Section 1.9. The data are given in data set `angio`. A plot of the data is shown in Figure 7.6.

The plot clearly suggests that the percentage bound is non-linearly related to the concentration of angiotensin II, but what form of relationship gives a suitable model? Initial attempts were made to linearise the relationship via transformation and it was found that, apart from the points at zero concen-

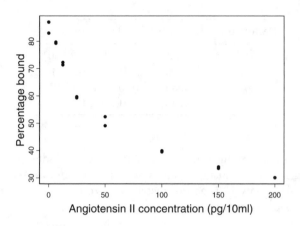

Figure 7.6 *Plot of the percentage bound against the concentration of angiotensin II.*

tration, the logit of percentage bound was strongly linearly related to the logarithm of concentration. It was then possible to re-work this finding in such a way that the points at zero could be accommodated. This led to the non-linear regression model.

$$v_i = \alpha + \frac{\beta}{\gamma + u_i^\delta} + e_i,$$

where α, β, γ and δ are unknown parameters and the e_i are independent $N(0, \sigma^2)$ random variables. This model was fitted to the data and it was found that δ was not significantly different from unity. The model was then re-expressed in order to reduce the correlations among the parameter estimates and to ensure the positivity of the parameters. Finally the non-linear regression model

$$v_i = \frac{e^\alpha + e^\beta u_i}{1 + e^\gamma u_i} + e_i \tag{7.6}$$

was fitted to the data using non-linear least squares and the results are given in Table 7.5. There are 13 degrees of freedom for error.

The estimated covariance matrix of $\hat{\theta}$, where $\theta = (\alpha, \beta, \gamma)$, is

$$\begin{bmatrix} 0.000131 & 0.001257 & 0.000755 \\ 0.001257 & 0.040292 & 0.019454 \\ 0.000755 & 0.019454 & 0.010013 \end{bmatrix}.$$

A plot of the data together with the fitted curve is shown in Figure 7.7 and this shows that the model provides a good fit to the data.

We now apply the three approaches discussed in Section 7.1.2. Working out the details of the estimative approach leads to the following formula for an

Table 7.5 *Estimates and approximate 95% interval estimates for the parameters of the model of (7.6)*

Parameter	Estimate	95% Interval
α	4.454	(4.431, 4.477)
β	−0.923	(−0.522, −1.324)
γ	−3.809	(−4.009, −3.609)
σ	1.64	(1.19, 2.64)

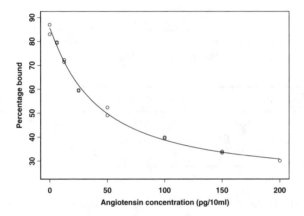

Figure 7.7 *Plot of the percentage bound against the concentration of angiotensin II together with the fitted curve corresponding to (7.6).*

approximate $100c\%$ calibrative interval for the concentration of angiotensin II u corresponding to a given value v for the percentage bound

$$\left[\frac{v - e^{\hat{\alpha}} + \hat{\sigma} z}{e^{\hat{\beta}} - (v + \hat{\sigma} z)e^{\hat{\gamma}}}, \frac{v - e^{\hat{\alpha}} - \hat{\sigma} z}{e^{\hat{\beta}} - (v - \hat{\sigma} z)e^{\hat{\gamma}}} \right],$$

where $z = N(0, 1; (1 + c)/2)$. In the Bayesian analysis, the prior distributions on α, β, σ and the unknown concentrations u_1, u_2, u_3 were taken to be independent with

$$\alpha \sim N(0, 10^6), \quad \beta \sim N(0, 10^6), \quad \gamma \sim N(0, 10^6),$$

$$\sigma \sim U(0, 100), \quad u_i \sim N(0, 10^6) \ (i = 1, 2, 3).$$

In the WinBUGS analysis three dispersed sets of initial values of α, β and γ were employed, with the other variables being generated randomly from the prior distributions, and a chain run from each of the sets. The chains were runs in Metropolis adaptive phase for 4,000 iterations and convergence was monitored during the next 10,000 runs. After 15,000 iterations the trace plots appeared to be stationary and the results were satisfactory according to the Brooks-Gelman-Rubin convergence statistics. There was, however, some autocorrelation among the variables, particularly the highly correlated β and γ, and also the trace plots for β and γ were rather under-dispersed within each chain even though the chains were overlapping and stationary. The fitted model appeared to be fine, with parameter estimates similar to the maximum likelihood estimates and the Monte Carlo error at each node was less than 5% of the node standard deviation. The chains were run for a further 5,000 iterations and then point estimates and highest posterior density intervals computed.

Table 7.6 *At three given values of percentage bound(PB), point estimates and 95% interval estimates of the corresponding concentrations of angiotensin II which would be obtained are given, based on the Estimative, Asymptotic and Predictive approaches*

PB	Estimative		Asymptotic		Predictive	
38	108.0	(86.9, 137.1)	108.0	(99.6, 116.3)	107.6	(84.2, 142.6)
55	37.7	(31.1, 45.6)	37.7	(34.7, 40.8)	38.1	(30.0, 48.7)
75	8.7	(5.8, 11.9)	8.7	(7.6, 9.8)	8.8	(5.3, 12.9)

The results are given in Table 7.6. The results obtained using the estimative and the predictive methods are fairly similar, with the predictive intervals being wider. The asymptotic intervals are noticeably narrower than those of the other two methods and this may simply be reflecting that the quadratic approximation on which they are based is not suitable in this example. The width of the predictive intervals vary from approximately 60 when the PB is 38 to 8 when the PB is 75. This reflects the shape of the calibration curve shown in Fig 7.6. Hence the determination of the concentration of Angiotensin II is much more precise for high values of percentage bound, where the curve is falling steeply, compared with low values, where the curve is flattening out.

7.6 Calibration of tobramycin

Samples of blood were taken from each of 20 patients and placed on a plate containing infected medium and on each plate the samples were exposed to tobramycin at six known concentrations which covered the range of interest. The clearance diameter was measured for each sample. For the ith patient data are available consisting of the set $\{(u_{ij}, v_{ij}) : (j = 1, \ldots, 6)\}$. The consultative question is:

Given a new blood sample of known clearance diameter, what is the corresponding unknown concentration of tobramycin?

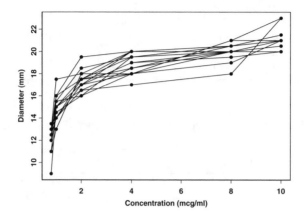

Figure 7.8 *Individual plots of clearance diameter against concentration of tobramycin.*

The data, which are available in data set `tobra`, are shown in Figure 7.8. Most of the patients' plots follow a similar pattern, with some variability from plot to plot. Some of the plots seem a little anomalous. For each patient the relationship between clearance diameter and concentration is non-linear. Various non-linear regression models provide roughly the same level of agreement between data and model and we consider here the Michaelis-Menten model. This non-linear regression model has two parameters and we allow them to be random in order to incorporate into the modelling the possibility that the relationship varies randomly from patient to patient; thus we consider the non-linear mixed-effects model

$$v_{ij} = \frac{a_i u_{ij}}{b_i + u_{ij}} + e_{ij}, \qquad (j = 1, \ldots, 6; \ i = 1, \ldots, 20) \qquad (7.7)$$

where the e_{ij}, a_i and b_i are mutually independent with $e_{ij} \sim N(0, \sigma_e^2)$, $a_i \sim N(\alpha, \sigma_a^2)$ and $b_i \sim N(\beta, \sigma_b^2)$. This model was fitted to the data using the *nlme* package and some relevant output is given in Table 7.7.

We see that the fixed-effects parameters α and β are quite precisely estimated and clearly significantly non-zero. The parameter σ_a is not well-determined and its interval suggests that having this parameter in the model is a case of over-fitting. The interval for the parameter σ_b is rather wide and the lower endpoint is close to zero, suggesting that this parameter may be unnecessary. In order to assess whether either of the variance components is required in the working model we compare the models (7.7) and (7.8). The

Table 7.7 *Point and interval estimates of the parameters of the model (7.7)*

Parameter	Estimate	95% Interval
α	21.681	(21.326, 22.037)
β	0.531	(0.486, 0.577)
σ_a	0.00171	(2.1×10^{-60}, 1.4×10^{54})
σ_b	0.0245	(0.00223, 0.271)
σ_e	0.980	(0.855, 1.125)

Table 7.8 *Point and interval estimates of the parameters of the model (7.8)*

Parameter	Estimate	95% Interval
α	21.675	(21.304, 22.044)
β	0.529	(0.482, 0.576)
σ_e	1.004	(0.893, 1.157)

asymptotic generalised likelihood ratio test has a P-value of 0.91. We therefore do not require to have random effects in the model and take as our working model the fixed-effects non-linear regression model

$$v_{ij} = \frac{\alpha u_{ij}}{\beta + u_{ij}} + e_{ij}, \qquad (j = 1,\ldots,6; i = 1,\ldots,20). \qquad (7.8)$$

Fitting this model to the data gives the output shown in Table 7.8. The fitted model is shown in Figure 7.9. The fit is fairly reasonable but could be improved, but this might require non-parametric methods.

In the Bayesian analysis, the prior distributions on α, β, σ and the unknown concentrations u_1, u_2, u_3 were taken to be independent with

$$\alpha \sim N(0, 10^6), \quad \beta \sim N(0, 10^6), \quad \sigma \sim U(0, 100), \quad u_i \sim U(0, 10) \ (i = 1, 2, 3).$$

We now consider how useful the three approaches are in determining the unknown concentration of tobramycin given three single values of 13, 15 and 17mm for the clearance diameter.

In the WinBUGS analysis three dispersed sets of initial values of α, β and σ of the variables were employed, with the other variables being generated randomly from the prior distributions, and a chain run from each of the sets. The chains were runs in Metropolis adaptive phase for 4,000 iterations, the results from the next 1,000 iterations were discarded and convergence was monitored during the next 10,000 runs. After 15,000 iterations the trace plots appeared to be stationary and the Brooks-Gelman-Rubin convergence statistics were satisfactory. The chains were run for a further 10,000 iterations and then

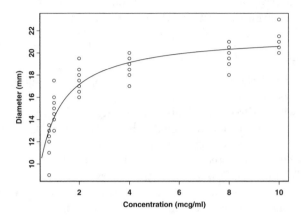

Figure 7.9 *Plot of clearance diameter against concentration of tobramycin together with the fitted curve corresponding to model (7.8).*

point estimates and highest posterior density intervals computed. Note that there is a complication in this analysis. Due to the fact that the assumption of an improper prior for u would lead to an improper posterior, it is essential to restrict the prior for the u_i's and in this example it has been assumed that they are uniform on the interval $(0,10)$, the range of concentrations used in the experiment. As the diameter increases beyond 17mm the calibrative intervals depend strongly on this prior assumption and they are very wide indeed – too wide to be useful in practice.

Table 7.9 *At three given values of the clearance diameter, point estimates and 95% interval estimates of the corresponding concentrations of tobramycin which would be obtained are given, based on the Estimative, Asymptotic and Predictive approaches*

Diameter	Estimative		Asymptotic		Predictive	
13	0.79	(0.55, 1.18)	0.79	(0.40, 1.57)	0.83	(0.56, 1.28)
15	1.19	(0.80, 1.91)	1.19	(0.60, 2.34)	1.28	(0.83, 2.19)
17	1.92	(1.19, 3.72)	1.92	(0.98, 3.79)	2.25	(1.30, 5.56)

The intervals are given in Table 7.9. If the asymptotic method is applied then the resulting intervals are far too narrow to be realistic. Therefore this method was applied to the logarithm of the unknown tobramycin concentrations and the intervals were back-transformed, resulting in rather wide intervals. The predictive and estimative intervals are quite similar when the diameter is 13mm and 15mm but a little different when the clearance diameter is 17mm. The intervals are wider as the clearance diameter increases and this is to be expected given the shape of the calibration curve in Figure 7.9.

7.7 Imprecision

When we considered the data on crown rump length and foetal maturity in Section 7.4 it was stated that foetal maturity was not known exactly but rather only to within three days. This is an example of imprecision within the context of a calibration problem; it could also be termed an issue of covariate measurement error. We now consider an approach which allows the effects of imprecision in either the direct measurement u or the indirect measurement v, or both, to be assessed. Suppose that the observed pair (u, v) are an imprecise version of the exact data values (x, y). We assume further that forms of stochastic relationship between the indirect measurements v and y and the direct measurements u and x are known, apart from some unknown parameters ϕ_1 and ϕ_2, to be $p(v|y, \phi_1)$ and $p(x|u, \phi_2)$, respectively, and that the model for the exact data is $p(y|x, \phi)$. Then we may express the model for the imprecise v given the imprecise u and unknown parameters $\theta = (\phi_1, \phi, \phi_2)$ as

$$p(v|u, \theta) = \int \int p(v|y, \phi_1)p(y|x, \phi)p(x|u, \phi_2)dydx. \qquad (7.9)$$

Given data D the components of θ could be estimated using maximum likelihood or via a Bayesian approach. If we assume a prior distribution $p(\theta)$ for θ we may convert this into a posterior distribution $p(\theta|D)$ and then form the predictive distribution using

$$p(v|u, D) \propto \int p(v|u, \theta)p(\theta|D)d\theta \qquad (7.10)$$

and then the calibrative density of u via

$$p(u|v, D) \propto p(v|u, D)p(u|D). \qquad (7.11)$$

We now illustrate this approach using the crown rump length data from Section 7.4. In this example the values of crown rump length are assumed to be known exactly, even though they are recorded to the nearest mm, and so there is imprecision only on the values of foetal maturity. We let x_{ij} denote the exact value of foetal maturity corresponding to the observed square root of crown rump length v_{ij}. We recall from Section 7.4 that $p(v_{ij}|x_{ij}, b_i, \phi_1)$ is

$$N(\alpha + \beta x_{ij} + b_i x_{ij}, \sigma_e^2).$$

We assume that $p(x_{ij}|u_{ij}, \sigma_x^2)$ is $N(u_{ij}, \sigma_x^2)$. It follows, by integrating x_{ij} out of the product of these density functions, that $p(v_{ij}|u_{ij}, b_i, \theta)$ is

$$N(\alpha + \beta u_{ij} + b_i u_{ij}, \sigma_e^2 + b_i^2 \sigma_x^2).$$

As in Section 7.4 we consider a Bayesian approach to this calibration problem for different assumed values of σ_x, namely 1, 3 and 5. We consider an individual referred woman whose foetus has a crown rump length measurement of $v_0 = 35$ mm at an unknown maturity of u days. In addition, we have a sequence of crown rump length measurements of $v_1 = 28$, $v_2 = 35$ and $v_3 = 48$ mm from this woman taken at 7-day intervals, with corresponding maturity values $u - 7$, u and $u + 7$ days. The following modelling assumptions are made.

$$v_{ij} \sim N(\alpha + b_i u_{ij}, \sigma_e^2 + b_i^2 \sigma_x^2),$$
$$b_i \sim N(\beta, \sigma_b^2),$$
$$\alpha \sim N(0, 10^6),$$
$$\beta \sim N(0, 10^6),$$
$$\sigma_e \sim U(0, 10),$$
$$\sigma_b \sim U(0, 10),$$
$$v_0 \sim N(\alpha + b'u, \sigma_e^2 + b'^2 \sigma_x^2),$$
$$v_1 \sim N(\alpha + b'(u_1 - 7), \sigma_e^2 + b'^2 \sigma_x^2),$$
$$v_2 \sim N(\alpha + b'u_1, \sigma_e^2 + b'^2 \sigma_x^2),$$
$$v_3 \sim N(\alpha + b'(u_1 + 7), \sigma_e^2 + b'^2 \sigma_x^2),$$
$$b' \sim N(\beta, \sigma_b^2),$$
$$u \sim N(0, 10^6),$$
$$u_1 \sim N(0, 10^6).$$

Table 7.10 *At four values of the imprecision standard deviation σ_x, point estimates and 95% highest posterior density estimates of the unknown foetal maturity are given based on (a) a single measurement and (b) a sequence of three measurements of crown rump length*

σ_x	Single measurement		Sequence of measurements	
	Estimate	Interval	Estimate	Interval
0	71.4	(67.4, 75.4)	72.2	(69.9, 74.6)
1	71.4	(65.8, 76.9)	72.2	(67.6, 76.8)
3	71.5	(64.9, 78.0)	72.2	(68.0, 76.5)
5	71.5	(61.7, 81.7)	72.2	(66.5, 78.1)

In WinBUGS the chain was run in Metropolis adaptive phase for 4,000 iterations and the results from a further 1,000 iterations were discarded. Sampling was continued for a further 10,000 iterations and, given satisfactory plots and convergence statistics, these results were used to compute the 95% highest posterior density intervals for u and u_1, which are given in Table 7.10 together with point estimates based on the posterior means. The case $\sigma_x = 0$ in which the imprecision is ignored has been included for reference.

As one might expect, the intervals for the unknown foetal maturity become increasingly wider as the extent of the imprecision increases, showing that taking account of the imprecision understandably results in greater uncertainty in the estimate of foetal maturity. The point estimates of foetal maturity are very stable in the presence of imprecision at the levels considered. In the practical context the foetal maturity is known to within 3 days. Taking this to mean that the imprecision standard deviation is approximately unity we conclude that the point estimates of maturity obtained by ignoring this imprecision is probably alright but the interval estimates are understating the level of uncertainty in the estimate by approximately 28% in the case of a single measurement and 49% when three replicates are taken. Clearly, the larger the imprecision standard deviation the greater the extent of this understatement of uncertainty.

7.8 Bibliographic notes

The general problem of indirect measurement by calibration and assay from the viewpoint of the predictive distribution is discussed in Aitchison and Dunsmore (1975). The problem of calibration is discussed by Brown (1982, 1993). The problem of non-linear calibration from a Bayesian perspective is discussed in Racine-Poon (1988).

There are many publications on the use of statistical aspects of radioimmunoassay techniques. We give a representative selection: Finney (1976), Healey (1972), Prentice (1976).

For details of the use of the reflectance meter in the diagnosis of neonatal hypoglycaemia, see Baxter (1974).

For further information of the use of ultrasound screening of the foetus and the measurement of crown-rump length see Robinson and Fleming (1975). For further details of the Michaelis-Menten model see Seber and Wild (1989).

7.9 Problems

Problem 7.1 Review the aldosterone assay problem of Section 7.2 considering the possibility of a weighted analysis and/or a transformation. Compare your analysis with that of Section 7.2 and decide which you would recommend to the clinic.

Problem 7.2 Two clinics using different methods of determining the amounts of a certain hormone in the blood have agreed to conduct a calibration experiment in which, for each of 24 patients, a blood specimen is divided into four aliquots, two being analysed by clinic A and the other two by clinic B. The results, reported in standard units, are set out in Table 7.11.

How would you report to the clinics in such a way that each clinic is able

Table 7.11 *Data for Problem 7.2*

Clinic	A		B	
Aliquot	1	2	3	4
	54	55	42	42
	141	176	101	136
	143	148	92	115
	503	588	341	344
	105	126	95	61
	73	70	78	43
	85	61	74	58
	219	280	183	180
	109	86	52	67
	1067	1093	765	605
	347	418	238	273
	276	251	159	211
	158	191	136	116
	248	280	222	227
	799	726	644	452
	23	25	15	14
	832	695	511	523
	136	156	99	85
	214	236	146	178
	592	395	372	445
	451	483	338	275
	39	46	30	24
	56	50	36	36
	351	330	354	184

to assess results from the other? Have you any comments to make on the reliability of such an exchange?

Problem 7.3 Refer to Problem 1.2 and prepare a report for the clinic on the questions of dosage assay which have been raised.

Problem 7.4 In a radioimmunoassay of aldosterone two vials at each of nine standard concentrations (pg/ml) were used and the proportions bound recorded, as set out below.

Dose (pg/ml)	Proportion bound
0	0.629, 0.629
6.25	0.584, 0.605
12.5	0.551, 0.571
25	0.507, 0.511
50	0.405, 0.411
75	0,311, 0.340
100	0,291, 0.312
150	0.231, 0.251
200	0.206, 0.196

On the same radioimmunoassay run two vials for each of four patients with unknown aldosterone concentrations were used and the corresponding proportions bound recorded as follows. You are asked to assess the aldosterone concentrations for these four patients.

Patient	Proportion bound
P1	0.352, 0.332
P2	0.314, 0.265
P3	0.537, 0.522
P4	0.210, 0.215

Problem 7.5 A clinic is faced with an unusual situation. For some time it has been deciding on treatment reasonably successfully on the basis of an expensive and slow technique of determining an (a, b, c) blood composition. The clinic now faces the possibility of introducing an autoanalyser for this purpose. A complication is that the autoanalyser recognises recent research which has identified a fourth part d of the composition of blood. The clinic recognises the obvious merits of the analyser, particularly with the possibility that the extra component may prove useful in the future but would like to be reassured that the four-part compositions available from it would provide reasonable assessments of the three-part compositions already in use. The clinic has conducted a calibration trial over the range of blood samples that occur in its work. For each of 32 blood samples aliquots were assigned to the existing method and the autoanalyser method, with results as recorded in Table 7.12.

How would you advise the clinic on this problem?

Problem 7.6 An inexpensive quick chromatographic method for determining the excretion rate (mg/24hr) of a certain steroid metabolite in urine has been developed. It is hoped that this method may in the future replace the long and costly, though accurate, bioassay technique currently used. The considerable

Table 7.12 *Data for Problem 7.5*

Existing method Percentages			Autoanalyser method Percentages			
a	b	c	a	b	c	d
14.1	20.2	65.7	16.0	16.9	63.7	3.4
31.0	51.2	17.8	27.6	40.1	15.1	17.2
28.7	43.9	27.4	26.8	37.4	26.1	9.7
23.9	49.4	26.7	20.8	34.7	22.6	21.9
23.9	54.4	21.7	23.5	39.3	18.6	18.6
9.1	50.5	40.4	10.7	38.5	35.7	15.1
16.3	54.5	29.2	14.6	39.8	21.7	23.9
14.0	73.8	12.2	9.5	34.1	6.7	49.7
17.0	74.8	8.2	12.0	42.1	5.7	40.2
23.5	47.1	29.3	22.4	36.2	24.9	16.5
20.6	55.6	23.8	18.4	37.5	20.1	24.0
19.0	71.5	9.5	15.2	43.8	6.7	34.3
26.5	35.4	38.1	25.0	28.0	40.1	6.9
24.9	45.8	29.3	24.5	38.2	26.6	10.7
12.6	54.5	32.9	11.9	42.7	28.9	16.5
29.2	41.2	29.6	27.4	37.0	24.8	10.8
14.1	63.1	22.9	12.4	37.0	18.0	32.5
31.9	44.2	23.9	33.1	39.0	22.9	5.0
15.4	65.5	19.1	18.1	45.9	19.1	16.9
17.2	43.6	39.2	18.0	32.7	40.6	8.7
19.4	34.2	46.4	17.1	29.4	43.6	9.9
20.0	52.5	27.5	16.8	35.2	18.6	29.4
11.1	23.5	65.4	12.2	19.8	63.7	4.3
20.8	52.5	26.7	24.6	38.0	24.3	13.1
12.7	53.1	34.2	12.3	35.8	29.1	22.8
20.7	51.5	27.8	21.3	36.4	26.1	16.2
14.0	70.8	15.2	12.1	44.4	10.2	33.3
11.5	37.3	51.2	12.8	28.3	43.0	15.9
13.4	66.3	20.3	10.8	35.5	13.6	40.1
21.1	56.4	22.5	18.5	35.0	16.3	30.2
23.4	50.9	25.7	20.6	36.6	19.3	23.5
18.5	51.9	29.6	21.1	44.3	27.1	7.5

past experience of such bioassays has shown that the excretion rates analysed are approximately normally distributed with mean 2 mg/24hr and standard deviation 0.5 mg/24hr. To explore the possibilities of the method, aliquots from a number of urine samples are available. The experimenter has made bioassay determinations on one aliquot from each urine sample and selected a subset which he felt gave adequate coverage of the range of excretion rates. Three other aliquots from each urine sample of this subset were then assigned to the chromatographic method and the results are tabled below.

Serial no of urine sample	Excretion rate (mg/24hr)	
	Bioassay method	Chromatographic method
1	0.50	0.80, 0.88, 0.98
2	1.00	1.07, 1.10, 1.10
3	1.20	1.20, 1.23, 1.35
4	1.40	1.36, 1.48, 1.49
5	1.60	1.52, 1.53, 1.56
6	1.80	1.63, 1.72, 1.82
7	2.00	1.76, 1.80, 1.88
8	2.20	1.95, 2.00, 2.02
9	2.40	2.01, 2.04, 2.18
10	2.60	2.16, 2.28, 2.29
11	2.80	2.31, 2.40, 2.42
12	3.00	2.45, 2.51, 2.52
13	3.50	2.82, 2.94, 3.01

Explore the possibilities of using the chromatographic method in the future. If the experimenter asks how the taking of more than three chromatographic determinations would affect the reliability of the method how would you respond?

CHAPTER 8

Diagnosis

8.1 Introduction

The general problem of differential diagnosis in clinical medicine has been well illustrated and motivated in previous chapters. In Chapter 1 data sets such as Conn's syndrome, Cushing's syndrome, haemophilia and non-toxic goitre were introduced. In Chapters 2–4 aspects and characteristics of the probability distribution of such data were discussed. In order to retain the logical sequence of the development of statistical concepts in clinical medicine through experience, observation and measurement which are fundamental to the data collection process, in this chapter we shall concentrate on what may be termed the standard statistical differential diagnosis problem.

This problem depends on the availability of a data set D which has arisen through experience, observation and measurement on patients who suffer from one of a set $\{u : u = 1, \ldots, k)$ of k disease types. The data in D consist of a set of measurements: the feature vector denoted by v on each patient along with the known disease type u for that patient. The data set

$$D = \{(u_i, v_i) : i = 1, \ldots, n\}$$

is commonly referred to as the training set.

We assume that D is homogeneous and complete in the sense that each case has been observed and measured in the same manner, for example that all patients arise from one specialist clinic, that the typing methods are stable, for example by post mortem or operation and that the features in v are measured on all patients so that the v_i are complete. There is no restriction on the nature of the features: they can be continuous or discrete.

The aim of the statistical diagnostic process is to employ the data set D as a vehicle for making a meaningful probability statement about a new patient with known feature vector v who has been ascertained to have one of the k disease types but so far the precise disease type u is unknown. We take the view that this statement should be a realistic and easily interpreted diagnostic aid to the clinical decision-making process. Inevitably the clinical decision will depend on the typing indicated and its uncertainty. A secondary but important consideration is that of past experience as discussed in Chapters 2–4. Has a case of this nature appeared before; in other words is the case typical of the experience in the training set D?

Statistical textbooks on medicine have a tendency to concentrate on so-called standard methods. The consulting statistician when first faced with the diagnosis problem might well think of it as an example of the standard classification problem in discriminant analysis. Thus a discriminant function (linear or otherwise) could be constructed based on modelling the conditional distribution of v on $u = j$ $(j = 1, \ldots, k)$ as, for example, multivariate normal. A new case is then allocated to disease type u depending on the value of the discriminant function score.

The imposition of this procedure on diagnostic data can be criticized immediately on the following grounds.

(i) The allocation procedure is based on long-run frequency considerations, namely the proportion of time cases are misclassified. From a clinical point of view this is unsatisfactory as it is the specific new undiagnosed patient who is of immediate concern and not some hypothetical performance over a long run of patients. What is best for the individual may differ from what is determined on the basis of a conceptual population of patients.

(ii) The procedure assumes that the conditional distributional forms for v on u are stable multivariate normal. We have seen from our discussion in Chapter 2 that this may be totally unjustified.

This line of reasoning leads us to the conclusion that as far as the individual patient is concerned, the best practice is to calculate realistic probabilities for the set of disease types as an aid to the clinical decision-making process. A secondary consideration will be a back-up assessment of how typical the new patient is of the past experience of patients in D.

8.2 Differential diagnosis in Conn's syndrome

The problem of differential diagnosis between adenoma and bilateral hyperplasia in Conn's syndrome with experience based on the data set conn has already been described in detail in Chapter 1. With disease type of the ith selected case denoted by u_i (1 for adenoma, 2 for bilateral hyperplasia) and the associated seven-dimensional feature vector denoted by v we thus have available a data set

$$D = \{(u_i, v_i) : i = 1, \ldots, n\}$$

for the selected cases $S_1, \ldots, S_n$, where $n = 31$. We now have a new patient R referred to the clinic, with recorded feature vector v and known to be suffering from Conn's syndrome but of unknown type u. The statistical problem is to arrive at a realistic diagnostic probability assessment for the referred patient based on the experience of D and the patient's own feature vector v.

In our discussion in Chapter 2 on the relation of the referral and selection processes in this differential diagnostic problem we saw that, because selection was made on the basis of feature vector v and not on syndrome type u, the appropriate connection between the referred patient R and a typical selected case S is

$$p_R(u|v) = p_S(u|v).$$

Our first step is to adopt a parametric maximal model for the conditional density function $p_S(u|v)$ and to fit this model using the techniques of Section 3.6. Since u is binary in nature the appropriate formulation is in terms of some form of binary regression model and we choose the logistic form. We shall see later that the normal form provides almost identical results.

8.2.1 Logistic form of binary regression analysis

A question that commonly arises when the covariate feature vector in such a regression analysis consists of continuous components is whether some transformation would enhance the effectiveness. There seems to be a tradition that there may be advantages in having the covariate cluster as ellipsoidal as possible. A simple way of achieving this might be to subject the components separately to the Box-Cox investigation for normality and to adopt such transformations. Statistical diagnosis with the binary regression model, however, does not depend on any distributional assumption of covariate vector variability. The main advantage that we see in making a transformation of the covariate vector to obtain an ellipsoidal cluster is in determining the relation of the covariate vector v of the referred case to past experience to ensure that we are not extrapolating in our diagnostic assessment. Since Q-Q plots indicated some evidence of non-normality, particularly in the potassium and aldosterone components, we have taken logarithms of all of the components in our analysis and verified that the resulting logged components are reasonably normally distributed. We can report that the diagnostic assessments using the untransformed components vary only slightly from those obtained here from the transformed components.

For the data set conn there is no complete separation in the full covariate space and the Newton-Raphson iterative procedure converges rapidly giving the following linear predictor:

$$-168.7 - 89.29 \log N - 22.88 \log K + 4.168 \log C$$
$$-1.76 \log R + 2.733 \log A - 35.64 \log D + 25.47 \log S$$

and with maximized loglikelihood -5.65.

The full lattice here consists of $128 \ (= 2^7)$ nodes but as shown in Table 8.1 examination of level 1, at which only one of the features enters the model, shows that the main contenders with possible diagnostic ability are potassium (K), carbonate (C) and renin (R). The sequence of investigation of these three features is shown in the lattice of Figure 8.1. Strict adherence to some fixed significance rule would have meant stopping at the first or second level. We have noted that at level 2 there is little to distinguish between the (K, C) and the (K, R) combinations and, since there appears to be an appreciable improvement in fit at level 3, we have taken the (K, C, R) combination as our working model. The maximized loglikelihood for this working model is -6.88 and the linear predictor is

$$-22.25 - 12.66 \log K + 12.72 \log C - 2.99 \log R, \tag{8.1}$$

Table 8.1 *Loglikelihoods of models in part of the lattice for Conn's data*

Level	Variable	Loglikelihood
0	Null	−20.16
1	logK	−10.08
	logC	−12.15
	logR	−14.44
	logA	−16.57
	logN	−18.42
	logS	−19.90
	logD	−20.00

with estimated covariance matrix of the estimator $\hat{\beta}$ given as follows.

	(Intercept)	logK	logC	logR
(Intercept)	1098.36	−89.19	−294.67	−16.27
logK	−89.19	57.47	3.70	5.06
logC	−294.67	3.70	88.19	0.67
logR	−16.27	5.06	0.67	5.60

As a first step in assessing the effectiveness of the working model as a tool for diagnosis we compute the predictive diagnostic assessments for the selected cases of the training set D. In making these assessments we use the leave-one-out technique. Table 8.2 provides the predictive assessments of $p(u|v, D)$ for the 31 cases. It will be seen that for adenoma cases A5 and A18 these assessments favour bilateral hyperplasia, and for bilateral hyperplasia cases B6, B7 and B9 the assessments favour adenoma. For this diagnostic problem we also show the estimative assessments, simply to bring out the fact that the predictive assessments are more conservative than the estimative assessments in the sense that they are always closer to the (0.5, 0.5) allocation associated with the greatest uncertainty. For the reasons set out in Chapter 3 we shall use only the more realistic predictive assessments.

This diagnostic picture can be communicated in the biplot of Figure 5.23, based on the standarized logarithmic values for the adenoma cases on which the positions of the bilateral hyperplasia cases have also been plotted. It is clear from this biplot that A5 and A18 are the adenoma cases most likely to be confused with the bilateral hyperplasia cases; it is clear also that cases B6, B7 and B9 are closest to the cluster of adenoma cases.

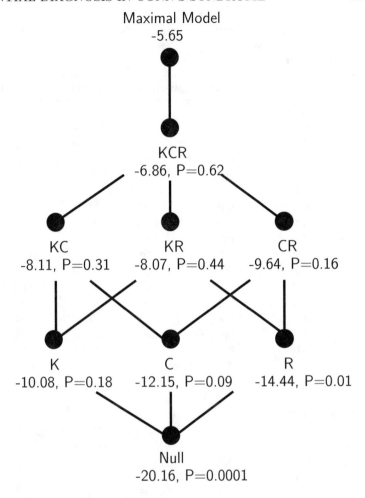

Figure 8.1 *Lattice of hypotheses for Conn's data. At each node is given the maximised loglikelihood and the P-value of the test of the model within the maximal model.*

8.2.2 Influential cases

Since the diagnostic objective is to obtain reliable assessments of $p(u|v, D)$ we follow the argument of Section 3.11 in attempting to identify influential cases in the selected set conn. More specifically we give in Table 8.3 the Kullback-Liebler influence measure providing for each case the difference in the assessments obtained by deleting and retaining the case. The cases that require investigation are A5, A18, B4 and B7. Cases A5, A18 and B7 have already been identified in the biplot of Figure 5.23 as cases which are within the overlap of the adenoma and bilateral hyperplasia cases in the covariate space. Case B4 has also been seen to be on the boundary of the bilateral

Table 8.2 *Diagnostic probability assessments for type 1(adenoma) of Conn's syndrome for the 31 cases of the training set*

Case no	Predictive	Estimative	Kernel	Bayesian
A1	0.86	1.00	0.98	0.85
A2	0.64	0.66	0.52	0.54
A3	0.92	1.00	1.00	0.82
A4	0.96	1.00	0.98	0.84
A5	0.02	0.01	0.14	0.24
A6	0.75	0.80	0.61	0.60
A7	0.92	0.99	0.91	0.76
A8	0.97	1.00	0.98	0.88
A9	0.98	1.00	1.00	0.95
A10	0.94	0.98	0.87	0.77
A11	0.94	1.00	0.92	0.81
A12	0.98	1.00	1.00	0.93
A13	0.95	1.00	0.97	0.83
A14	0.78	0.81	0.66	0.61
A15	0.93	1.00	0.99	0.84
A16	0.94	0.99	0.91	0.77
A17	0.98	1.00	1.00	0.95
A18	0.41	0.38	0.37	0.47
A19	0.98	1.00	1.00	0.94
A20	0.91	0.97	0.80	0.72
B1	0.03	0.00	0.23	0.12
B2	0.19	0.09	0.28	0.32
B3	0.23	0.23	0.40	0.39
B4	0.41	0.35	0.48	0.41
B5	0.19	0.09	0.31	0.34
B6	0.53	0.54	0.53	0.48
B7	0.62	0.66	0.51	0.50
B8	0.09	0.04	0.24	0.27
B9	0.62	0.64	0.57	0.52
B10	0.14	0.08	0.29	0.31
B11	0.05	0.01	0.19	0.20

hyperplasia biplot of Figure 5.23. In discussions with the consulting clinicians there seemed to be no good reason for excluding any of these cases and they have been retained in all subsequent analyses.

Table 8.3 *Kullback-Liebler influence for 31 cases of the training set for Conn's syndrome*

Case no	Influence	Case no	Influence	Case no	Influence
A1	0.0000	A11	0.0000	B1	0.0000
A2	0.0048	A12	0.0000	B2	0.0027
A3	0.0000	A13	0.0000	B3	0.0018
A4	0.0000	A14	0.0034	B4	0.0301
A5	0.0525	A15	0.0000	B5	0.0025
A6	0.0023	A16	0.0001	B6	0.0172
A7	0.0001	A17	0.0000	B7	0.0534
A8	0.0000	A18	0.0338	B8	0.0003
A9	0.0000	A19	0.0000	B9	0.0076
A10	0.0001	A20	0.0002	B10	0.0009
				B11	0.0000

8.2.3 Normal form of binary regression analysis

We can report here that use of the normal form for the binary regression model leads through lattice inspection to the same form of working model with linear predictor

$$-11.17 - 6.94 \log K + 6.67 \log C - 1.64 \log R.$$

Note that the ratios of the coefficients in this normal form to those in the logistic form are 0.50, 0.55, 0.52, 0.55, and so approximately conforming to the approximation $\Psi(t) = \Phi(0.59t)$ of Section 3.6. The ratios of the corresponding standard errors of these estimated coefficients are 0.54, 0.52, 0.54, 0.55, respectively, showing a similar conformity with the approximate relationship between logistic and normal forms. The predictive diagnostic assessments and atypicalities for this normal form do not differ from those of the logistic form by more than 0.02.

Weighted kernel diagnostic assessments

We now compare the use of the working model of logistic binary regression form with that of the weighted kernel method of Section 4.8 for obtaining a direct assessment of the diagnostic probabilities $p(u|v, D)$. Here $v = [v_1, v_2, v_3] = [\log K, \log C, \log R]$ and we use the binomial kernel

$$K(u_i|u_j) = \begin{cases} \lambda & (u_i = u_j), \\ 1 - \lambda & (u_i \neq u_j). \end{cases}$$

For the weighting factors we take

$$G(v, z) = 1 - \exp\{-d(v, z)/\mu\},$$

where

$$d(v, z) = \sum_{j=1}^{3} (v_j - z_j)^2 / s_j^2$$

and s_j is the estimated standard deviation of the jth component v_j in the data set conn. The pseudo-loglikelihood $l(\lambda, \mu)$ is easily computed for any given (λ, μ) and the maximizing values (λ, μ) are readily obtained by a search technique. For this data set we obtain $\lambda = 1$, the upper limit of the possible range, and $\mu = 0.065$. These values can be used to compute the kernel diagnostic assessments for the training set conn using the leave-one-out principle to avoid resubstitution bias. These are shown in Table 8.2 and there is clearly broad agreement in the inferences which would be drawn from the predictive and the Bayesian assessments.

8.2.4 Diagnostic assessments for new cases

The diagnostic working model using the linear predictor of (8.1) can now be applied to the cases of Clinic 2 to obtain the predictive diagnostic assessments $p(u = 1 | v, D)$ shown in Table 8.4 for the 43 new cases recorded in newconn. We recall that these assessments will be appropriate even if the selection and referral process differs from that of Clinic 1. Application of the weighted kernel method investigated above yields the diagnostic assessments also shown in Table 8.4. Also shown in the table are the extrapolation indices relative to the adenoma and to the bilateral hyperplasia experience.

First we note that the pattern of weighted kernel assessments is in broad agreement with the predictive assessments and we therefore confine our comments to the predictive assessment. Cases C1–C17 have predictive diagnostic probabilities varying between 0.61 and 0.98 and favouring adenoma, now known to be the true type. Moreover the extrapolation indices with respect to adenoma for these cases are all less than 1 except for C17 for which the excess over 1 is really negligible. Of the predictive assessments for D1–D4 only those for D1 and D3 favour the true type, bilateral hyperplasia. Here again no extrapolation difficulty arises. Of the cases E1–E22 of unknown type at the time of assessment we see that the extrapolation indices associated with the favoured type are all less than 1 except for cases E7 and E21. The reasons for these extrapolation warnings are easily identified. For case E7 the K value equals the maximum (in the bilateral hyperplasia group) and the C value is greater than the overall maximum; for case E21 the R value is greater than the overall value. For both of these cases the diagnostic assessment hardly distinguishes between adenoma and hyperplasia.

As we have already stated the complete separation problem of maximum likelihood estimation does not arise for this data set. We have, however, purely for illustrative purposes, applied the Bayesian approach for handling complete separation as described in Section 4.3. The resulting linear predictor based on

Table 8.4 *Diagnostic probability assessments for type 1(adenoma) for 43 cases of Conn's syndrome*

| Case no | Predictive | Kernel | Bayesian | Extrapolation index | |
				Adenoma	Hyperplasia
C1	0.93	0.99	0.82	0.53	6.05
C2	0.83	0.96	0.71	0.63	5.20
C3	0.98	1.00	0.95	0.41	8.28
C4	0.61	0.56	0.53	0.32	0.77
C5	9.95	0.93	0.79	0.00	2.51
C6	0.84	0.72	0.65	0.10	1.07
C7	0.97	0.99	0.90	0.21	5.48
C8	0.60	0.60	0.54	0.42	1.23
C9	0.85	0.94	0.72	0.47	4.07
C10	0.96	0.98	0.86	0.08	4.08
C11	0.92	0.89	0.75	0.22	2.25
C12	0.62	0.64	0.55	0.45	1.80
C13	0.97	0.99	0.86	0.27	4.30
C14	0.98	1.00	0.94	0.58	8.50
C15	0.76	0.88	0.65	0.61	3.77
C16	0.88	0.96	0.75	0.42	4.48
C17	0.87	0.99	0.77	1.07	8.49
D1	0.17	0.30	0.34	0.70	0.22
D2	0.79	0.63	0.61	0.14	0.80
D3	0.06	0.26	0.22	0.94	0.22
D4	0.56	0.55	0.52	0.37	0.94
E1	0.95	1.00	0.87	0.79	6.53
E2	0.44	0.46	0.46	0.52	1.16
E3	0.09	0.19	0.24	1.19	0.39
E4	0.29	0.36	0.40	0.71	0.31
E5	0.03	0.13	0.12	1.41	0.68
E6	0.05	0.16	0.21	1.02	0.23
E7	0.46	0.62	0.50	3.89	3.64
E8	0.30	0.36	0.40	1.50	1.40
E9	0.03	0.17	0.13	1.39	0.61
E10	0.81	0.93	0.69	0.73	4.52
E11	0.95	0.93	0.71	0.51	3.82
E12	0.15	0.32	0.31	0.72	0.08
E13	0.08	0.20	0.24	0.88	0.04
E14	0.22	0.29	0.36	1.34	0.67
E15	0.25	0.32	0.38	0.84	0.60
E16	0.76	0.79	0.63	0.42	2.26
E17	0.15	0.27	0.32	0.63	0.02
E18	0.30	0.37	0.40	0.77	0.73
E19	0.78	0.67	0.61	0.21	0.84
E20	0.03	0.10	0.12	1.51	0.72
E21	0.39	0.48	0.44	1.14	2.76
E22	0.90	0.96	0.76	0.39	4.08

the normal form of binary regression is

$$-9.82 - 4.19 \log K + 4.89 \log C - 1.02 \log R$$

and the resulting predictive assessments are presented in Tables 8.2 and 8.4. As we would expect these assessments based on the vague prior distribution on β are more conservative than those based on maximum likelihood methodology, reflecting the smaller values of the coefficients in the linear predictor. The Bayesian assessments are, however, broadly of the same pattern as the maximum likelihood assessments.

8.2.5 Reliability curves for new cases

We cannot overemphasize the good sense of investigating the reliability curves, as described in Section 3.11, for assessing how reliable a particular differential diagnosis is. To illustrate this we provide in Figure 8.2 the reliability curves for six of the new patients to demonstrate the variability in the firmness of the diagnosis. Patient C1 is a clear cut case of adenoma. Patient C4 whose differential diagnosis is also adenoma has a curve clearly indicating unreliability. Patient C6 is a fairly clear case of adenoma but with a reliability curve less convincing than patient C1. Cases D1 and E12 have curves suggesting reliable diagnoses of bilateral hyperplasia, with D1's diagnosis firmer than that of E12. Finally E22 has a very unreliable diagnosis placing roughly equal emphasis of the two forms of Conn's syndrome. We can report that overall the differential diagnosis of Conn's syndrome as described above is reliable, with most of the reliability curves similar to those for patients C1, C6, D1 and E12.

8.2.6 General comments on the effectiveness of the diagnostic system

It must be fairly clear that although the experience of data set conn can be of use in helping in the differential diagnostic process in Conn's syndrome there remain a number of cases where either the evidence points to the wrong type or where the predictive assessment is split fairly evenly between the two types. It can be reported that at the time of the use of the diagnostic system built on this experience there appeared to be no other diagnostic tools available and so it certainly played a helpful role for the cases where the inference was clear. A postscript to this work allows us to emphasize the ephemeral nature of much of statistical diagnosis. Put simply there is now a technique whereby blood samples can be extracted from the neighbourhood of each adrenal gland. If the aldosterone concentrations in these samples are approximately equal we have a case of bilateral hyperplasia. If the concentrations are different, then we have a case of an adenoma. Moreover the side with the higher concentration identifies the adrenal with the adenoma, a highly desirable piece of information in subsequent surgery.

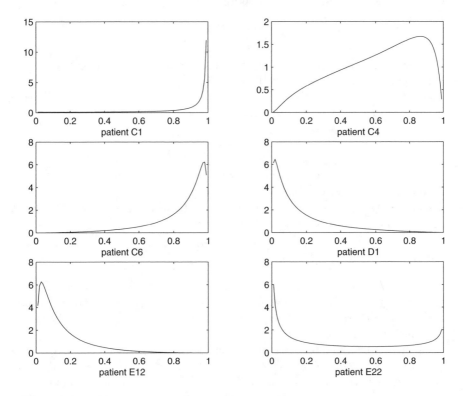

Figure 8.2 *Reliability curves for a selection of new Conn's syndrome patients.*

8.3 Screening of rheumatoid arthritis patients

The reliable diagnosis of Keratoconjunctivitis sicca (KCS) in patients with rheumatoid arthritis by an opthalmic specialist is not always available at a rheumatic clinic. In such circumstances the question arises as to whether it is possible to use non-specialists and ten binary features (presence or absence of certain symptoms) of patients to differentiate between cases of KCS and non-KCS.

Data set `kcs` shows these binary features in 77 rheumatoid arthritis patients, A1–A40 with KCS type and B1–B37 with no KCS. This data set was obtained by an opthalmic specialist first screening a group of rheumatoid arthritis patients for KCS. Once the members A1–A40 of this KCS group had been identified a group B1–B37 of similar size of patients with no KCS was taken as controls. Selection of these cases has thus been made on the basis of disease type u (1 for KCS, 2 for non-KCS) with subsequent recording of the 10-dimensional multivariate binary feature vector v. The objective is thus to use the information in this data set D to arrive at a diagnostic assessment

$p(u|v, D)$ for a new referred rheumatoid arthritis patient R or, equivalently, the odds

$$\frac{p_R(u = 1|v, D)}{p_R(u = 2|v, D)}.$$

In terms of our analysis of the relationship between referral and selection in Chapter 2 we see that we have the following alternatives.

Method 1 We may use the data set kcs to model the conditional distribution $p_S(v|u)$ and then arrive at odds for the referred patient R by the relationship

$$\frac{p_R(u|v)}{p_R(u^*|v)} = \frac{\pi(u)}{\pi(u^*)} \frac{p_S(v|u)}{p_S(v|u^*)}$$

where $\pi(u)/\pi(u*)$ is the true odds of KCS to non-KCS in the population of rheumatoid arthritis patients.

Method 2 We may model the conditional distribution $p_S(u|v)$ and arrive at odds for the referred patient R by the relationship

$$\frac{p_R(u|v)}{p_R(u^*|v)} = \frac{p_S(u|v)}{p_S(u^*|v)} \left\{ \frac{\pi(u)}{\pi(u^*)} \middle/ \frac{s(u)}{s(u^*)} \right\},$$

where $s(u)/s(u*)$ is the ratio of the selection rates of cases within the KCS and non-KCS groups. We note that factor $\{\pi(u)/\pi(u^*)\}/\{s(u)/s(u^*)\}$ in method 2 is simply a correction for the possible difference between the true incidence and the selection odds ratios.

For method 1 there is a lack of parametric models between the usually unrealistic independent binary model with its 10 parameters and the full multinomial model with its embarrassingly large number 1023 of parameters. An alternative non-parametric approach is the multivariate kernel method already applied in Section 4.8 in its simplest form with one common smoothing parameter within each group.

For method 2 a simple parametric model in the form of logistic binary regression is available and this can be compared with a non-parametric weighted kernel method, as for the differential diagnosis problem of Conn's syndrome.

We shall report all our analyses on the basis that $\pi(u)/\pi(u*) = 1$ and $s(u)/s(u*) = 1$. The adjustments for other values are obvious.

8.3.1 Logistic binary regression model

In order to investigate whether all the binary features are relevant to the diagnostic problem we first fit the maximal logistic model with covariate vector the 10-dimensional binary vector and investigate the associated lattice of hypotheses. There is no problem of complete separation here and the resulting maximal model has an estimated linear predictor

$$-4.02 + 4.45v_1 + 2.10v_2 + 1.14v_3 + 4.68v_4 + 3.48v_5$$
$$+0.80v_6 - 0.77v_7 + 2.37v_8 - 1.83v_9 + 0.92v_{10}$$

and the maximized loglikelihood is -10.37. The complete lattice here has

1024 nodes, but exploration of the lower part of this soon shows that the features v_6, v_7, v_9, v_{10} are, individually, not the strongest contenders for entry to a working model; see Table 8.5.

Table 8.5 *Loglikelihoods of models in part of the lattice for the KCS data*

Level	Variable	Loglikelihood
0	Null	−54.32
1	v1	−28.27
	v2	−31.32
	v3	−36.52
	v4	−31.34
	v5	−43.65
	v6	−48.12
	v7	−52.59
	v8	−45.03
	v9	−50.84
	v10	−46.91

Examination of the loglikelihoods in the lattice suggests that a reasonable working model may be based on the subset $(v_1, v_2, v_4, v_5, v_8)$ of the binary feature vector. The estimated linear predictor for this working model is

$$-4.14 + 3.68v_1 + 2.73v_2 + 4.45v_4 + 3.55v_5 + 2.93v_8$$

with maximized loglikelihood -11.09. For the asymptotic likelihood ratio test of this model within the maximal model the test statistic is 1.44 on 5 degrees of freedom ($P = 0.92$). The estimated covariance matrix of the parameter estimator is as follows.

	(Intercept)	v1	v2	v4	v5	v8
(Intercept)	1.40	−1.19	−0.79	−1.17	−1.27	−0.90
v1	−1.19	2.19	0.46	1.01	1.00	0.81
v2	−0.79	0.46	2.19	0.45	0.73	-0.20
v4	−1.17	1.01	0.45	2.58	1.02	0.69
v5	−1.27	1.00	0.73	1.02	2.47	0.81
v8	−0.90	0.81	-0.20	0.69	0.81	3.55

Table 8.6 *Diagnostic probability assessments for KCS for the 40 KCS cases of the training set*

Case no	Predictive	Weighted kernel	Multivariate binary kernel
A1	0.973	0.943	0.997
A2	0.998	0.993	1.000
A3	0.997	0.990	1.000
A4	0.998	0.993	1.000
A5	0.988	0.974	0.999
A6	0.973	0.943	0.997
A7	0.961	0.925	0.997
A8	0.988	0.974	0.999
A9	0.998	0.993	1.000
A10	0.278	0.113	0.197
A11	0.996	0.989	1.000
A12	0.961	0.925	0.997
A13	0.997	0.990	1.000
A14	0.998	0.992	1.000
A15	0.866	0.311	0.833
A16	0.988	0.974	0.999
A17	0.643	0.340	0.813
A18	0.994	0.975	1.000
A19	0.991	0.895	0.996
A20	0.988	0.974	0.999
A21	0.242	0.090	0.148
A22	0.997	0.990	1.000
A23	0.973	0.943	0.997
A24	0.996	0.989	1.000
A25	0.996	0.989	1.000
A26	0.431	0.154	0.288
A27	0.998	0.993	1.000
A28	0.988	0.974	0.999
A29	0.886	0.516	0.867
A30	0.988	0.974	1.000
A31	0.881	0.714	0.930
A32	0.997	0.990	1.000
A33	0.932	0.409	0.845
A34	0.988	0.974	0.999
A35	0.065	0.767	0.991
A36	0.996	0.989	1.000
A37	0.997	0.990	1.000
A38	0.802	0.652	0.916
A39	0.004	0.024	0.017
A40	0.881	0.714	0.930

Table 8.7 *Diagnostic probability assessments for KCS for the 37 non-KCS cases of the training set*

Case no	Predictive	Weighted kernel	Multivariate binary kernel
B1	0.504	0.260	0.355
B2	0.024	0.056	0.029
B3	0.323	0.167	0.303
B4	0,024	0.056	0.029
B5	0.423	0.123	0.347
B6	0.024	0.056	0.029
B7	0.024	0.056	0.029
B8	0.024	0.056	0.029
B9	0.024	0.056	0.029
B10	0.024	0.056	0.029
B11	0.323	0.167	0.303
B12	0.024	0.056	0.029
B13	0.024	0.056	0.029
B14	0.024	0.056	0.029
B15	0.024	0.056	0.029
B16	0.024	0.056	0.029
B17	0.024	0.056	0.029
B18	0.024	0.056	0.029
B19	0.480	0.241	0.309
B20	0.024	0.056	0.029
B21	0.024	0.056	0.029
B22	0.024	0.056	0.029
B23	0.024	0.056	0.029
B24	0.480	0.241	0.309
B25	0.504	0.260	0.366
B26	0.024	0.056	0.029
B27	0.024	0.056	0.029
B28	0.024	0.056	0.020
B29	0.024	0.056	0.029
B30	0.024	0.056	0.029
B31	0.724	0.322	0.557
B32	0.024	0.056	0.020
B33	0.024	0.056	0.029
B34	0.024	0.056	0.029
B35	0.024	0.056	0.029
B36	0.024	0.056	0.029
B37	0.024	0.056	0.029

Tables 8.6 and 8.7 show the predictive assessments for KCS on a leave-one-out basis for the 77 cases of the training set kcs, together with the Kullback-Liebler measure of influence. The cases for which the predictive assessment favours the wrong diagnosis are A10, A21, A26, A39 and B31 and these are associated with influence measures in excess of 1. It is not difficult to identify peculiarities of these cases which may account for their influence. It is clear that overall KCS cases have more presences of symptoms than the non-KCS cases. Of all the KCS cases there are just four with number of features present at most 2 and these are A10, A21, A26 and A39 with 1, 1, 2, 0 presences, respectively. Among the non-KCS cases, B31 is the only case with feature 4 present, with $v_4 = 1$. Among the other KCS cases only A17 has an influence measure in excess of 1, possibly explained by having only two presences, and it is interesting that this is associated with a very uncertain diagnostic assessment. Of the other non-KCS cases, B1, B5, B19, B24, B25 are very uncertainly diagnosed and have influence measures in excess of 1. Of these cases B5 has by far the largest influence measure of 2.72 and this can probably be explained by the fact that B5 is the only non-KCS case with feature 8 present. There is no reason to suspect anything unusual in the original observation of these cases and so there is no justification for excluding them from the data set.

8.3.2 Weighted kernel diagnostic assessments

The weighted kernel method for assessing $p_S(u|v)$ follows similar lines to that of Section 8.2 for the differential diagnosis of Conn's syndrome. To compare with the logistic binary regression model above we consider only the binary features $(v_1, v_2, v_4, v_5, v_8)$. Again we use the binomial kernel

$$K(u_i|u_j) = \begin{cases} \lambda & (u_i = u_j), \\ 1 - \lambda & (u_i \neq u_j). \end{cases}$$

For the weighting factors we take

$$G(v, z) = 1 - \exp\{-d(v, z)/\mu\},$$

where

$$d(v, z) = \sum_{j=1}^{10} (v_j - z_j)^2$$

is simply the number of disagreements in the binary features of v and z. The pseudo-loglikelihood $l(\lambda, \mu)$ is easily computed for any given (λ, μ) and the maximizing values (λ, μ) are readily obtained by a search technique. For this data set we obtain $\lambda = 0.994$ and $\mu = 0.497$ with maximized logarithm of the pseudolikelihood equal to -19.85. With these values the kernel diagnostic assessments for the training set using the leave-one-out principle are shown in Tables 8.6 and 8.7. There is clearly broad agreement in the inferences which would be drawn from the predictive logistic and the kernel assessments.

Table 8.8 *Diagnostic probability assessments for KCS on predictive, weighted kernel and multivariate binary kernel bases for all symptom combinations*

Symptom combination					Predictive	Weighted kernel	Multivariate binary kernel
1	2	4	5	8			
0	0	0	0	0	0.023	0.055	0.028
0	0	0	0	1	0.312	0.102	0.200
0	0	0	1	0	0.388	0.210	0.229
0	0	0	1	1	0.803	0.308	0.776
0	0	1	0	0	0.560	0.276	0.371
0	0	1	0	1	0.880	0.628	0.902
0	0	1	1	0	0.935	0.636	0.896
0	0	1	1	1	0.980	0.805	0.993
0	1	0	0	0	0.262	0.144	0.224
0	1	0	0	1	0.728	0.612	0.883
0	1	0	1	0	0.803	0.429	0.834
0	1	0	1	1	0.952	0.708	0.989
0	1	1	0	0	0.892	0.779	0.942
0	1	1	0	1	0.978	0.901	0.996
0	1	1	1	0	0.984	0.894	0.996
0	1	1	1	1	0.995	0.970	1.000
1	0	0	0	0	0.412	0.227	0.268
1	0	0	0	1	0.818	0.450	0.856
1	0	0	1	0	0.897	0.666	0.900
1	0	0	1	1	0.965	0.901	0.995
1	0	1	0	0	0.944	0.640	0.921
1	0	1	0	1	0.981	0.886	0.996
1	0	1	1	0	0.991	0.933	0.997
1	0	1	1	1	0.995	0.983	1.000
1	1	0	0	0	0.831	0.736	0.930
1	1	0	0	1	0.962	0.946	0.997
1	1	0	1	0	0.974	0.955	0.997
1	1	0	1	1	0.991	0.790	1.000
1	1	1	0	0	0.988	0.976	0.999
1	1	1	0	1	0.996	0.990	1.000
1	1	1	1	0	0.997	0.990	1.000
1	1	1	1	1	0.998	0.993	1.000

Table 8.9 *Diagnostic probability assessments for KCS, for the test cases C1-C23, and for not-KCS, for the test cases D1-D17, based on the predictive and weighted kernel methods*

Case no	Predictive	Weighted kernel
C1	0.88	0.98
C2	0.95	0.98
C3	0.93	0.98
C4	0.93	0.98
C5	0.92	0.97
C6	0.95	0.94
C7	0.97	0.98
C8	0.84	0.96
C9	0.94	0.98
C10	0.92	0.98
C11	0.98	0.98
C12	0.97	0.98
C13	0.93	0.98
C14	0.98	0.87
C15	0.96	0.98
C16	0.92	0.94
C17	0.78	0.74
C18	0.94	0.84
C19	0.97	0.98
C20	0.86	0.94
C21	0.96	0.98
C22	0.98	0.97
C23	0.98	0.97
D1	0.67	0.95
D2	0.73	0.93
D3	0.43	0.78
D4	0.73	0.93
D5	0.83	0.93
D6	0.77	0.93
D7	0.96	0.91
D8	0.96	0.91
D9	0.77	0.93
D10	0.96	0.91
D11	0.96	0.91
D12	0.83	0.93
D13	0.96	0.91
D14	0.73	0.93
D15	0.96	0.91
D16	0.96	0.91
D17	0.77	0.93

8.3.3 Multivariate binary kernel diagnostic assessments

In Section 5.6 we have already carried out the multivariate binary kernel density estimation of $p_S(v|u)$ separately for the 40 KCS cases (u = 1) and the 37 non-KCS cases (u =2) and for the full 10-dimensional binary feature vector. In our analysis above we arrived at a working model confined to the features $(v_1, v_2, v_4, v_5, v_8)$ and so for comparison purposes we report briefly the results of applying this kernel method to the subset of binary features. The estimates of λ for the A group (KCS) and the B group (non-KCS) are $\lambda_A = 0.806$ and $\lambda_B = 0.972$ with the resulting maximized logarithms of the pseudo-likelihood equal to -127.65 and -37.65 respectively. The resulting diagnostic assessments in favour of KCS are shown in Tables 8.6 and 8.7. On the whole and making allowances for the unspecified selection ratio, assumed to be 1 in our presentation here, these assessments are broadly similar to those of the predictive logistic assessments, with the greatest discrepancies being with the influential cases identified above. These greater discrepancies are probably the result of the kernel method forcing some peaking on these apparently isolated cases.

8.3.4 Diagnostic assessments for new cases

For a working model involving five binary features it is possible to enumerate the resulting diagnostic assessments in tabular form and these are collected in Table 8.8. We emphasize that these assessments, intended for use on new cases, differ from those of Tables 8.6 and 8.7 in that they are based on the full data set kcs, whereas the previous assessments were based on the leave-one-out principle.

The data set newkcs is a set of test data, with 23 cases C1–C23 of known KCS type and 17 cases D1-D17 of known non-KCS type. Probability assessments based on the predictive and weighted kernel methods are given in Table 8.9.

Note that the extrapolation indices can again be evaluated here, and there is no evidence that in the application of the system there is any case of extrapolation.

8.4 Genetic counselling and haemophilia

The problem of the genetic counselling, briefly introduced in Section 1.10, of a referred woman R who may be a haemophilia carrier is how to marshall the information w from the woman's family tree and the result $v = (v_1, v_2)$ of her coagulation tests to provide some quantitative assessment of her unknown status u, carrier ($u = 1$) or non-carrier ($u = 2$). The objective is to obtain a realistic assessment of the conditional probabilities $p_R(u|v, w)$ as diagnostic assessments. Information about the pattern of variability of the coagulation measurements for a selected set of 43 women, C1–C20 selected because of their known carrier status and D1–D23 selected from normal, presumed non-carrier, women hospital workers. The patient has, of course, been referred for counselling on the basis of the family tree w with subsequent determination of her coagulation measurement v, whereas the 43 women in data set `haemo` providing past experience of coagulation variability have been selected on the basis of their known status u. In our detailed study of the relationship of referral to selection in this problem of genetic counselling in Chapter 2 we arrived at the following basis for assessing the relevant odds:

$$\frac{p_R(u|v,w)}{p_R(u^*|v,w)} = \frac{p_R(u|w)}{p_R(u^*|w)} \frac{p_S(v|u)}{p_S(v|u^*)},$$

where we use u, u^* to shorten the notation $u = 1, u = 2$.

We emphasize here that for the moment we are considering a situation where the only person in the family tree who has undergone the coagulation tests is the referred patient. There are then two stages to our task. First, the use of our genetic knowledge and the family tree w allows us to obtain diagnostic assessments $p_R(u|w), p_R(u^*|w)$ for the referred patient R, prior to the use of her coagulation test results. Secondly, we have to use the data set `haemo` to obtain assessments of the two conditional distributions of the bivariate measurement v for each of the statuses: carrier and non-carrier; in other words we require to assess $p_S(v|u, D)$ from the experience of C1–C20 and $p_S(v|u^*, D)$ from D1–D23.

8.4.1 Analysis of the family tree

Such trees clearly start with the nearest antecedent, who is a known carrier, traced back through the distaff side of the family: mother, maternal grandmother, mother of maternal grandmother, and so back. From such a starting point, the only branches of the family tree which provide information on the status of the referred patient are those leading to normal males. Moreover in the evaluation of conditional probabilities of normal sons only the assumed status of the mother of these sons need be retained in the conditioning. The probabilistic argument can be best illustrated by a simple example.

Illustrative example A referred woman R, actually new case N15 from data set `newhaem`, knows that her maternal grandmother G was a carrier. Her mother M has n_M normal sons, she herself has already n_R normal sons, and she has a sister S with n_S normal sons. We wish to calculate, on the basis of all this information, the probability that the referred patient R is a carrier.

We use $c_P(\bar{c}_P)$ to denote the event that person P is a carrier (non-carrier) and n_P to denote the event that person P has n_P normal sons. We can then easily evaluate the probabilities of joint events such as $(c_M, c_R, c_S, n_M, n_R, n_S)$

conditional on the knowledge that G is a known carrier. For example,

$$p(c_M, \bar{c}_R, c_S, n_M, n_R, n_S | c_G)$$

$$= p(c_M | c_G) p(n_M | c_G) p(\bar{c}_R | c_M) p(n_R | \bar{c}_R) p(c_S | c_M) p(n_S | c_S)$$

$$= \tfrac{1}{2} \cdot (\tfrac{1}{2})^{n_M} \cdot \tfrac{1}{2} \cdot 1 \cdot \tfrac{1}{2} \cdot (\tfrac{1}{2})^{n_S}$$

$$= (\tfrac{1}{2})^{n_M + n_S + 3}.$$

By similar arguments we arrive at the following complete set of joint probabilities:

$$p(c_M, c_R, c_S, n_M, n_R, n_S | c_G) \ = \ (\tfrac{1}{2})^{n_M + n_R + n_S + 3},$$

$$p(c_M, c_R, \bar{c}_S, n_M, n_R, n_S | c_G) \ = \ (\tfrac{1}{2})^{n_M + n_R + 3},$$

$$p(c_M, \bar{c}_R, c_S, n_M, n_R, n_S | c_G) \ = \ (\tfrac{1}{2})^{n_M + n_S + 3},$$

$$p(c_M, \bar{c}_R, \bar{c}_S, n_M, n_R, n_S | c_G) \ = \ (\tfrac{1}{2})^{n_M + 3},$$

$$p(\bar{c}_M, \bar{c}_R, \bar{c}_S, n_M, n_R, n_S | c_G) \ = \ (\tfrac{1}{2}),$$

with the other impossible joint events having probability 0. By simple conditional probability arguments we arrive at the relevant conditional probability $p(c_R | c_G, n_M, n_R, n_S)$ as

$$\frac{(\tfrac{1}{2})^{n_M + n_R + n_S + 3} + (\tfrac{1}{2})^{n_M + n_R + 3}}{(\tfrac{1}{2})^{n_M + n_R + n_S + 3} + (\tfrac{1}{2})^{n_M + n_R + 3} + (\tfrac{1}{2})^{n_M + n_S + 3} + (\tfrac{1}{2})^{n_M + 3} + \tfrac{1}{2}}.$$

For the referred woman of our original example we have

$$n_M = 2, \quad n_R = 1, \quad n_S = 3,$$

so that the relevant probability $p(u|w)$ of being a carrier is 0.032 and the complementary probability of being a non-carrier $\pi(u^*|w)$ is 0.968.

8.4.2 Analysis of the data set of coagulation measurement

The pattern of variability of the coagulation data of haemo has been studied in detail from parametric and non-parametric views in Section 5.3.2. In the parametric study we decided that the separate distributions of the bivariate coagulation measurements are adequately described by bivariate lognormal models for $p_S(v|u), p_S(v|u^*)$ leading to predictive assessments of logStudent form for the referred patient R, as in Section 5.3.2. The values of these density functions corresponding to the referred woman's coagulation measurements (95, 90) are 0.0362 and 1.349, with odds ratio 0.268 from Table 5.4. Hence the odds against of this referred patient being a carrier are estimated to be 113 to 1.

8.5 Cushing's syndrome

We consider the differential diagnosis of the two disease types adenoma (type 1) and bilateral hyperplasia (type 2). The observation available on each patient of known type, 7 of type 1 and 27 of type 2, is a 7-dimensional vector of urinary excretion rates (mg/24h) of seven steroid metabolites. Despite the fact that there is considerable univariate overlap in the ranges of the two types, as shown in Table 8.10, application of maximum likelihood estimation reveals that there is complete separation in the 7-dimensional space.

Table 8.10 *Ranges of steroid metabolite measurements (mg/24h) for two types of Cushing's syndrome*

Steroid metabolite	Type 1 Range	Type 2 Range
Tetrahydrocortisol	1.600–6.405	3.205–19.905
Allotetrahydrocortisol	0.005–0.405	0.005– 3.305
Tetrahydrocortisone	1.905–4.105	3.805–15.705
Reichstein's compound U	0.005–0.245	0.005– 0.165
Cortisol	0.195–0.425	0.155– 1.125
Cortisone	0.055–0.205	0.085– 0.605
Tetrahydro-11-desoxycortisol	0.325–4.405	0.025– 2.405

This complete separation persists if we use the logarithms of the data, a transformation that is suggested by the skewness of each of the measurements. Despite this complete separation the overlap of the ranges and the small sample size of 34 relative to the vector dimension 7 suggests that it would be unwise to claim the extreme diagnostic probabilities of 1 and 0 assigned by maximum likelihood. Application of the Bayesian method with the fair prior described in Section 4.3 and the logged data gives the estimated linear predictor as

$$4.09 - 0.602v_1 - 0.194v_2 - 1.89v_3 + 0.12v_4 + 0.44v_5 - 0.19v_6 + 0.55v_7,$$

where $v_1, \ldots, v_7$ denote the logarithms of the seven measurements. In the associated predictive diagnostic assessments of the original cases using the leave-one-out technique, all the type 2 cases are assigned probabilities in favour of type 2 in the range 0.77 to 0.996. The type 1 cases have diagnostic probabilities for type 1 of 0.81, 0.71, 0.85, 0.40, 0.91 and 0.90. The misclassified case has steroid metabolite measurements

$$6.405 \quad 0.325 \quad 3.805 \quad 0.165 \quad 0.425 \quad 0.205 \quad 0.325,$$

four of which are at the boundaries of the type 1 range or nearly so. Thus we see that the problem of complete separation, as far as assigning realistic diagnostic probabilities for future referred patients is concerned, has been overcome by taking a Bayesian approach and particularly by adopting the fair prior advocated in Section 4.3.

8.6 Bibliographic notes

Clinical diagnosis is a special form of the wider concept of taxonomy, and probably the first attempt at a statistical model for the problem of classification was the much quoted paper by Fisher (1936) on the distinction between different varieties of Iris. The application of the emerging linear discriminant approach was applied to the diagnosis of lung cancer by Hollingsworth (1959). The use of the predictive method for multivariate normal discrimination is considered by Geisser (1964) and Dunsmore (1966), and the predictive format also emerges in a likelihood ratio approach by Anderson (1984). The distinction between estimative and predictive methods was highlighted in Aitchison and Dunsmore (1975), Aitchison and Kay (1975) and Aitchison, Habbema and Kay (1977).

For further details of the Keratoconjunctivitis sicca data see Anderson et al. (1972) and for discussion of multivariate binary kernel modelling and its application see Aitchison and Aitken (1976). For other methods of kernel density estimation see Lauder (1983).

8.7 Problems

Problem 8.1 A baby is said to be dysmature if its weight at birth is below a certain level. In an attempt to diagnose during pregnancy whether or not a dysmature baby will be born the biparietal diameter (in cms) of the baby is measured by an ultrasonic technique. Extensive study has shown that at a certain time during pregnancy the distribution of biparietal diameter is normal with mean 5.7 cm and standard deviation 0.3 cm for dysmature babies and with mean 6.1 cm and standard deviation 0.4 cm for normal babies. A suggested diagnostic procedure classifies a baby as dysmature if the biparietal diameter is less than 5.85 and as normal otherwise. Evaluate the two probabilities of misclassification for such a procedure.

If it is thought necessary to ensure that only 1 in 100 dysmature babies should be wrongly classified what critical level of biparietal diameter should be used? Comment on this alternative procedure.

If it is known that 10 per cent of all babies are dysmature, what proportion of babies will be misclassified under the two procedures?

Problem 8.2 A thirty-four year old married woman, Mrs R, knows that her great-grandmother on the distaff side (her mother's mother's mother) was a carrier of haemophilia because Mrs R had a haemophiliac great uncle. Mrs R has a normal brother and her maternal aunt (her mother's sister) has two normal sons (cousins of Mrs R). Mrs R already has a daughter.

Mrs R has recently consulted a genetic counsellor and has undergone two coagulation index tests A and B which may help in assessing probabilities of whether or not Mrs R is a carrier. The counsellor has information on the ages and A and B coagulation indices of 20 known carriers and 20 apparently normal women. These are provided in the table below.

Table 8.11 *Data for Problem 8.2*

Carriers		Non-carriers	
A	B	A	B
309	355	131	490
199	383	151	594
199	476	295	314
236	493	136	364
249	421	171	431
270	393	164	327
325	402	315	450
294	408	206	447
126	438	124	285
299	537	120	337
307	455	323	398
295	539	337	303
343	349	316	316
273	335	111	249
202	552	185	380
239	460	186	421
77	485	222	279
283	422	160	283

Mrs R's coagulation scores were recorded as 203 for A and 406 for B.

(i) On the basis of all the above information how should the counsellor assess the probability that Mrs R is a carrier?

(ii) Mrs R is also seeking advice for her sixteen year old daughter who has A and B coagulation scores of 280 and 487. What genetic counselling advice would you provide for the daughter?

(iii) Mrs R now asks you if the information on her daughter in any way affects your genetic counselling assessment in (i). What answer would you provide?

Problem 8.3 A clinician is investigating the pattern of hormone levels in patients suffering from two mutually exclusive forms A and B of a hormone imbalance syndrome. The table below (Type 1: healthy, 2: form A, 3: form B) shows the levels (milli-equivalents per litre) of nine hormones H1-H9 in 11 healthy persons and in 9 forms of A and 5 forms of B syndrome patients. The hormones are known to be produced only by three endocrine glands, the adrenal, the pituitary and thyroid glands, according to the following scheme.

Adrenal:	H1-H6
Pituitary:	H7-H8
Thyroid:	H9, but also some of H6 and H8

You are asked by the clinician to help him in his attempts to describe the pattern of variability in these hormone levels. In particular he is interested in ways in which the pattern differs in the three categories, healthy, A and B, and whether any such differences may provide some indication of which glands are responsible for the different forms of the syndrome.

Case	H1	H2	H3	H4	H5	H6	H7	H8	H9	Type
1	48	12.6	8.6	21	4.3	2.5	53	1.6	26	1
2	74	8.3	8.2	19	6.8	5.4	50	2.7	24	1
3	58	9.7	7.4	27	5.7	11.8	41	0.9	14	1
4	52	4.4	5.4	37	6.1	6.9	49	1.3	8	1
5	76	9.0	9.4	28	7.4	2.6	45	2.0	17	1
6	52	12.2	7.2	25	5.0	3.0	42	2.3	22	1
7	51	4.2	5.4	25	5.5	11.6	43	2.0	16	1
8	54	7.0	7.0	27	4.4	9.0	37	1.8	12	1
9	72	9.0	6.2	26	3.3	2.7	48	3.1	29	1
10	95	5.1	9.4	22	5.6	5.1	46	4.4	20	1
11	62	11.2	8.2	20	6.2	4.0	35	1.9	23	1
12	55	1.2	1.0	9	0.7	0.2	80	7.1	10	2
13	42	5.4	3.2	9	1.3	1.4	107	4.8	25	2
14	53	10.2	5.6	13	6.0	2.4	65	1.4	24	2
15	46	10.4	7.4	12	7.8	6.4	46	1.0	21	2
16	29	11.1	5.8	10	4.8	0.3	76	7.0	25	2
17	37	9.1	5.4	21	7.0	3.6	68	2.6	40	2
18	34	5.6	3.0	12	3.7	1.2	94	6.8	17	2
19	51	4.1	4.2	18	7.6	3.6	82	4.4	17	2
20	24	4.5	2.4	10	3.6	0.7	106	7.4	19	2
21	99	8.9	6.6	21	5.7	6.8	53	3.1	39	3
22	56	2.7	5.6	19	2.6	7.0	79	10.1	39	3
23	49	4.5	5.8	15	2.5	4.0	69	5.5	40	3
24	34	3.3	2.2	5	7.0	17.0	51	6.1	48	3
25	39	3.0	6.2	9	6.8	8.4	55	7.6	43	3

Problem 8.4 A question has arisen as to whether it may be possible to determine the category A or B of an ear infection quickly from seven easily elicited symptoms, $s1$-$s7$, rather than delay for a laboratory assessment. Details of the symptoms, present (1) or absent (0), for 25 category A and 20 category B infected patients are given below.

Examine the possibility of differentiating between the two categories of infection with these symptoms, including the question of whether they are all necessary for reasonable differentiation.

How would you apply your findings to the five new cases C1–C5 with symptom combinations given in the tables below?

Category	s1	s2	s3	s4	s5	s6	s7
A	1	0	1	1	0	0	0
A	0	0	0	0	1	0	0
A	1	1	0	0	0	0	0
A	1	0	0	0	1	0	0
A	1	0	1	0	0	0	0
A	0	0	1	0	0	0	0
A	1	1	1	0	1	0	1
A	0	0	1	0	1	1	0
A	1	0	1	0	1	0	0
A	1	0	0	0	0	1	0
A	1	1	0	0	0	1	0
A	1	0	0	1	0	1	1
A	0	0	1	0	1	0	0
A	1	1	1	0	1	0	0
A	0	1	1	0	0	1	0
A	1	0	0	1	1	0	1
A	1	0	0	0	0	1	1
A	1	0	0	1	1	1	1
A	0	0	1	0	0	0	0
A	1	0	1	0	0	0	1
A	0	0	0	1	0	0	1
A	0	1	1	1	0	0	0
A	1	0	0	0	1	0	1
A	1	1	1	0	1	0	0
A	1	0	0	0	1	0	1

Category	$s1$	$s2$	$s3$	$s4$	$s5$	$s6$	$s7$
B	1	0	1	0	0	1	1
B	0	0	1	0	0	1	1
B	0	1	1	1	0	1	1
B	1	1	1	1	1	1	1
B	1	1	1	0	0	1	0
B	0	1	1	0	0	0	0
B	0	0	0	0	0	1	0
B	0	1	0	0	0	0	1
B	0	1	1	1	0	0	1
B	0	1	1	0	0	1	1
B	1	1	0	0	0	1	0
B	1	1	0	0	1	0	1
B	0	1	1	0	1	1	1
B	0	1	0	1	0	1	1
B	1	0	1	1	0	1	1
B	0	1	1	0	0	1	1
B	0	1	0	0	0	1	1
B	0	0	1	0	0	1	1
B	1	0	0	0	0	1	0
B	0	0	0	1	0	0	1

Category	$s1$	$s2$	$s3$	$s4$	$s5$	$s6$	$s7$
C1	0	1	1	1	0	1	1
C2	1	0	1	0	0	0	0
C3	1	1	1	0	1	1	1
C4	0	0	1	0	0	1	1
C5	1	0	1	1	1	0	0

Problem 8.5 Clinicians are having difficulty in distinguishing between two forms X and Y of a rare blood disease. Certain cells in the blood can be classified as being one of three different types A, B, C and the clinicians hope that this information may help with this form of differential diagnosis. These proportions have been determined for forty patients, 20 of each form, as they have come into the clinic, and are set out below.

	Form X			Form Y	
A	B	C	A	B	C
0.51	0.27	0.22	0.29	0.29	0.42
0.43	0.27	0.30	0.30	0.28	0.42
0.44	0.30	0.26	0.18	0.26	0.56
0.47	0.34	0.19	0.25	0.49	0.26
0.42	0.48	0.10	0.20	0.54	0.26
0.33	0.49	0.18	0.31	0.46	0.23
0.53	0.38	0.09	0.23	0.27	0.50
0.51	0.18	0.31	0.24	0.37	0.39
0.51	0.34	0.15	0.24	0.25	0.51
0.43	0.22	0.35	0.34	0.29	0.37
0.49	0.20	0.31	0.39	0.27	0.34
0.42	0.36	0.22	0.36	0.21	0.43
0.48	0.35	0.17	0.42	0.43	0.15
0.62	0.29	0.09	0.21	0.41	0.38
0.53	0.27	0.20	0.27	0.39	0.34
0.52	0.22	0.26	0.13	0.23	0.64
0.64	0.16	0.20	0.22	0.32	0.46
0.47	0.16	0.37	0.15	0.19	0.66
0.56	0.20	0.24	0.17	0.54	0.29
0.56	0.27	0.17	0.17	0.25	0.58

You have been asked to investigate the diagnostic potential of such data.

If you develop a diagnostic system based on these data how would you report on the following new cases?

Case no	A	B	C
1	0.40	0.26	0.34
2	0.50	0.26	0.24
3	0.17	0.14	0.69
4	0.34	0.24	0.42
5	0.27	0.21	0.52

Problem 8.6 A new syndrome with forms A and B has been discovered. A clinic wishes to avoid the existing long, costly and disturbing process of differential diagnosis and is investigating the possibility of the use of five simple diagnostic tests (a, b, c, d, e) as an alternative to the existing diagnostic procedure. For the 31 patients, 17 with form A and 14 with form B, recently referred to the clinic, the five tests have been carried out and the results in standard units are recorded below.

Form A	a	b	c	d	e
	15	27	192	805	33
	64	17	159	1185	20
	77	26	640	1027	51
	56	11	385	415	21
	64	42	202	951	17
	27	13	207	627	40
	35	19	244	500	20
	43	26	359	779	61
	94	31	841	775	26
	50	27	262	383	21
	207	77	274	146	21
	81	79	272	428	19
	21	47	316	811	42
	54	30	400	539	9
	48	17	519	1529	24
	79	20	213	452	19
	64	11	186	1082	60

Form B	a	b	c	d	e
	55	8	127	234	29
	41	18	39	375	15
	34	9	130	93	51
	6	37	44	141	117
	37	25	105	316	35
	20	14	36	262	59
	31	13	172	283	27
	29	11	232	481	21
	17	37	281	240	39
	54	15	244	103	22
	43	16	60	351	28
	29	8	152	197	22
	67	21	166	98	16
	106	97	35	622	14

You have been asked to investigate fully the possibility of the use of these tests for differential diagnostic purposes and have been asked to report to the clinic in terms the doctors will understand.

Problem 8.7 It is suspected that help in the differential diagnosis of three forms I, II, III of a malignancy may be provided by determination of a three-part composition (a, b, c) of tissue from a biopsy. In the study so far conducted of 36 patients referred to a clinic the percentages of these parts have been determined for patients with known form: 10 of form I, 12 of form II and 14 of form III, as recorded below.

Form I Percentages			Form II Percentages			Form III Percentages		
a	b	c	a	b	c	a	b	c
38	41	21	38	55	8	26	44	30
47	39	14	51	42	7	28	27	45
27	50	23	56	35	9	36	23	40
53	25	23	37	45	18	35	32	33
46	21	33	47	43	9	22	14	64
23	34	42	36	52	12	38	27	35
55	26	19	29	58	13	23	23	54
45	27	29	24	70	6	24	21	54
55	33	12	40	50	10	25	18	57
45	34	21	38	50	13	30	17	53
			45	46	8	18	19	62
			51	40	9	34	33	33
						25	21	53
						44	17	39

You have been asked to study this data set and to offer recommendations as to its value. It would be helpful if your report could include diagrammatic evidence to support your conclusions.

Problem 8.8 A special feature of the diagnostic situation in Problem 1.3 is that the feature vector consists of a mixture of binary and compositional data. You are challenged to investigate the differential diagnostic problem and to provide a full report for the clinic.

Problem 8.9 Review and prepare a report on Problem 1.6.

CHAPTER 9

Special Aspects of Diagnosis

9.1 Introduction

In Chapter 8 we developed the basic techniques required for statistical diagnosis in the simple standard situation where there is: a single clinic; complete, precise though possibly mixed feature vector v; disease type ascertained with certainty and a well-defined relationship between selection of past cases and referral of a new patient. In this chapter we consider realistic non-standard situations in diagnosis which can be regarded as extensions or deviations from the above. We consider the following situations.

Diagnostic system transfer: a calibration problem. Under what circumstances is it valid to use a diagnostic data set from one clinic to assess new undiagnosed cases in another?

Clinic amalgamation: a calibration problem. If diagnostic data are available from more than one clinic on a given set of diseases, how can they be combined to produce a more efficient diagnostic system, taking into account the interplay of referral and selection? In relation to this and the preceding question, how can we cope with features which are either measured in one clinic but not in the other, or features which are not identical but related, for example through calibration by an assay technique?

Imprecision in the feature vector. For a single clinic how do we deal with imprecise features in v?

Missing features. For a situation with a single clinic how do we deal with missing values in some feature vectors?

Uncertainty in ascertainment of type. How do we arrive at diagnostic techniques in a clinic where the typings are uncertain and all the diagnostic information we have about the type u of a case is a composite diagnosis giving $\mathrm{pr}(u = j)\ (j = 1, \ldots, k)$?

We shall attempt to answer these questions systematically against the background of specific cases. The emphasis will be based on direct modelling of $p(u|v)$ mainly by parametric methods as this will be seen to be the most relevant technique. Where appropriate, non-parametric techniques will be cited and also indirect modelling via $p(v|u)$. In other words, the emphasis will be on what are robust methods of most use in specific practical situations rather than an academic catalogue of all possible methodologies.

9.2 Diagnostic system transfer

The system transfer problem arose from two particular and related problems in diagnosis. For differentiating between two types of Conn's syndrome a statistical diagnostic system had been developed for a particular Clinic A (see Section 8.2). After use of the system for some years the clinic has changed its method of measurement of one of the features, plasma concentration of the hormone aldosterone, from a double isotope assay to a less expensive, more efficient radioimmunoassay. Any new case of Conn's syndrome will therefore have this hormone measured by the new method only. Since the patients forming the diagnostic training set have been discharged or are undergoing treatment which affects the hormone concentration it is impossible to find the radioimmunoassay counterparts of their original double isotope assay measurements in order to construct a new diagnostic system directly from these patients. Fortunately, however, although the concentration of hormone depends on the type of syndrome the conditional distributions relating one hormone determination to the other are known not to depend on type or indeed on whether the patient has the particular syndrome. We can therefore investigate the possibilities of calibrating from the new to the old by measuring hormone concentration by both methods on portions of blood from a number of people not in the training set and not suffering from the disease; see Section 7.2. Such pairs of observations are available on 72 blood samples. It is tempting to suppose that all that is then necessary is to plot a scatter diagram, fit some form of regression line and, for a given radioimmunoassay measurement, to read off from the regression line the corresponding 'calibrated' value of double isotope determination, and finally to use this directly in the original statistical diagnostic system devised for clinic A. Unfortunately such a method, though simple, takes no account of the unreliability of the calibrated value. It is our purpose in this section to analyse the extent to which this naive calibration method may differ from the full approach which takes full account of this unreliability.

Another problem arose when requests were received from another clinic B to process data from its patients through the statistical diagnostic system devised for clinic A. Uncritical application of the system to data from clinic B on its patients can give rise to serious failures with a subsequent loss of confidence in the system in both clinics. The reason for such failures is almost invariably that the clinics use different methods of determining some or all of the features on which the statistical diagnosis is based. Again the circumstances and the methods in the particular example were such that calibration information could be obtained from blood samples on other patients. Thus statistically these system transfer problems are identical, clinic B being interpreted as different from clinic A and with different methods of measurement, or as clinic A after it has changed to its new methods of measurement.

We suppose for simplicity that the methods of measurement of all features differ from clinic A to clinic B. The data available for this system transfer problem arise from three sources. First, diagnostic data

$$D_A = \{(u_i, v_i) : i = 1, \ldots, n\}$$

from clinic A consisting of known types u_i and known feature vectors v_i of n of its patients forming the diagnostic training set. Secondly, calibration data

$$C_{AB} = \{(y_{Aj}, y_{Bj}) : j = 1, \ldots, k\}$$

consisting of determinations of feature vectors made by both clinics on k individuals, y_{Aj} referring to measurement by clinic A and y_{Bj} the corresponding measurement by clinic B. Thirdly, for a new case of unknown type u, we have observed the feature vector v_B by the methods of clinic B. The problem then is to model the situation so as to obtain a realistic assessment of the conditional probabilities $p(u|v_B, D_A, C_{AB})$, the plausibilities to be attached to the possible disease types for this new case on the basis of the diagnostic and calibration data and the patient's own feature vector.

Our first step in the modelling is to postulate a sensible probabilistic mechanism for the generation of a complete record (u, v_A, v_B) for an individual case, where u is the type of the case and v_A and v_B are the feature vectors of this case as measured in clinics A and B, respectively. Postulating such a model does not imply either that the complete records must be available in the data set or that we contemplate the determination of complete records for new cases. This basic model provides a conceptual link between the patient's type and the two clinics' methods of measurement. It simply consists of formulating the joint distribution of (u, v_A, v_B) in terms of conditional distributions together with assumptions concerning separability of parameters and independence of data sets. To provide an operational model we must pay attention to a number of interrelated factors.

(i) The model should allow an expression of our understanding of the type-feature relationship in clinic A.

(ii) It should allow an adequate description of the nature of the calibration experiment.

(iii) It must allow a derivation of a likelihood function for the observed data C_{AB}, D_A and v_B.

(iv) It must allow the fulfilment of the purpose of the investigation, in our case, the assessment of the probabilities $p(u|v_B, C_{AB}, D_B)$.

We now consider six assumptions of a model for the system transfer problem, discuss their relevance and then deduce from the assumptions the appropriate method of calibrated diagnostic assessment.

Assumption 1. Any case has associated with it a unique type belonging to a set U of possible types, and possesses a feature vector belonging to a set V_A or V_B of possible feature vectors depending on whether the features are observed in clinic A or clinic B. *Assumption* 2. The model is parametric with parameter set Ω, so that the model corresponding to $\omega \in \Omega$ is specified by the density function

$$p(u, v_A, v_B|\omega) \quad (u \in U, v_A \in V_A, v_B \in V_B).$$

Assumption 3. In the conditional specification

$$p(u|\omega)p(v_A|u,\omega)p(v_B|u,v_A,\omega)$$

of $p(u,v_A,v_B|\omega)$ the parameter ω and the parameter set Ω can be factored
into $\omega = (\psi,\theta,\delta)$ and $\Omega = \Psi \times \Theta \times \Delta$ in such a way that they are separable:

$$p(u,v_A,v_B|\omega) = p(u|\psi)p(v_A|u,\theta)p(v_B|u,v_A,\delta).$$

Assumption 4. We have $p(v_B|u,v_A,\delta) = p(v_B|v_A,\delta)$. *Assumption* 5. Given
ψ,θ,δ and the type u of the new case from clinic B the data sets C_{AB}, D_A
and v_B are independent. *Assumption* 6. There is prior independence in that
$p(\psi,\theta,\delta) = p(\psi)p(\theta)p(\delta)$.

In the clinical setting our first assumption is standard in statistical diagnosis, asserting that the disease types have been defined so as to be mutually
exclusive and exhaustive, and that symptoms, signs and the results of diagnostic tests constituting a feature vector can be obtained for each patient. Our
second assumption merely acknowledges that we are adopting a parametric
model.

In the third assumption the separation of ψ and θ follows the usual assumption adopted in diagnostic models which recognise ψ as an incidence
parameter and θ as a structural parameter, in the sense that it reflects the
possible dependence of the feature variability on the disease type. The separation of δ from θ and ψ is also often reasonable. Its only implication is that
if we know u and v_A then the distribution of v_B can be indexed by a separate
parameter. For example, in the case where $p(v_A,v_B|u,\omega)$ is multivariate nor-
mal, this can always be achieved by θ referring to the marginal mean vectors
and covariance matrices and δ to the familiar and separable parameters of the
regression distributions of v_B on v_A.

The fourth assumption is one which will require careful scrutiny in any
particular application. It asserts that the calibration relationship does not
depend on type. In the case of Conn's syndrome, although a patient's plasma
concentration of a substance such as aldosterone certainly depends on type,
the relationship of radioimmunoassay determination to double isotope assay
determination is one which holds irrespective of type or indeed irrespective of
whether the blood sample comes from a patient with Conn's syndrome. All
that was necessary therefore was to select a range of blood samples to meet the
obvious calibration requirements that they cover the set of future values likely
to arise, and to make determinations by both methods on portions of these
samples. If this assumption does not hold then we may be in great difficulty.
For example, if v_A were the concentration, measured in mg/dl, of a hormone
in urine and v_B were the urinary excretion rate, measured in mg/day, and
if patients with type 1 had a tendency to retain body fluid compared with
patients of type 2, then the relationship of v_B to v_A would clearly depend
on type. To assess the density functions $p(v_B|v_A,u,\delta)$ we would require to be
able to observe the features in both clinics for patients of each possible type,
and this may be physically impossible. It is then only realistic to admit that

no reliable system transfer can be achieved and that the only course open is to start building up a new diagnostic training set within clinic B.

Since the three data sets, C_{AB}, D_A and the feature vector v_B of the new case from clinic B, are associated with completely different sets of individuals in our practical situations the fifth assumption automatically applies.

Our final assumption is common in such Bayesian formulations and asserts that any prior information concerning ψ, θ and δ arises from independent sources. The vague priors that we adopt in practice to ensure no overstatement of odds satisfy this assumption. Its great merit is that of mathematical tractability by ensuring, with Assumptions 3 and 5, that the posterior distribution for these parameters separates in exactly the same way as the prior.

The consequences of these assumptions can easily be worked through and we give a brief outline of the main steps. First, note that we can effectively ignore the parameter ψ in the argument due to the separability assumptions and the fact that its role is to perform incidence rate adjustment. Then the essential step in forming the likelihood $L(u, \theta, \delta | v_B, D_A, C_{AB})$ is to note that

$$
\begin{aligned}
p(v_B | u, \theta, \delta) &= \int_{V_A} p(v_B | v_A, u, \theta, \delta) p(v_A | u, \theta, \delta) dv_A \\
&= \int_{V_A} p(v_B | v_A, \delta) p(v_A | u, \theta) dv_A
\end{aligned}
\tag{9.1}
$$

by Assumptions 3 and 4. The likelihood can thus, by Assumption 5, be expressed in the form

$$
p(v_B | u, \theta, \delta) p(D_A | \theta) p(C_{AB} | \delta).
$$

Assumption 6 about the factorisation of the prior distribution then ensures that the posterior distribution can be expressed in the form

$$
p(u, \theta, \delta | v_B, D_A, C_{AB}) \propto p(v_B | u, \theta, \delta) p(\theta | D_A) p(\delta | C_{AB}),
$$

invoking the equal incidence assumption. Integration with respect to θ and δ then gives

$$
\begin{aligned}
p(u | v_B, D_A, C_{AB}| &\propto \int_{\Theta} \int_{\Delta} p(v_B | u, \theta, \delta) p(\theta | D_A) p(\delta | C_{AB}) d\theta d\delta \\
&\propto \int_{V_A} p(v_B | v_A, C_{AB}) p(v_A | u, D_A) dv_A
\end{aligned}
\tag{9.2}
$$

by (9.1), where

$$
p(v_B | v_A, C_{AB}) = \int_{\Delta} p(v_B | v_A, \delta) p(\delta | C_{AB}) d\delta,
\tag{9.3}
$$

$$
p(v_A | u, D_A) = \int_{\Theta} p(v_A | u, \theta) p(\theta | D_A) d\theta,
\tag{9.4}
$$

are the predictive calibrative and diagnostic distributions.

The mathematical problem involved in calibrated diagnosis is thus the evaluation of the convolution-type integral in (9.1), and this is seldom standard since the calibrative distribution $p(v_B|v_A, C_{AB})$ may involve v_A in a complicated way.

We now describe the implementation of the modelling on the basis of normality assumptions and then consider an application to Conn's syndrome. Suppose that $p(v_A|u, \theta)$ is $N^1(\mu_u, \sigma^2)$ and $p(v_B|v_A, \delta)$ is $N^1(\alpha + \beta v_A, \gamma^2)$, and that we adopt vague priors for the parameters. Then we have the predictive calibrative density function

$$p(v_B|v_A, C_{AB}) = St^1 \left[k - 2, a + bv_A, c^2 \{ 1 + 1/k + (v_A - \bar{y}_A)^2/S_A \} \right],$$

where a, b are the usual regression estimates, c^2 is the residual mean squared error, $\bar{y}_A$ and S_A are the mean and corrected sum of squares of the y_{Aj} and, as a basis of predictive diagnosis,

$$p(x_A|u, D_A) = St^1 \left[n - 1, m_u, s^2(1 + n_u^{-1}) \right],$$

where n_u is the number of x_{Ai} of type u, m_u their mean and s^2 the usual pooled sample variance. In contrast the effect of applying naive calibration and estimative diagnosis is to replace $p(v_B|u, D_A, C_{AB})$ by a normal distribution $N^1(a + bm_u, b^2 s^2)$.

The integral in (9.1) cannot be evaluated directly in terms of known functions but we can obtain a useful approximation for comparison purposes by first determining the mean and variance associated with this integral by the usual iterated expectation method and then using a normal approximation with this mean and variance. This results in a normal distribution with the same mean $a + bm_u$ as the naive-calibration estimative-diagnostic method but the variance is

$$f_n(1 + n_u^{-1})b^2 s^2 + f_k c^2 \left\{ 1 + k^{-1} + \frac{(m_u - v_A)^2 + s^2 f_n(1 + n_u^{-1})}{S_A} \right\}, \quad (9.5)$$

where $f_r = (r - 2)/(r - 4)$, instead of the $b^2 s^2$ of the naive-calibration estimative-diagnostic method, and the differences between these terms could well translate into appreciable differences between the methods in practice.

We have considered the situation where all of the features are measured differently between clinics A and B but often there will be a number of features, such as age, for which we may safely assume that observation or measurement will lead to the same value in both clinics. We can thus partition v_A into two subvectors $(v_A^{(1)}, v_A^{(2)})$, where only $v_A^{(2)}$ requires calibration. Then C_{AB} need contain calibrative information only on the subvectors $y_{Aj}^{(2)}, y_{Bj}^{(2)}$ while D_A still contains information on the whole vector v_{Ai}. Then if v_B is the complete feature vector of a new patient observed in clinic B we have as the basis of our diagnostic assessment the counterpart of (9.1) that $p(u|v_B, C_{AB}, D_A)$ is proportional to

$$p(v_A^{(1)} = v_B^{(1)}|u, D_A) \int_{V_A^{(2)}} p(v_B^{(2)}|v_A^{(2)}, C_{AB}) p(v_A^{(2)}|u, v_A^{(1)} = v_B^{(1)}, D_A) dv_A^{(2)}.$$

$$(9.6)$$

We can now illustrate with reference to Conn's syndrome the consequences of neglecting the full statistical problem of calibrating for diagnosis. Clinic B is clinic A after it has switched from double isotope assay determination $v_A^{(2)}$ to radioimmunoassay determination $v_B^{(2)}$ of plasma concentration of aldosterone, the techniques of determining the other seven features $v_A^{(1)}$ remaining the same, so that $v_B^{(1)} = v_A^{(1)}$. For multivariate normality considerations we work throughout in terms of transformed data and use the natural logarithms of the feature observations. The calibrative experiment with a random selection of 72 blood plasma samples provides the set C_{AB} of data from which we determine $p(v_B^{(2)}|v_A^{(2)}, C_{AB})$ using predictive methods as

$$St^1 \left\{ 70, 0.647 + 0.749 v_A^{(2)}, 0.187 + 0.00194(v_A^{(2)} - 2.70)^2 \right\}.$$

The other factor in the integrand of (9.4) can be easily obtained for a particular case. Using a new undiagnosed case for which

$$p(v_A^{(2)}|u = 1, v_A^{(1)}, D_A) = St^1(19, 3.42, 0.483), \tag{9.7}$$

$$p(v_A^{(2)}|u = 2, v_A^{(1)}, D_A) = St^1(10, 2.74, 0.0583). \tag{9.8}$$

We compare the naive and predictive calibration methods within the framework of predictive diagnosis. For both methods the first factor of (9.6) takes the same seven-dimensional Student form, so that the difference in the methods lies in the treatment of the second factor. The naive calibration method replaces the second factor of (9.8) by

$$p(v_A^{(2)} = \hat{v}_A^{(2)}|v_A^{(1)}, u, D_A),$$

where $\hat{v}_A^{(2)} = (v_B^{(2)} - 0.647)/0.749$ is the naive calibrate corresponding to $v_B^{(2)}$.

For the particular case under discussion this naive method leads to odds of 310 to 1 in favour of adenoma. The predictive calibration method requires the numerical evaluation of the integral associated with the second factor in (9.6) and this may be easily achieved by numerical integration and this leads to odds of 2 to 1 on adenoma. The difference between these two sets of odds would lead to quite different treatments for the patient. This case has been used simply as a convenient and dramatic means of illustrating the contrast in the naive and predictive calibration methods of resolving the system transfer problem in diagnosis. For it the assay method was in fact identical to that used in the training set so that the above analysis is only a pointer to what might happen. In the analysis of 43 new cases in data set newconn, where the assay methods differed from that of the training set, the odds assigned by the naive and predictive calibrative methods are shown in Figure 9.1. We note here that the 'variance parameters' of the conditional feature distributions in (9.7) and (9.8) associated with the published case are substantially different. The same is true for the conditional feature distributions of these 43 new cases. There are obviously appreciable departures from the line of equal odds assessments. Where both naive and predictive odds both exceed, or are both below, unity by a substantial factor such differences would have little effect

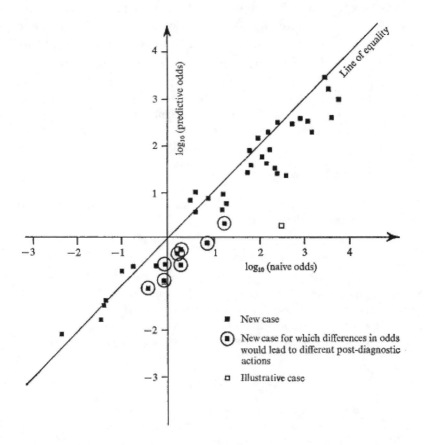

Figure 9.1 *Comparison for 43 new cases of Conn's syndrome of the predictive diagnostic odds as determined by naive and by predictive calibration. (Taken from Aitchison, J. Biometrika, **64**, 470, 1977, [Oxford University Press] with permission.)*

on the treatment of the case. Although there is no case displaying as extreme a difference as the illustrative case, there do remain eight cases, identified by open circles in Figure 9.1, where the naive and predictive calibrative methods are sufficiently different to lead to important differences in the assessment of the next step in the clinical management.

9.3 Clinic amalgamation

Suppose that two or more clinics wish to pool their diagnostic data in order to construct a more reliable diagnostic system than any one clinic could produce by itself. Indeed when the differential diagnosis of a set of rare diseases is involved it may be impossible for any one clinic to obtain enough cases to make construction of a diagnostic system a feasible proposition. When methods of measurement of diagnostic features differ from clinic to clinic or have changed over time within a clinic we then have a calibrative problem of diagnosis which we can conveniently term the *clinic amalgamation problem*. The nature of the clinic amalgamation problem can be clearly seen from its very simplest form involving only two clinics, labelled 1 and 2, and faced with the problem of differential diagnosis between just two mutually exclusive disease types, say types 1 and 2. We suppose that we have two independent training sets D_1 and D_2 in the two clinics, with

$$D_i = \{(u_{ij}, v_{ij}) : j = 1, 2, \ldots, n_i\},$$

where u_{ij} denotes the disease type and v_{ij} the feature vector of the jth case in the ith clinic. Moreover we have available also a calibrative set of data C_{12}, assumed independent of D_1 and D_2, with

$$C_{12} = \{(y_{1j}, y_{2j}) : j = 1, \ldots, n\},$$

where y_{1j} and y_{2j} are associated measurements on the jth calibrative case by the methods of measurement in clinics 1 and 2 respectively. In what follows we adopt the diagnostic paradigm, in which emphasis is laid on the assumed stability of the conditional distribution of type for given feature vector, rather than the sampling paradigm adopted in Section 9.2, where emphasis is laid on the assumed stability of the conditional distribution of feature vector for given type. Since, as we shall see later, the clinic amalgamation model contains the system transfer model as a special case we will obtain a diagnostic paradigm version of the system transfer model as an alternative to the sampling paradigm version of system transfer.

Our objective is, in general, to provide each clinic with a diagnostic system for use with its own method of measurement. Since modelling of the links between the two clinics depends on the nature of the calibration experiment we take this aspect as our starting point. If the calibration is a natural one, in the sense that the measurements used occur naturally in bivariate form, we have sufficient information to adopt a symmetrical approach, postulating conditional parametric models $p(v_1|v_2, \gamma_1)$ and $p(v_2|v_1, \gamma_1)$ for calibrating from v_1 to v_2 and from v_2 to v_1 respectively, where $\gamma_1 \in \Gamma_1$ and $\gamma_2 \in \Gamma_2$ are the indexing parameters for the two classes of calibrative models. Because of this symmetry we need only show the construction of a diagnostic system for clinic 1. Clinic 1 wishes to relate disease type u to its own feature measurements v_1 through a diagnostic paradigm $p(u|v_1, \delta_1)$, where $\delta_1 \in \Delta_1$ is the indexing parameter of the class of diagnostic models. To use the diagnostic data D_2 from clinic 2 for the construction of the diagnostic system for clinic 1 we require to obtain from the calibrative and diagnostic models for clinic 1, namely $p(v_1|v_2, \gamma_1)$ and $p(u|v_1, \gamma_1)$, an induced model

$$p(u|v_2, \gamma_1, \delta_1) = \int_{V_1} p(u|v_1, \delta_1) p(v_1|v_2, \gamma_1) dv_1 \tag{9.9}$$

for the explanation of the variability of the data D_2 in terms of the clinic 1 parameters γ_1 and δ_1.

We can then focus our attention on the likelihood function for γ_1 and δ_1 for given calibrative and diagnostic data C_{12}, D_1, D_2 which is

$$\prod_{j=1}^{n_1} p(u_{1j}|v_{1j}, \delta_1) \prod_{j=1}^{n_2} p(u_{2j}|v_{2j}, \gamma_1, \delta_1) \prod_{j=1}^{n} p(y_{1j}|y_{2j}, \gamma_1)$$
$$= L_1(\delta_1) L_2(\gamma_1, \delta_1) L_3(\gamma_1) \qquad (9.10)$$

in an abbreviated notation which emphasises the extent of the dependence of the three factors on the parameter components γ_1 and δ_1.

We may then make an assessment of the diagnostic probabilities within clinic 1 by first obtaining from the likelihood and with, if necessary, vague priors on γ_1 and δ_1 the posterior distribution $p(\gamma_1, \delta_1|C_{12}, D_1, D_2)$ for γ_1 and δ_1. Then, for a new case of unknown type but with known feature vector v_1 measured in clinic 1, we compute the diagnostic assessment

$$p(u|v_1, C_{12}, D_1, D_2) = \int_{\Delta_1} p(u|v_1, \delta_1) p(\delta_1|C_{12}D_1, D_2) d\delta_1, \qquad (9.11)$$

where the marginal density function $p(\delta_1|C_{12}, D_1, D_2)$ is obtained by integrating out γ_1 in the full posterior distribution. The provision of an appropriate system for clinic 2 follows exactly the same procedure with v_1 and v_2 interchanged and γ_2 and δ_2 replacing γ_1 and δ_1.

We now consider the implications of adopting particular parametric forms for the calibration and diagnostic components of our model. For the diagnostic paradigm for clinic 1 we adopt the normal distribution function form with argument a linear form of the feature vector:

$$\mathrm{pr}(u = 1|v_1, \delta) = 1 - \mathrm{pr}(u = 2|v_1, \delta) = \Phi(v_1 \delta^T), \qquad (9.12)$$

where Φ is the standard univariate normal distribution function and allowing the first component of v_1 to be 1 for the usual purpose of simplified notation and yet recognising the necessity of a constant term in the linear form $v_1 \delta^T$. Note that for simplicity we have now dropped the suffix notation in the parameters γ and δ. For the calibrative paradigm we adopt the normal linear regression model

$$p(v_1|v_2, \gamma) = \phi(v_1|v_2 A, B). \qquad (9.13)$$

With these particular normal linear forms (9.12) and (9.13) the awkwardness of modelling, namely the multiple integration of Equation 9.9 involved in formulating the induced diagnostic paradigm for clinic 2, is easily resolved by reduction to a one-dimensional integral through the transformation $x = v_1 \delta^T$, giving

$$\mathrm{pr}(u = 1|v_2, \gamma, \delta) = \int_{-\infty}^{\infty} \Phi(x)\phi(x|v_2 A\delta^T, \delta B\delta^T)dx = \Phi(v_2 \epsilon^T), \qquad (9.14)$$

where $\epsilon = A\delta^T / \sqrt{(1 + \delta B\delta^T)}$. Thus the induced diagnostic paradigm for clinic 2 is also of the normal linear form in (9.12) with parameter ϵ instead of δ.

The simple forms of the (9.12)–(9.14) provide an easily computable likelihood function from which, by the Newton-Raphson iterative technique expressible in a modified probit analysis form, we can arrive at maximum likelihood estimates (c, d) for (γ, δ) and also at the information matrix inverse J. The details are omitted here. By the standard Bayesian counterpart of maximum likelihood large sample theory we adopt the approximate posterior normal forms

$$p(\gamma, \delta | C_{12}, D_!, D_2) = \phi^2(\gamma, \delta | c, d; J)$$

and

$$p(\delta | C_{12}, D_1, D_2) = \phi^1(\delta | d, G),$$

where G is the appropriate submatrix of J.

For a new case of unknown type but with known feature vector v_1 measured in clinic 1 we have, by (9.11), the diagnostic assessment

$$\begin{aligned}
\mathrm{pr}(u = 1 | v_1, C_{12}, D_1, D_2) &= \int_\Delta \Phi(v_1 \delta^T) \phi(\delta | d, G) d\delta \\
&= \Phi\{v_1 \delta^T / \sqrt{(1 + v_1 G v_1^T)}\}. \quad (9.15)
\end{aligned}$$

In Section 9.2 we considered a system transfer approach to dealing with the problem which arose in the context of Conn's syndrome due to the change in the method used to measure the concentration of the hormone aldosterone. Since the new method of measurement is now used on all new cases the designation of 'clinics' using the new and old methods of measurement as clinic 1 and 2, respectively, means that we need only aim for diagnostic assessments of the form in (9.14) for new cases in clinic 1. The original training set D_2 (conn) in clinic 2 consists of 20 cases of type 1 and 11 cases of type 2 with an eight-dimensional feature vector, and clinic 1 has now, on the basis of cases diagnosed by the system transfer method and with type subsequently confirmed histpathologically, another training set D_1 (newconn) consisting of 17 cases of type 1 and 4 cases of type 2. In the analysis considered here we use only the three most discriminating of the eight features, namely the plasma concentrations of potassium, renin and aldosterone, the last of which is the feature involved in the calibration aspect of the problem. The calibration data C_{12} relevant here is that described in Section 9.2. We rewrite (9.12) using the superscript 1 to denote that part of the feature vector not requiring calibration and superscript 2 for that part requiring calibration as

$$\mathrm{pr}(u = 1 | v_1, \delta) = \Phi(\delta_0 + v_1^{(1)} \delta_1^T + v_1^{(2)} \delta_2^T) \quad (9.16)$$

and confine the calibration regression model to the appropriate component by writing

$$p(v_1^{(2)} | v_2^{(2)}, \gamma, \delta) = \phi(v_1^{(2)} | \alpha + \beta v_2^{(2)}, \sigma^2). \quad (9.17)$$

Then (9.14) provides the basis for handling the diagnostic data D_2 (conn) in clinic 2 by becoming

$$\mathrm{pr}(u = 1 | v_2, \gamma, \delta) = \Phi \left[\{ \delta_0 + v_2^{(1)} + \delta_2 (\alpha + \beta v_2^{(2)}) \} / \sqrt{(1 + \delta_2^2 \sigma^2)} \right]. \quad (9.18)$$

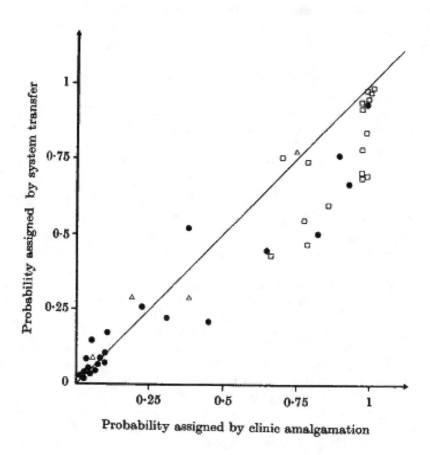

Figure 9.2 *Comparison of type 1 probabilities assigned by full clinic amalgamation and system transfer methods:* □, *clinic 1 case of known type 1;* △, *clinic 1 case of known type 2;* •, *new case in clinic 1 of unknown type. (Taken from Aitchison, J. Biometrika,* **66**, *364, 1979, [Oxford University Press] with permission.)*

The full clinic amalgamation method, the system transfer method and the naive calibration method were each applied to obtain diagnostic assessments for the 21 training cases in clinic 1, by resubstitution, and for 22 new cases of unknown type. Figure 9.2 provides, for each of these 43 cases, a comparison of probabilities of type 1 assigned by the clinic amalgamation and system transfer methods. Note that on the whole the full clinic amalgamation method gives assessments of greater firmness than the system transfer method and in a number of cases the differences are substantial.

It is not possible to show the results of the naive calibration method on the same diagram since there is practically no difference from those of the full clinic amalgamation method. An explanation of this finding has two aspects. First, naive calibration here is directed towards producing a diagnostic system for clinic 1 in contrast to the assessment for a new case in clinic 1 as in system transfer. The calibration experiment is sizeable and so produces reasonably reliable estimates of the regression parameters. Although for transfer of a single case the naive calibrate has an appreciable unreliability, ignoring this unreliability may yet produce, because of averaging over a number of cases, a satisfactory diagnostic system for clinic 1. Secondly, since new cases have features measured in clinic 1 there is no need for any additional calibration technique to be applied to the diagnostic assessment stage, in contrast to the situation in system transfer where each new case requires individual calibration.

9.4 Imprecision in the feature vector

We have assumed so far that the components recorded in the feature vector v are precise. This is not always the case. For a variety of reasons features can be imprecise; for example there may be physiological variability in the determination of a feature such as blood pressure, assessment may be by an assay technique with a quantifiable imprecision, or there may be imprecision arising from observer error. Later in this section we investigate how imprecision in the determination of the steroid metabolite features in the differential diagnosis of Cushing's syndrome, where the coefficient of variation in the determinations is quoted as 20 per cent, affects the reliability of the diagnoses. Also earlier in this chapter we have been investigating essentially imprecision problems which arise from a need to calibrate certain features between different clinics; we have already considered imprecision within the context of calibration in Sections 7.7 and 9.2. In view of this we introduce into our statistical modelling of imprecision an extra degree of generality which will serve to simplify our approach to these calibration problems.

We observe a feature vector v subject to imprecision which is related in probabilistic fashion to a true underlying feature vector y for that individual. Due to the fact that the observed feature vectors v could arise from different clinical sources, with varying degrees of imprecision and possible selection on the observed v or related factors, we again concentrate development on the conditional density $p(u|y, \delta)$ for precise cases. This can be justified by the fact that the imprecise feature v is related to the precise y for an individual through the imprecision model $p(y|v, \gamma)$, and the conditional form $p(u|v, \delta)$ for the observed v is related to $p(u|v, \gamma, \delta)$ by

$$p(u|v, \gamma, \delta) = \int_Y p(u|y, \delta)p(y|v, \gamma)dy,$$

which is clearly stable in terms of selection on v. We first consider the situation where there are just two types and where the feature measurements are continuous.

9.4.1 Parametric modelling for two types

We have seen in Chapter 8 in terms of practical results there is nothing to choose between normal and logistic forms for the modelling of the conditional distribution of $p(u|y, \delta)$. Here for reasons of tractability we choose the normal form. Specifying the model for precise y as $\mathrm{pr}(u = 1|y, \delta) = \Phi(y\delta^T)$, we have

$$\mathrm{pr}(u = 1|v, \gamma, \delta) = \int_Y \Phi(y\delta^T)p(y|v, \gamma)dy.$$

Realistic modelling of the error distribution $p(y|v, \gamma)$ together with consideration of tractability suggest a normal form. Looking back to our use of this modelling in calibrative situations we may specify

$$p(y|v, \gamma) = \phi(y|vA, B), \tag{9.19}$$

the multivariate normal regression model with $\gamma = (A, B)$. Then

$$\mathrm{pr}(u|v, \gamma, \delta) = \Phi\left\{ \frac{vA\delta^T}{\sqrt{(1 + \delta B\delta^T)}} \right\}. \tag{9.20}$$

The choice of $A = I$ is appropriate if v is quoted as an estimate of y with computed variance B or, in the multivariate situation, estimated covariance matrix B. We have retained the more general A since information about y is sometimes obtained through some indirect form of measurement such as calibration and assay. In general, individual cases of the training set will have A_i and B_i $(i = 1, \ldots, n)$ differing from each other and from the A and B of a new case, so that the precise form of the diagnostic model in (9.20) varies from case to case.

We note that $B = 0$ corresponds to the case of a precise feature vector with (9.20) reducing to $\Phi(y\delta^T)$. The obvious inequality

$$|\Phi(v\delta^T) - \tfrac{1}{2}| \leq |\Phi\left\{ vA\delta^T \big/ \sqrt{(1 + \delta B\delta^T)} \right\} - \tfrac{1}{2}|$$

confirms the intuitive modelling requirement that knowledge of inaccurate v rather than true y must lead us to diagnostic probabilities which are closer to 0.5, the diagnostic assessment expressing the greatest uncertainty.

The likelihood problem is easily resolved for the normal model since the integrals take an explicit and easily computable form. It is tempting to hope that the problems of taking account of imprecision are thereby automatically resolved but we shall see that imprecision in clinical situations can cause substantial, and at times insurmountable, further difficulties. Since we shall assume that the parameters A and B are known or assumed from factors outside the diagnostic problem we shall drop $\gamma = (A, B)$ from the notation.

The likelihood for a given data set $D = \{(u_i, v_i) : i = 1, \ldots, n\}$ is given explicitly by

$$L(\delta|D) = \prod_{i=1}^{n} p(u_i|v_i, \delta),$$

where

$$\mathrm{pr}(u_i = 1|v_i, \delta) = \Phi(v_i\epsilon_i), \quad p(u_i = 2|v_i, \delta) = 1 - \Phi(v_i\epsilon_i),$$

and

$$\epsilon_i = \frac{A_i\delta}{\sqrt{(1 + \delta B_i\delta^T)}}.$$

To arrive at diagnostic assessments for new cases some simple form for $p(\delta|D)$ must be obtained. We assume the applicability of the Bayesian form of large-sample maximum likelihood theory; in other words, δ is assumed to be approximately multivariate normally distributed as $N\{\hat{\delta}, V(\hat{\delta})\}$, where $\hat{\delta}$ is the maximum likelihood estimate and $V(\hat{\delta})$ the usual asymptotic estimate of the covariance $V(\delta)$, evaluated at $\hat{\delta}$. The algorithm to obtain $\hat{\delta}$ and $V(\hat{\delta})$ by the Newton-Raphson method is only slightly more complicated than a straight-forward binary regression in probit analysis form, each iterative step being expressible in weighted regression form. Write

$$s_i = \frac{v_i A_i\delta}{\sqrt{(1 + \delta B_i\delta^T)}}, \qquad \omega = \frac{\phi^2}{\Phi(1 - \Phi)}$$

and define the weights w_i as $\omega(s_i)$, and the regressor vector X_i and the regressand Y_i by

$$\begin{aligned} X_i &= (1 + \delta B\delta^T)^{-\frac{3}{2}} \left\{ (1 + \delta B_i\delta^T)v_i A_i - v_i A_i\delta B_i\delta^T \right\}, \\ Y_i &= s_i + \{2 - u_i - \Phi(s_i)\}/\phi(s_i). \end{aligned}$$

The iterative relation determining the rth iterate is

$$\delta^{(r)} = \left(\sum_i w_i X_i^T X_i \right)^{-1} \left(\sum_i X_i^T Y_i \right),$$

where the right-hand side is evaluated at the $(r-1)$th iterate $\delta^{(r-1)}$. At convergence $\delta = \delta^{(r)}$ and $V(\delta)$ is the inverse matrix, the first factor of the right-hand side.

For a new case with an exact feature vector, and so with $B = 0$, this multiple integral can be evaluated explicitly to give

$$\mathrm{pr}(u = 1|y, D) = \Phi \left[\frac{yA\delta^T}{\sqrt{(1 + yAV(\hat{\delta})A^T y^T)}} \right].$$

For a new case with $B \neq 0$ there is no closed form for

$$p(u = 1|y, D) = \int_\Delta \Phi \left[\frac{yA\delta^T}{\sqrt{(1 + \delta B\delta^T)}} \right] \phi\{\delta|\hat{\delta}, V(\hat{\delta}\}d\delta. \qquad (9.21)$$

This problem is identical to the probabilistic assessment for the system transfer problem, a useful 'control variate' approximation being given by the control term

$$\Phi\left[\frac{yA\delta^T}{\sqrt{(1+\hat{\delta}B\hat{\delta}^T+yAV(\hat{\delta})A^Ty^T)}}\right], \tag{9.22}$$

which can be improved by addition of the integral

$$\int F(\delta)\phi\{\delta|\hat{\delta},V(\hat{\delta})\}d\delta,$$

where

$$F(\delta)=\Phi\left\{\frac{yA\delta^T}{\sqrt{(1+\delta B\delta^T)}}\right\}-\Phi\left\{\frac{yA\delta^T}{\sqrt{(1+\hat{\delta}B\hat{\delta}^T)}}\right\}.$$

Application to the differential diagnosis of Cushing's syndrome

We provide here an illustration of this modelling to an imprecision problem involving Cushing's syndrome and data set cush. We confine attention here to the problem of differentiating between the two benign forms, adrenal adenoma (type 1) and adrenal hyperplasia (type 2). Such differentiation is of practical importance because the treatments are quite different for the two types. A training set of 7 type 1 and 27 type 2 cases is available, with each case, for our limited illustration, having a two dimensional feature vector, consisting of urinary excretion rates of two steroid metabolites, allo-tetrahydrocortisol and tetrahydrocortisone, determined by the paper chromatography method which has a 20% coefficient of variation. To take account of a coefficient of variation equal to c the error model in (9.19) takes the form

$$p(v|y,S)=\phi[v|y,\{c\times\mathrm{diag}(y)\}^2], \tag{9.23}$$

where diag(y) is the diagonal matrix whose diagonal elements are the components of the vector y.

We reemphasize that our main purpose here is to investigate for new cases the extent to which admission of this factor of imprecision alters the diagnostic assessments which we would obtain using the excretion rates as if they were precise. A general study of the effects of imprecision requires the evaluation of the multiple integral in (9.21) for various degrees of imprecision in the training set and in the new case. To avoid any possible confounding of imprecision effects with the accuracy of the approximation in (9.22), we can conveniently approach the general study in two stages. At the first stage we ask what is the effect of recognizing imprecision only in the training set, with $B=0$ for a new case, when (9.21) takes the exact form in (9.22). The second stage is then simply to let B increase from zero and to use (9.22) or a Monte Carlo technique.

To study the first stage, (9.20) with the error distribution in (9.23) has been fitted by the iterative procedure with coefficient of variation $c=0$, that is considering the training set as accurate, and then with increasing values of c up to 5 per cent. For each c, after convergence, the predictive diagnostic probabilities were determined for 40 new cases. For all cases but one the diagnostic probabilities changed substantially as illustrated by typical cases in Figure 9.3, the probabilities moving towards one-half.

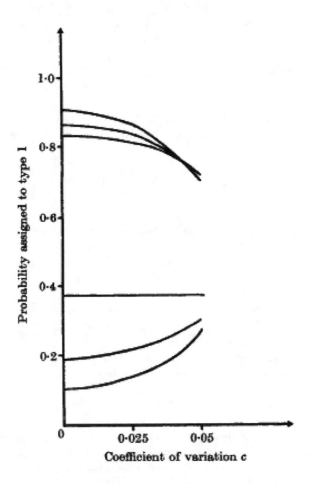

Figure 9.3 *Changes in the diagnostic probabilities of typical cases as the coefficient of variation increases. (Taken from Aitchison, J. and Lauder I.J. Biometrika, **66**, 479, 1979, [Oxford University Press] with permission.)*

At the second stage we investigated the additional effect of increasing the coefficient of variation for a new case up to 5 per cent using the approximation in (9.22). The further reduction in the diagnostic probabilities was smaller than 2 per cent in all cases. The investigation was restricted to a maximum coefficient of variation of 5 per cent instead of the actual 20 per cent. As the coefficient of variation increases past 5 per cent it becomes increasingly difficult to obtain convergence by the Newton-Raphson iterative process.

A second application of dealing with the issue of imprecision involves an alternative to the clinic amalgamation problem for Conn's syndrome. Here, two clinics wish to amalgamate their training sets but one of the features, plasma concentration of aldosterone, is determined by different techniques in the two clinics. In presenting this example to illustrate the new methods, we have used the same three logged features for the differential diagnosis of the two types of Conn's syndrome as in Section 8.2. In brief, the training set is here considered to consist of 21 cases from clinic 1, with 17 of type 1 and 4 of type 2, whose feature measurements, by the latest method, are regarded as exact; and 31 cases from clinic 2 with 20 of type 1 and 11 of type 2, whose first feature, because of its calibration to the first clinic standard, is imprecise but whose other two feature measurements are exact. The B_i and S_i then take the forms

$$B_i = I_4, \quad S_i = 0 \quad (i = 1, \ldots, 21),$$

$$B_i = \begin{bmatrix} a & b & 0 \\ 0 & 0 & I_2 \end{bmatrix}, \quad S_i = \mathrm{diag}\{0, \mathrm{c}\{\mathrm{d} + \mathrm{e}(\mathrm{v} - \mathrm{f})^2\}, 0, 0\} \quad (i = 22, \ldots, 52),$$

where a and b are the calibration regression coefficients, c is the residual mean square of the calibration regression, $d = 32/31$, $e = 1/S_{uu}$, $f = \bar{u}$ and v is the aldosterone measurement in clinic 2; see Section 7.1.1 under the heading 'Predictive approach'. Our approach here thus completely separates out the calibration problem from the diagnostic one, producing a single training set with a mixture of precise cases and imprecise, calibrated cases, whereas the approach adopted in Section 9.3 retains the two training sets using a calibration paradigm as the binding element. Where the calibration experiment is large, as in the present problem, the two approaches are likely to give similar results.

Here new cases are measured by the new technique so that $B = I_4, S = 0$ and only the first stage, involving the effects of imprecision in the training set, need be considered. The degree of imprecision in this example is represented by c and so we can again study the effects of ignoring the imprecision by setting $c = 0$ as well as to its actual value $c = 0.184$. For both assumptions about c, there were no practical problems of numerical convergence in fitting the cumulative normal model and (9.22) was applied to obtain the predictive diagnostic probabilities for 22 new cases. The differences between the odds assigned on a basis of ignoring imprecision and those taking account of the calibration imprecision are negligible. This is in sharp contrast to the substantial differences in the application to Cushing's syndrome. A possible explanation is that precise cases are sufficiently frequent in the combined training set to prevent the imprecise, calibrated cases from causing much of an effect at their actual degree of imprecision. If, however, we let the degree of imprecision increase well beyond its actual value, up to $c = 1$, the odds do change by a factor of 3 in a substantial number of cases. From this result it is fairly safe to conclude that it is the frequency and the magnitude of imprecision that dually affect the assessments.

9.5 Missing features: non-toxic goitre

Data are available in the data set `goitre` on three types of goitre: Hashimoto's disease (type 1), simple goitre (type 2) and thyroid cancer (type 3). There are 40, 40 and 28 complete cases for types 1, 2, 3, respectively. Four features are recorded for each case. Feature v_1 is the continuous variable "erythrocyte sedimentation rate", feature v_2 is the binary variable "recent increase in size" recorded as 0 (no) or 1 (yes), feature v_3 is the ordinal variable 'consistency' recorded as 1, 2 or 3 according to an observed firm, hard or soft consistency, and feature v_4 is the binary variable 'tracheal deviation or compression on X-ray' recorded as 0 (no) or 1 (yes). In addition to the complete cases there are 31 incomplete cases, with 4 involving v_4 and 27 of them involving variables v_1 and v_2. We first perform an analysis based on the 108 complete case records.

We have the data

$$D = \{(u_i, v_i) : i = 1, \ldots, 108\},$$

where $u_i = (u_{ij}, j = 1, \ldots, 3)$, with $u_{ij} = 0$ or 1 and $\sum_{j=1}^{3} u_{ij} = 1$ and $v_i = (v_{ij}, j = 1, \ldots, 4)$, with v_{ij} denoting the observation made of the jth feature on the ith subject, with the variables v_2 and v_4 binary and the others taken to be continuous. Then the model $p(u|v)$ takes the form of a multinomial logistic regression model. The full lattice of possible models is rather large in this problem and so we present only some of the models and comparisons. Given that there are two binary explanatory factors and two covariates the most general maximal model M_3 may be written as

$$M_3 : \quad u_i|v \sim Mu(1, \psi_{ijrs}),$$

where

$$\psi_{ijrs} = \frac{\phi_{ijrs}}{\sum_{j=1}^{3} \phi_{ijrs}},$$

with

$$\log(\phi_{ijrs}) = \rho_{jrs} + \sigma_{jrs} v_{i1} + \tau_{jrs} v_{i3},$$

subject to the corner-point constraints

$$\rho_{1rs} = \sigma_{1rs} = \tau_{1rs} = 0 \qquad (r = 1, 2, s = 1, 2).$$

Of the many sub-models in the lattice we present results only for the following:

$$
\begin{aligned}
M_0 : \quad & \rho_{jrs} = \alpha_j, \quad \sigma_{jrs} = \tau_{jrs} = 0, \\
M_1 : \quad & \rho_{jrs} = \alpha_j + \gamma_j v_{i2}, \quad \sigma_{jrs} = \beta_j, \quad \tau_{jrs} = \delta_j, \\
M_2 : \quad & \rho_{jrs} = \alpha_j + \gamma_j v_{i2} + \epsilon_j v_{i4}, \quad \sigma_{jrs} = \beta_j, \quad \tau_{jrs} = \delta_j,
\end{aligned}
$$

Table 9.1 *Comparison of some sub-models with the maximal model M_3 on the basis of asymptotic likelihood ratio tests*

Model	Deviance	Dimension	TS(df)	P
M_3	90.1	24		
M_2	105.1	10	15.0(14)	0.37
M_1	107.1	8	17.0(16)	0.38
M_0	234.5	2	144.4(22)	$< 10^{-7}$

subject to the constraints $\alpha_1 = 0$, $\beta_1 = 0$, $\gamma_1 = 0$, $\delta_1 = 0$ and $\epsilon_1 = 0$.

The details of the formal comparisons of models M_0, M_1 and M_2 within the maximal model M_3 are given in Table 9.1. Clearly model M_1 is not rejected and in fact this is the simplest of the sub-models which fails to be rejected and so we adopt this as our working model in further analysis.

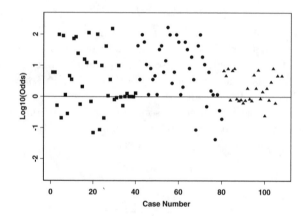

Figure 9.4 *Log_{10} odds in favour of the correct type for each of the 108 patients in the training set. The types of the patients are indicated by squares (type 1), circles (type 2) and triangles (type 3).*

We may obtain estimated probabilities for each of the three types of goitre for each patient. They were computed on a leave-one-out basis and the results are shown in Figure 9.4 in the form of $\log_{10}$ odds in favour of the correct type for each patient, labelled by type. We see that the estimated probabilities in favour of the known type are fairly strong in several cases but doubtful in other cases. If one were to consider the results from the viewpoint of classification of patients into their correct type then using the Bayes classifier the leave-one-out estimate of misclassification rate with future patients is 26%, and the conditional estimates for the three types of goitre are 30%, 13% and 39%, respectively.

We now deal with all the cases by including those with missing data and assume that the missing values are completely missing at random. There are 112 complete case records on variables v_1-v_3 and a further 21 cases in which the value of v_1 is missing and a further 6 cases in which v_2 is missing. We adopt a Bayesian approach to the imputation of the missing values and use WinBUGS. We need to consider how to impute these missing values. Using the 112 complete records we build a linear model to predict v_1 using the variables v_2, v_3 and u and we also adopt a logistic regression model to predict v_2 given v_1, v_3 and u. These models are then used to predict the missing values in the incomplete case records. At each iteration a missing value is imputed from the posterior distribution of the missing node given the current values of all connected variables in the model. Then using all 139 case records, including the imputations, the multinomial logistic regression model M_1 is used to predict u. For a referred patient with covariate vector $z = (1, z_1, z_2, z_3)$ we wish to estimate the posterior probability that she belongs to the jth type given the data. If we let $\theta_j = (\alpha_j, \beta_j, \gamma_j, \delta_j)$ and $\theta = (\theta_1, \theta_2, \theta_3)$ we may write this probability for $j = 1, 2, 3$ as

$$\int_\Theta \frac{\exp(\theta_j z^T)}{\sum_{r=1}^3 \exp(\theta_r z^T)} p(\theta|\text{data}) d\theta,$$

which is the posterior mean of the probability that the referred patient belongs to type j. We compute these integrals using WinBUGS. Independent non-informative priors were assumed for the parameters.

In the WinBUGS analysis three chains were run from dispersed initial values of the parameters. The chains were run for 4,000 iterations in Metropolis adaptive phase and the results from the next 1,000 iterations were discarded. Convergence was monitored during the next 5,000 iteration and on the basis of trace plots, autocorrelation plots and the Brooks-Gelman-Rubin convergence statistics the chains appeared to be in equilibrium. The sampling was continued for a further 5,000 iterations and these results used. As there was some degree of autocorrelation it was also checked that the Monte Carlo error was less than 5% of the estimated standard deviation of the output at each node. The posterior probabilities were computed for five referred patients and the results are given in Table 9.2.

Simple goitre can be ruled out for patient N1 and this patient would appear to be suffering from either Hashimoto's disease or thyroid cancer. It seems likely that patient N2 has cancer of the thyroid, patient N3 has simple goitre and patient N5 has Hashimoto's disease. Thyroid cancer can be ruled out for patient N4 and it is more likely that this patient suffers from Hashimoto's disease rather than simple goitre but the probabilities are quite close.

Table 9.2 *Diagnostic assessments of five referred patients with non-toxic goitre*

Patient	v_1	v_2	v_3	Probabilities
N1	33	1	1	(0.52, 0.00, 0.48)
N2	15	1	2	(0.09, 0.02, 0.89)
N3	4	0	3	(0.01, 0.99, 0.00)
N4	10	0	1	(0.58, 0.41, 0.01)
N5	18	0	1	(0.94, 0.05, 0.01)

9.6 Uncertainty of type

In situations where the type information on patients is uncertain, the training set consists of cases each with the feature vector again of the d-dimensional form v but with composite diagnosis $w = (w_1, \ldots, w_k)$, where

$$w_j = p(u = j) \quad (j = 1, \ldots, k).$$

For example, the composite diagnosis w may be a consensus of the opinions of a group of clinicians. General modelling considerations here again involve the effect of selection $s(v)$ on v and how the training set D can be employed to give a realistic firm diagnostic statement $p(u|v)$ for a new case with feature vector v. Selection arguments now lead to $p(w|v)$ as the stable estimable form in v. The special feature of this situation is the composite or compositional form of w, but we have seen in Section 4.2 how to deal appropriately with such compositions. For direct modelling of $p(w|v)$ we can clearly use a logistic normal regression type model $L^{k-1}(vB, \Sigma)$. Since $\text{pr}(u = j|w) = w_j$ we obtain the following form for the diagnostic assessment of a new case:

$$p(u = j) = \int_{S^{k-1}} w_j \lambda^{k-1}(w|vB, \Sigma) dw,$$

where λ^{k-1} is the density function of the $(k-1)$-dimensional logistic-normal distribution. This integral can be transformed to more familiar multivariate form by the additive logratio transformation $z = \text{alr}(w)$:

$$p(u = j|v) = \int \psi_j(w) \phi^{k-1}(z|vB, \Sigma) dz, \tag{9.24}$$

where $\psi_j(w)$ is the logistic function

$$\frac{\exp(w_j)}{\sum_{r=1}^{k} \exp(w_r)}.$$

We note that this is essentially the same as first transforming w by a logratio transformation $z = \text{alr}(w)$ and then imposing a multivariate normal regression model on z for given v. The multivariate regression theory of Section 3.4 applies to the estimation of B and Σ, yielding $\hat{B}$ and $\hat{\Sigma}$. The estimative

Table 9.3 *Kernel functions for uncertain typing*

1. Dirichlet:

$$K(w, w') = \frac{\Gamma(k - 1 + 1/\lambda)}{\Gamma(1 + w'_1/\lambda) \cdots \Gamma(1 + w'_k/\lambda)} w_1^{w'_1/\lambda} \cdots w_k^{w'_k/\lambda}$$

2. Logistic Normal:

$$K(w, w') = (w_1 \cdots w_k)^{-1} \phi_{k-1}(v|w', \lambda^2 T),$$

$$v_j = \log(w_j/w_k), \qquad V_j = \log(w'_j/w'_k),$$

$$T = (n - 1)^{-1} \sum_{i=1}^{n} (V_i - \bar{V})(V_i - \bar{V})^T.$$

T cannot be taken as diagonal in this instance. To ensure invariance of K under permutations of the components of w, the above form is appropriate.

approach takes

$$p(z|v, D) = \phi(z|v\hat{B}, \hat{\Sigma})$$

and arrives at an estimative diagnostic assessment. A predictive assessment may be obtained by assuming vague priors on B and Σ and from Property 3.10 we have

$$p(z|v, D) = St^{k-1} \left[n - c, v\hat{B}, \{1 + v(V^T V)^{-1}v^T\}\hat{\Sigma} \right]. \tag{9.25}$$

For discrete or mixed features or when the multivariate normality of $p(z|v)$ is questionable kernel methods can be used. The development follows the weighted kernel arguments of Section 4.8 to give

$$p(w|v) = \sum_{i=1}^{n} K_1(w, w_i)w(v, v_i),$$

where K_1 is the Dirichlet kernel of Table 9.3, and

$$p(z|v) = \sum K_2(z, z_i)w(v, v_i),$$

with K_2 the logistic normal kernel of Table 9.3 and w a weighting function.

Good approximate analytic reduction for $p(u|v)$ when $k = 2$ can be obtained from

$$p(u = 1|v) = \sum_{i=1}^{n} \psi(v'_i)w(v, v_i),$$

$$v'_i = v_i/\sqrt{1 + \lambda^2 \sigma_r^2/c^2} \quad (k > 2),$$

but requires integration in the logistic case. The use of the Dirichlet kernel is more complicated computationally, but explicit assessments for $k \geq 2$ are

Table 9.4 *Probabilistic assessments of the electrocochleography cases by the estimative parametric approach (E), the kernel method (K1) and the discrete kernel method (K2) for groups 1 and 2, with probability of type 1 given for cases 1-23 and probability of type 2 shown for cases 24-48*

Case	E	K1	K2	Case	E	K1	K2
1	.83	.87	.90	24	.39	.22	.21
2	.83	.87	.90	25	.70	.45	.45
3	.73	.85	.87	26	.76	.83	.85
4	.70	.76	.77	27	.87	.87	.90
5	.74	.68	.69	28	.68	.87	.90
6	.87	.87	.90	29	.47	.13	.10
7	.80	.87	.90	30	.47	.18	.16
8	.43	.58	.58	31	.56	.18	.15
9	.75	.87	.90	32	.58	.42	.42
10	.39	.13	.11	32	.58	.42	.42
11	.74	.87	.90	33	.58	.42	.42
12	.56	.76	.78	34	.79	.87	.90
13	.60	.57	.58	35	.86	.87	.90
14	.88	.87	.90	36	.88	.87	.90
15	.63	.86	.90	37	.52	.55	.55
16	.72	.87	.90	38	.93	.87	.90
17	.88	.87	.90	39	.83	.87	.90
18	.46	.32	.31	40	.65	.38	.37
19	.78	.87	.90	41	.55	.78	.80
20	.61	.61	.62	42	.88	.87	.90
21	.55	.25	.23	43	.55	.24	.22
22	.71	.87	.90	44	.93	.87	.90
23	.90	.87	.90	45	.78	.87	.90
				46	.57	.87	.90
				47	.42	.47	.45
				48	.86	.87	.90

given by

$$p(u = j|v) = \sum_{i=1}^{n} E(w_{ij})w(v, v_i)$$

with

$$E(w_{ij}) = (w_{ij}/\lambda + 1)/(k + 1/\lambda),$$

where λ is a smoothing parameter.

When v is discrete or consists of mixed features, the weight function W can be modified as appropriate. If the w_i constitute a small set of values, then

modelling the V_i as a discrete set can be accomplished by the kernel method
to give

$$p(u|v) = \Sigma Z(u, v_i) w(v, v_i)$$

with $Z(w, w_i) \propto K(w, w_i)$, such that

$$\sum_i Z(w, w_i) = 1.$$

The parametric and kernel methodology was applied to data set hearing:
the electrocochleography data. Four measurements of auditory dysfunction
were recorded for each of 93 patients. Each patient belonged to one of four
groups: normal hearing, conduction hearing loss, Menière's disease and hair-
cell damage, with sample sizes 23, 25, 26, 19, respectively. The assessment
vectors u_i were composite but constant within each group. The application
of the continuous normal model for $p(z|v)$ is therefore open to question. The
kernel model can be used as a tool to ascertain the robustness and consequent
validity of the parametric approach for this particular application.

The estimative method and both kernel methods were applied to attempt
to form a diagnostic assessment of the patients in groups 1 and 2 on a
leave-one-out basis and the results are displayed in Table 9.4. The assessed
probabilities are generally similar across all three methods but there are ex-
ceptions, for example patients 10, 21, 29 and 43 in which the estimative and
kernel methods tend to disagree.

In the above analysis only two groups were compared. We now apply the
predictive approach using data from all four groups and we produce diagnostic assessments for three referred patients. We use WinBUGS to compute
the probability defined in (9.24). In this application WinBUGS is being used
in direct simulation mode simply to compute an expectation of the logistic
functions with respect to the predictive distribution in (9.25). The first 1,000
iterations were discarded and estimates were based on the output of the next
5,000 iterations. The results are given in Table 9.5. None of the diagnostic
assessments is particularly clear. Patients N1, N2 and N3 are most likely to
belong to groups 4, 3 and 1, respectively.

Table 9.5 *Diagnostic assessments of three referred patients*

Patient	Type 1	Type 2	Type 3	Type 4
N1	0.10	0.29	0.05	0.56
N2	0.09	0.22	0.64	0.05
N3	0.48	0.15	0.29	0.08

9.7 Cushing's syndrome

The challenge of developing a diagnostic method to deal with the tree-like
nature of the decision-making in the management of patients with Cushing's
syndrome was described in Section 1.10 and an approach was formulated in
Section 5.4. The nature of the tree-like structure of the types is shown in
Figure 9.5.

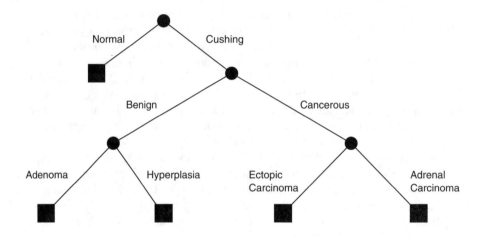

Figure 9.5 *The diagnostic structure of patient management in Cushing's syndrome.*

At the first stage a patient is either normal or has one of the forms of
Cushing's syndrome. Secondly, if the patient has Cushing's syndrome is it
a benign or cancerous form? Thirdly, if the form is benign is it due to an
adenoma or is it bilateral hyperplasia? Fourthly, if the form is cancerous is the
carcinoma ectopic or adrenal? The clinician could, given sufficient evidence,
stop at a particular node and not traverse the whole tree of possibilities. We
now apply the method introduced in Section 5.5 and produce full diagnostic
probability trees for three referred patients. For Cushing's syndrome the tree
has three levels, five terminal nodes and four branch nodes and we now give
the likelihood factors for the four branch nodes.

$$
\begin{aligned}
&\text{Node 1} \quad \prod_{r=1}^{n_1} F(v_{r1}; \beta_1) && \times \quad \prod_{t=2}^{5} \prod_{r=1}^{n_t} [1 - F(v_{rt}; \beta_1)] \\
&\text{Node 2} \quad \prod_{t=2,3} \prod_{r=1}^{n_t} F(v_{rt}; \beta_2) && \times \quad \prod_{t=4,5} \prod_{r=1}^{n_t} [1 - F(v_{rt}; \beta_2)] \\
&\text{Node 3} \quad \prod_{r=1}^{n_2} F(v_{r2}; \beta_3) && \times \quad \prod_{r=1}^{n_3} [1 - F(v_{r3}; \beta_3)] \\
&\text{Node 4} \quad \prod_{r=1}^{n_4} F(v_{r4}; \beta_4) && \times \quad \prod_{r=1}^{n_5} [1 - F(v_{rt}; \beta_4)]
\end{aligned}
\tag{9.26}
$$

In practical terms one can perform a logistic regression for each of the four branch nodes in the tree. At node 1 we attempt to distinguish a normal case (type 1) from a Cushing case (types 2–5) and use the data from all cases in the training set but now binary-coded as either type 1 or not type 1. At the second node we attempt to distinguish a benign case (types 2 or 3) from a cancerous case (types 4 or 5), but now using the training data only for types 2-5 with each case now binary-coded as either a combined 2–3 type or a combined 4–5 type, and so on for the other nodes. We use the most promising four of the fourteen steroid metabolites (tetrahydocortisone, Reichstein's compound U, cortisol and pregnenetriol) as features and we use the same four at each node, although it is easy to incorporate different subsets at each node.

The data were logged and then standardised. Logistic regressions were run for each node and it was found that the probabilities were very close to 0 or 1, indicating problems due to complete or near-complete separation of the feature vectors. Therefore we used the fair prior which was introduced in Section 4.3 as a prior for the β parameters at each of the branch nodes. Diagnostic probabilities were computed for three referred patients using WinBUGS. The initial values of the prior parameters β were generated randomly from the prior distribution. The usual diagnostic checks were conducted and the results from iterations 5,001 to 10,000 were used for the estimation of the diagnostic probabilities and also the model parameters β. For each node the code given below was used with the relevant data for the node in question. The b[i] are the β parameters in the logistic regression, x1–x4 denote the four features used in the model and z[j,k] denotes the value of the kth feature for the jth referred patient. The prior on β is multivariate normal with mean vector mu and precision matrix prec and p[j] is the probability of the 'type' coded 1 for the jth referred patient. The values of x1–x4, z, mu and prec are input as data.

```
model {

for(i in 1:N) {
 y[i]~dbin(phi[i],1)
logit(phi[i])<-b[1]+b[2]*x1[i]+b[3]*x2[i]+b[4]*x3[i]+b[5]*x4[i]}

b[1:5]~dmnorm(mu[1:5], prec[1:5,1:5])

for(j in 1:M)
 { t[j]<-b[1]+b[2]*z[j,1]+b[3]*z[j,2]+b[4]*z[j,3]+b[5]*z[j,4]
 p[j]<-exp(t[j])/(1+exp(t[j])) }
 }
```

The diagnostic trees are shown in Figures 9.6, 9.7 and 9.8.

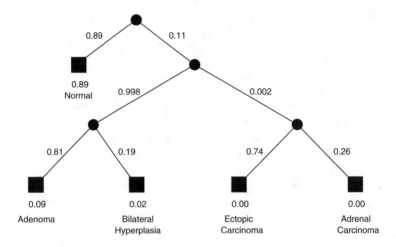

Figure 9.6 *Diagnostic probability tree for referred patient N1. The unconditional probabilities for each type are printed at the terminal nodes. All probabilities are rounded to two decimal places.*

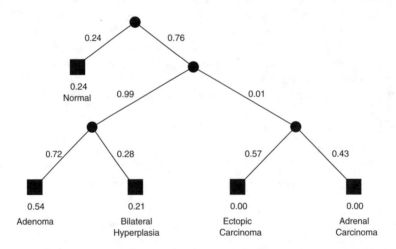

Figure 9.7 *Diagnostic probability tree for referred patient N2. The unconditional probabilities for each type are printed at the terminal nodes. All probabilities are rounded to two decimal places.*

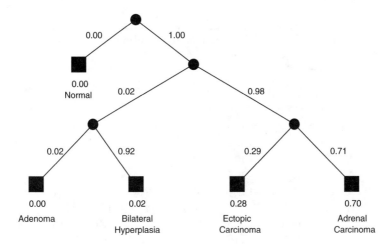

Figure 9.8 *Diagnostic probability tree for referred patient N3. The unconditional probabilities for each type are printed at the terminal nodes. All probabilities are rounded to two decimal places.*

9.8 Bibliographic notes

The modelling and applications of diagnostic system transfer and clinic amalgamation are developed in Aitchison (1977, 1979). The implications of imprecision in feature vectors is discussed in Aitchison and Lauder (1979). The problem of missing features is dependent on the basic concept of the EM algorithm first formally and generally developed in Dempster, Laird and Rubin (1977) though its origins date back to many special situations.

Details of modelling when the cases of the training set are imprecisely diagnosed are contained in Aitchison and Begg (1976) and a method of updating a diagnostic system using unconfirmed cases is found in Titterington (1976). For further details of the illustration discussed in Section 9.6, see Hermans et al. (1975). The tree analysis of the differential diagnosis of Cushing's syndrome is, we believe, new, though related to the latent variable models of Lauder (1981).

For an early consideration of situations where the feature vectors are of mixed type, for example binary and continuous, see Krzanowski (1975).

9.9 Problems

Problem 9.1 A clinic is attempting to resolve a difficult problem in differential diagnosis between two types A and B and has determined the composition of a group of metabolites in urine as a possible source of separation. These six-part compositions are reproduced in Table 9.6 for 20 patients of known type A

Table 9.6 *Data for Problem 9.1*

Patient	Proportions of metabolites					
	X1	X2	X3	Y1	Y2	Y3
A1	0.173	0.359	0.232	0.040	0.035	0.159
A2	0.114	0.188	0.314	0.106	0.057	0.218
A3	0.129	0.147	0.112	0.109	0.169	0.331
A4	0.060	0.170	0.539	0.022	0.071	0.135
A5	0.078	0.404	0.303	0.071	0.052	0.089
A6	0.052	0.176	0.250	0.108	0.094	0.317
A7	0.120	0.175	0.317	0.091	0.157	0.138
A8	0.059	0.251	0.176	0.128	0.127	0.256
A9	0.079	0.170	0.315	0.040	0.157	0.235
A10	0.102	0.103	0.328	0.082	0.121	0.261
A11	0.031	0.116	0.572	0.036	0.062	0.181
A12	0.068	0.153	0.403	0.056	0.076	0.241
A13	0.143	0.221	0.207	0.073	0.112	0.241
A14	0.024	0.229	0.219	0.079	0.132	0.314
A15	0.160	0.222	0.320	0.107	0.076	0.111
A16	0.080	0.086	0.291	0.079	0.094	0.367
A17	0.151	0.091	0.375	0.077	0.182	0.121
A18	0.060	0.195	0.302	0.049	0.109	0.283
A19	0.048	0.159	0.174	0.061	0.038	0.519
A20	0.064	0.133	0.416	0.071	0.094	0.221
B1	0.042	0.144	0.183	0.184	0.085	0.360
B2	0.059	0.086	0.373	0.294	0.056	0.128
B3	0.070	0.100	0.138	0.118	0.110	0.463
B4	0.018	0.127	0.100	0.313	0.080	0.359
B5	0.057	0.147	0.115	0.165	0.167	0.346
B6	0.033	0.080	0.136	0.185	0.117	0.446
B7	0.048	0.139	0.105	0.079	0.148	0.477
B8	0.052	0.153	0.090	0.204	0.088	0.410
B9	0.102	0.154	0.200	0.073	0.078	0.390
B10	0.055	0.116	0.079	0.366	0.075	0.306
B11	0.033	0.080	0.030	0.218	0.098	0.537
B12	0.087	0.118	0.083	0.114	0.144	0.453
B13	0.067	0.061	0.084	0.422	0.118	0.246
B14	0.034	0.063	0.079	0.288	0.098	0.436
B15	0.150	0.074	0.253	0.147	0.059	0.314
B16	0.026	0.100	0.113	0.138	0.137	0.484
B17	0.057	0.100	0.159	0.204	0.029	0.448
B18	0.023	0.078	0.114	0.152	0.026	0.603
B19	0.058	0.266	0.099	0.122	0.080	0.374
B20	0.020	0.082	0.198	0.395	0.041	0.261

and 20 patients of known type B. The metabolites are of two distinct forms X and Y.

You are consulted by the clinic and asked three questions.

(a) Are the metabolite compositions of any diagnostic value and how should the metabolite information be used in any differential diagnosis of new patients?

(b) The Y-form metabolites are costly and time-consuming to separate and so it would be very helpful to know whether simply measuring the X-forms and the total Y-form would provide a reasonable differential diagnostic procedure. How would you answer this question?

(c) One clinician even conjectures that total X-form and total Y-form might prove sufficient for diagnostic purposes. What is your view of this conjecture?

Problem 9.2 Refer to problem 8.2. You have now been told that the diagnostic tests a-e are not precise but are subject to coefficients of variation of 5, 3, 10, 10 and 5 per cent, respectively. How does this information alter your report to the clinic?

Problem 9.3 Refer to Problem 8.3. Suppose that after you have submitted your report to the clinic it becomes obvious that there is some degree of imprecision in the determination of the three-part compositions. How would you go about eliciting the extent of such imprecision and how might you incorporate it into your modelling?

Problem 9.4 Clinic A has devised a differential diagnostic system between two disease types a and b based on four diagnostic blood tests I - IV conducted on 15 patients with known type a and 17 patients with known type b. The data (in standard units) on which the system has been based are set out in Table 9.7.

Clinic B is also engaged in this differential diagnosis problem and has collected similar data on its patients but is not yet in a position to construct its own diagnostic system. Moreover, while its methods of carrying out tests III and IV are identical with those of clinic A there is considerable doubt about the comparability of tests I and II with those of clinic A. To resolve this problem aliquots of 25 blood samples have been assigned to both clinics A and B for comparison of the results of tests I and II. The results of this calibrative experiment are set out in Table 9.8.

On the basis of all this information investigate the possibility of transferring clinic A's diagnostic system to the situation in clinic B, and prepare a full report of your findings for the two clinics.

Problem 9.5 Refer to Problem 9.4. Clinic C, which has developed an independent differential diagnostic system based on the data below, has contacted clinic A with a view to amalgamating their systems. Again only the methods of recording tests I and II are in doubt, and a calibrative experiment, similar to that between clinics A and B, has been conducted for clinics A and C with

Table 9.7 *Data for Problem 9.4*

Type a				Type b			
I	II	III	IV	I	II	III	IV
56	72	95	48	72	54	70	57
58	51	71	43	90	49	75	61
36	55	76	42	71	67	70	53
46	72	84	41	66	65	81	46
41	86	90	35	75	58	85	51
72	74	78	37	57	56	79	45
59	65	80	42	69	50	100	43
72	69	92	49	75	40	74	40
66	71	74	38	67	43	79	37
65	91	95	52	68	47	57	50
53	69	94	36	72	56	70	55
63	80	80	47	74	62	58	51
46	69	92	33	88	62	74	50
52	61	98	36	91	47	63	50
53	73	89	39	77	68	69	46
				56	65	67	63
				74	76	74	48

Table 9.8 *Data for Problem 9.4*

Clinic A		Clinic B		Clinic A		Clinic B	
I	II	I	II	I	II	I	II
56	95	62	82	98	75	107	76
94	67	106	63	73	48	84	44
95	75	107	77	65	61	73	59
75	69	85	64	72	65	79	65
73	70	78	70	82	72	90	73
91	65	100	65	84	80	98	74
75	68	83	66	82	53	93	48
76	81	89	76	74	67	80	63
95	75	107	71	70	62	76	60
83	55	91	51	92	62	102	58
100	73	111	67	105	74	117	72
72	98	74	95	104	85	110	77
74	69	76	68				

Table 9.9 *Diagnostic data for clinic C*

| | Type a | | | | Type b | | |
I	II	III	IV	I	II	III	IV
47	69	93	46	64	41	74	50
48	65	100	38	61	79	61	57
53	83	81	34	40	61	81	47
46	87	79	55	40	66	77	59
46	70	105	44	70	77	81	43
57	83	82	33	60	69	85	49
38	67	66	46	66	75	69	47
55	96	90	43	57	55	71	35
62	62	77	40	64	53	74	45
53	63	84	45	52	66	81	49
46	86	80	38	72	58	84	47
50	84	84	41	68	54	78	55
56	72	93	32				

the results recorded in Tables 9.9 and 9.10. You are asked to report to clinics A and C as to how they may use their combined data for a differential diagnostic system. Clinic B asks you to investigate whether this amalgamated data could be used to improve diagnosis within clinic B.

Table 9.10 *Calibrative data between clinics A and C*

| Clinic A | | Clinic C | | Clinic A | | Clinic C | |
I	II	I	II	I	II	I	II
77	76	72	82	82	62	73	67
53	79	44	82	57	58	52	61
61	58	51	61	34	81	33	83
55	70	49	72	53	84	49	85
68	67	62	69	80	74	74	80
82	63	71	66	56	67	51	72
44	96	38	100	61	67	53	65
67	67	62	71	58	62	50	66
53	62	48	65	63	75	54	78
74	79	66	82	48	78	42	83

Problem 9.6 A clinic faced with distinguishing between two forms A and B of a disease, only verifiable at post mortem, is attempting to define an 'expert system' based on 32 surviving cases. On the basis of assessments by all the available clinicians and on the results of four diagnostic tests the clinic has, for each case, placed consensus probabilities on forms A and B. These probabilities together with the diagnostic test results (in standard units) are recorded below.

Probabilities		Test results			
A	B	1	2	3	4
0.53	0.47	76	59	61	55
0.74	0.26	69	50	67	54
0.96	0.04	81	38	82	58
0.26	0.74	71	73	62	72
0.76	0.24	83	44	76	64
0.28	0.72	66	61	63	49
0.88	0.12	83	30	74	61
0.25	0.75	76	74	83	43
0.75	0.25	88	60	69	56
0.27	0.73	58	101	80	50
0.74	0.26	84	44	85	69
0.16	0.84	70	72	68	57
0.75	0.25	77	44	60	59
0.21	0.79	78	79	83	63
0.87	0.13	65	57	76	50
0.12	0.88	72	76	90	70
0.83	0.17	76	50	76	64
0.38	0.62	58	58	58	54
0.74	0.26	77	53	84	60
0.27	0.73	65	70	80	59
0.23	0.77	62	58	72	51
0.06	0.94	49	75	59	49
0.85	0.15	79	48	59	52
0.06	0.94	54	62	65	64
0.75	0.25	82	55	72	61
0.07	0.93	63	64	81	46
0.80	0.20	103	59	66	50
0.06	0.94	47	76	72	59
0.11	0.89	47	84	77	59
0.83	0.17	86	51	92	65
0.05	0.95	64	76	62	58
0.12	0.88	62	60	87	66

You have been asked to express your views on this diagnostic assessment system and report to the clinic.

Table 9.11 *Data for Problem 9.7*

	a1	a2	a3	c1	c2	c3	c4
Form A	1	1	1	9	6	70	15
	0	1	1	21	14	28	37
	0	1	1	21	13	28	38
	x	1	0	11	7	62	21
	0	0	1	11	8	58	23
	0	1	0	x	11	56	33
	0	0	1	11	7	62	20
	1	x	x	8	6	86	x
	0	1	1	16	10	38	36
	0	1	1	18	12	31	39
	1	1	1	6	4	80	10
	1	0	0	x	x	50	50
	0	1	x	21	14	14	51
	0	0	1	12	8	54	26
	0	0	1	19	13	28	40
	0	0	1	17	11	41	32
	0	0	1	20	12	34	33
	1	1	1	18	12	39	31
	0	1	1	11	8	58	23
	1	0	1	12	8	56	24
	1	1	0	18	13	34	35
	1	x	x	21	14	26	39
Form B	1	1	0	33	16	30	21
	1	0	0	36	16	19	29
	0	1	0	28	14	30	28
	1	1	0	39	18	12	30
	0	0	x	x	19	52	29
	1	0	0	28	15	33	24
	1	0	1	25	11	44	20
	1	0	0	19	15	47	19
	1	0	0	33	17	21	29
	0	0	1	30	16	24	30
	1	1	1	53	x	47	x
	0	1	0	25	13	40	21
	x	1	x	18	11	46	25
	1	0	0	24	12	38	27
	1	0	0	31	14	31	24
	1	1	1	21	11	49	19

Problem 9.7 In a diagnostic problem similar to that of Problem 1.5 a clinic has recorded similar binary and compositional data on 22 patients with form A and 16 patients with form B. Unfortunately there are missing data problems. For some patients some of the symptoms have not been elicited and for some of the compositions some parts have not been obtained, in which case only the subcompositions formed from the recorded parts are available. In the data reported in Table 9.11 an x denotes the missing items.

Investigate whether these data provide a means of constructing a reasonable differential diagnostic system.

CHAPTER 10

Prognosis and Treatment

10.1 Introduction

The role of diagnosis in clinical medicine can be regarded as a preliminary phase in which an attempt is made to discover the category or type of the subsequent decision problem of patient management that next faces the clinician. Our emphasis on this diagnostic phase has been conditioned not only by its obvious importance in current medical thinking but also because it is at present the best quantified phase of most medical problems. Let us now turn our attention to the complex of less well quantified concepts and actions which are usually considered under the headings of prognosis and treatment.

The main objective tool by which clinicians have attempted to compare and assess treatments is undoubtedly the controlled clinical trial. Since much has already been written and the concepts and practice of such trials are well known, together with the question of ethics and the relative effectiveness of sequential and fixed-size trials, we do not deal with the subject here. One general point concerning controlled clinical trials does however provide the motivation for our subsequent formulation of the decision problem, and we can here illustrate it by a simple example. Suppose that in a clinical trial to compare two treatments $t1$ and $t2$, 200 patients are allocated randomly, 100 to each treatment, that a check is made of the similarity of the composition of the two groups and that the usual double blind requirements of management of patients and assessment of treatment are met. Suppose that the results of the trial are as follows:

		Treatment	
		t_1	t_2
	Success	50	70
Outcome			
	Failure	50	30

The standard statistical analysis would then test the null hypothesis of no difference between the treatments by a standard chi-squared test. A significant difference between the treatments would thus be revealed and, if the sole criterion is to maximise the proportion of successful treatments, the accompanying recommendation would be that treatment t_2 should be used.

If we have to choose between using treatment t_1 for all patients and using treatment t_2 for all patients we may be convinced that treatment t_2 is to be preferred. But we may not have made fully effective use of all the information available. For example, consider the conceptual classification of patients into four mutually exclusive groups $g_{11}, g_{10}, g_{01}, g_{00}$, where the suffices i and j are assigned for each patient by the following criterion:

$i = 1$ if treatment t_1 would be successful with the patient, $= 0$ otherwise,

$j = 1$ if treatment t_2 would be successful with the patient, $= 0$ otherwise.

It is of course impossible to assign a patient to these groups but the concept allows us to make the following points. If $p(g_{ij})$ denotes the proportion of patients in group g_{ij} in the trial then the only restrictions determined by the results are:

$$p(g_{11}) + p(g_{10}) = 0.5$$
$$p(g_{11}) + p(g_{01}) = 0.7$$

It is clear that these can be satisfied by a number of specifications lying between two extremes:

$$p(g_{11}) = 0.5, \quad p(g_{10}) = 0, \quad p(g_{01}) = 0.2, \quad p(g_{00}) = 0.3$$

and

$$p(g_{11}) = 0.3, \quad p(g_{10}) = 0.2, \quad p(g_{01}) = 0.5, \quad p(g_{00}) = 0.$$

If the first configuration is the case then we cannot improve on the overall success rate 0.7 envisaged by the recommendation whereas if the second configuration is the case and if we could identify patients in the various groups we could clearly attain complete success with all patients. We ought therefore to investigate the patients in the four treatment response categories to discover whether there are any features that distinguish among them. For example if the distributions of gender (M and F) in the patients were as follows:

		Treatment	
		t_1	t_2
	Success	50F	50M & 20F
Outcome			
	Failure	50M	30F

then it would surely be sensible to consider allocating males to treatment t_2 and females to treatment t_1.

Thus we consider shifting the emphasis in clinical trials and consequently in prognosis from the customary question posed 'which treatment is best?' to 'which treatment is best for which patient?' In our illustrative example we see that for the latter question to be answerable we require to know for each patient in the clinical trial the triplet (v, t, s), where $v \in V$ denotes an observation on a set V of potentially useful indicating features (in our example, gender), where $t \in T$ denotes the treatment assigned in the trial, here t_1 or t_2, and $s \in S$ is an observation on a recognised set S of response features (here success or failure).

A clinical trial will have achieved its purpose if it provides us with a clear picture of the variability of s for given t and v. For this is simply the quantification of the medical concept of prognosis for a patient in 'present condition'

v if put on treatment t, a concept that is clearly necessary however implicitly it may remain in the formal decision process. To investigate its possible quantification we may consider some suitable parametric form labelled by the parameter $\delta \in \Delta$, say

$$p(s|t, v, \delta) \quad (s \in S),$$

for the prognosis distributions, and use the data

$$D = \{(v_i, t_i, s_i) : i = 1, \ldots, n\}$$

from the clinical trial to obtain, in the same kind of way as for the diagnostic assessment, the predictive forms of the prognosis distributions

$$p(s|t, v, D).$$

There have been some recent attempts to tackle this kind of problem quantitatively in an estimative rather than predictive way such that the statistical technique is indistinguishable from estimative diagnosis. An example of more sophisticated model-building is implicit in the discussion of prognosis and the effects of treatment is illustrated by an example. Suppose that plots of cumulative survival percentages against blood pressure for patients on different treatments support different straight line fits and suggest that the basic family of prognostic distributions, with s the logarithm of survival time and v a measure of current blood pressure, are well characterised by normal distributions with mean $\alpha_t + \beta_t v$ and variance σ_t^2. It is easy to visualise circumstances in which it will be desirable to give different treatments at different current blood pressure levels; for example, if the α_t are the same but the β_t are different.

The discussion on clinical trials in terms of which treatment for which patient and the stratification introduced typified by the above blood pressure example leads to the following formulation of the assessment of prognosis. The prognostic model may be written as

$$p(s|t, u, v)p(u|v),$$

where v is the feature vector of concomitant variables for the patient; u is the current status of the patient, for example disease type; t is the course of action to be considered, for example do nothing or assign a specific treatment; s is the measure of success or the prognostic index, for example, survival or death, survival time, or cure or no cure.

Thus we can identify two stages in the prognostic development.

1. Assessment of the patient status u given v through $p(u|v)$, the diagnostic stage.

2. Assessment of the prognostic distribution $p(s|t, u, v)$.

We see immediately that stage 1 is formally equivalent to the problem of differential diagnosis discussed in Chapters 8 and 9. The prognostic process may terminate at this stage as a straightforward risk analysis. At stage 2, which may indeed be the main aim of the investigation, modelling and assessment of $p(s|t, u, v)$ are required. In the blood pressure example u is blood pressure range and v is age and we obtain the separate estimates of the survival curves $p(s|u, v)$.

In the simplest cases $p(s|t, u, v)$ reduces to $p(s)$, the lifetime probability density function, which can be estimated by various methods. When covariates or concomitant variables v are observed along with different treatments our interest centres on $p(s|t, v)$.

10.2 A prognostic study of paediatric head injury

Before we investigate more complicated modelling of prognosis we report a straightforward application which involves the complete specification

$$p(s|t, u, v)p(u|v).$$

Table 10.1 gives the frequencies of the combinations of four binary variables observed in children who suffer from injury to the skull. The frequencies are given for two groups corresponding to different types of injury. For group one the injury is serious (haematoma or brain swelling) and hospitalised treatment is required. For group two the injury is not serious and hospitalisation is not necessary. In terms of our prognostic model we have

$$v = (v_1, v_2, v_3, v_4), \quad v_i = 1 \text{ or } 0, 1 \leq i \leq 4,$$

$u = 1$ (serious), $u = 2$ (not serious), $t =$ treatment ($\equiv$ action), to hospitalise ($t = 1$), or not ($t = 2$), and finally s is the measure for prognosis which may be summarised as

Prognosis	Good	Poor
$u = 1, t = 1, v$	$\checkmark$	
$u = 1, t = 2, v$		$\checkmark$
$u = 2, t = 1, v$	$\checkmark$ (but resources wasted)	
$u = 2, t = 2, v$	$\checkmark$	

In terms of our prognostic formulation, we require to allocate to treatment $t = 1$ for large values of the likelihood ratio $\lambda_v = \mathrm{pr}(u = 1|v)/\mathrm{pr}(u = 2|v)$. The problem of determining the cut-off point λ such that allocation is to $t = 1$ for $\lambda_v \geq \lambda$ depends on the sampling and selection of the data set.

For random sampling ($p(u), p(v|u)$ observed), or selected sampling ($p(v|u)$ only observed), the rule can be based on the magnitudes of $p(V_\lambda|u = 2)$, and $p(V_\lambda^*|u = 1)$ or the odds ratio

$$\frac{\mathrm{pr}(u = 1|V_\lambda)}{\mathrm{pr}(u = 2|V_\lambda)} \bigg/ \frac{\mathrm{pr}(u = 1|V_\lambda^*)}{\mathrm{pr}(u = 2|V_\lambda^*)} ,$$

where

$$V_\lambda = \{v : \frac{\mathrm{pr}(u = 1|v)}{\mathrm{pr}(u = 2|v)} \geq \lambda\}.$$

The suggested cut-off point in Table 10.1 is based on this form of argument. Note that for random sampling $\mathrm{pr}(u = 2|V_\lambda) = 0.55$, which could be regarded

Table 10.1 *Paediatric head injury*

(1)	(2)	(3)	(4)=$\frac{(2)}{159}$	(5) =$\frac{(3)}{9691}$	(6)	(7)	(8)
	Frequency					Cumulative	
ISEV	A+B	C+D	Relative Frequency		Ratio $\frac{(4)}{(5)}$	relative frequency	
	(t=1)	(t=2)	A+B	C+D	= λ_x	A+B	C+D
1111	6	3	.03774	.00031	122.000	.03774	.00031
1110	7	5	.00403	.00052	85.300	.08177	.00083
1101	28	22	.17610	.00227	77.600	.25787	.00310
1100	46	16	.28931	.00165	175.000	.54718	.00475
1011	2	7	.01258	.00072	17.400	.55976	.00547
1010	7	9	.04403	.00093	47.400	.60379	.00640
0111	1	3	.00629	.00031	20.300	.61008	.00671
0101	9	12	.05660	.00124	45.700	.66668	.00795
0110	1	4	.00629	.00041	15.200	.67297	.00836
1001	12	69	.07547	.00712	10.600	.74844	.01548
1000	22	89	.13836	.00918	15.100	.88680	.02466
0100	10	58	.06289	.00598	10.500	.94969	.03064
0011	1	11	.00629	.00114	5.500	.95598	.03178
.....	.....	.....	....	....	....	....	....
0001	3	4241	.01887	.43762	0.043	.97485	.46940
0010	0	40	.00000	.00413	0.000	.97485	.47353
0000	4	5102	.02516	.52647	0.048	1.00000	1.00000
	159	9691					

I: impaired consciousness	A: haematoma
S: skull fracture	B: brain swelling
E: epilepsy	C: groups II, III, IV
V: vomiting	$\cdots$: Proposed value for λ defining
	X_λ above the line
1: symptom present	
0: symptom absent	

as a high wastage rate, but is unavoidable under this decision structure given the incidence rates $p(u)$. For sampling with selection on v,

$$\mathrm{pr}(u = 1|v)/\mathrm{pr}(u = 2|v)$$

is stable, but the odds-ratio is not estimable, and the decision has to be based somewhat arbitrarily on the relative magnitudes of the λ_u.

It is interesting to note that these data are complete in terms of the complete sample space V being observed. If not all values are observed, the following are possibilities.

(i) For natural or separate sampling, form kernel density estimates of the $p(v|u)$ and proceed as before for complete data.

(ii) For v–selected data, proceed to the logistic formulation, compute the λ_v in estimative/predictive fashion and proceed as for complete selected data.

10.3 Prognosis and cervical cancer

In the hope of improving the survival prospects for patients who have cancer of the uterus, a trial was conducted to compare the efficacy of two treatments: treatment A, in which patients were treated in a hyperbaric oxygen chamber as well as receiving radiotherapy, and treatment B which consisted of radiotherapy alone. The data are available in data set `cancer`.

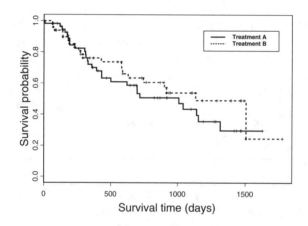

Figure 10.1 *Kaplan-Meier estimates of survival probability under treatments A and B.*

Each patient was randomly allocated to receive treatment A or treatment B. The survival time (in days) was recorded, with the survival times of patients who were lost to follow-up or who were still alive at the end of the study being right-censored. No information is available on relevant factors or covariates. Kaplan-Meier estimates of the survival functions are given in Figure 10.1. For survival times in the range 300-1500 days treatment B shows a higher survival probability than treatment A. Applying the log-rank test (chi-squared = 0.8, P=0.37) shows that this observed difference in survival probability over time is not statistically significant. Thus the hoped-for improved prognosis of patients on treatment A is not realised and so patients would be expected to have a similar prognosis on either of the treatments. An estimated survival curve, with pointwise confidence intervals, is given in Figure 10.2 and is based on the pooled data. Hence the prognosis of each patient within previous experience could be summarised as follows: the probability of survival falls fairly rapidly over time and it is estimated that patients have a 67% chance (56% to 76%) of surviving 500 days, a 50% chance (39% to 61%) of surviving 1000 days and only a 26% chance (0.08% to 49%) of surviving 1500 days. Without relevant factors or covariates it is not possible to make more specific conclusions for a given referred patient.

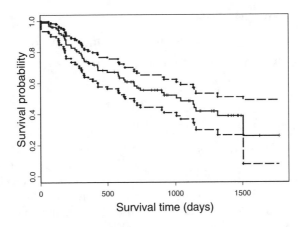

Figure 10.2 *Estimated survival curve and pointwise 95% confidence intervals based on the pooled survival data.*

10.4 Kidney function

A nephrologist is interested in the possible relationship of the dosage of a new drug NEP required to stabilise kidney function in a certain group of patients to certain measurable concentrations in each patient. Data are available in data set **kidney** from each of a selected set of patients with regard to sex, creatinine, cholesterol and triglyceride concentrations, the stabilising dose of NEP and the absence/presence of side effects. The measurements are given in standard units. The nephrologist is interested in two questions, namely (a) to what extent may it be possible to predict the stabilising dose of NEP for a patient from information on sex and the creatinine, cholesterol and triglyceride concentrations? and (b) to what extent is the incidence of side effects dependent on sex, triglyceride and stabilising dosage? In particular, the nephrologist has just examined a female patient and creatinine, cholesterol and triglyceride concentrations of 2.50, 300 and 120 were recorded; what may be said about her stabilising dose of NEP and what is the chance that there may be some side effect?

10.4.1 Prediction of NEP dose

Several linear models were fitted to the data, with NEP dosage as the response variable and the other variables apart from side-effects as the explanatory variables. The triglyceride concentrations were logged. We denote the observations obtained from the ith patient by v_i, u_{1i}, u_{2i}, u_{3i} and u_{4i}, representing the values of sex, creatinine, cholesterol and log(triglyceride), respectively. We assume that

$$v_i | u \sim N(\theta_i, \sigma^2)$$

and consider the maximal model

$$M_3: \qquad \theta_i = \mu + \alpha u_{1i} + \beta_1 u_{2i} + \beta_2 u_{3i} + \beta_3 u_{4i} + \beta_{11} u_{1i} u_2 + \beta_{21} u_{1i} u_{3i} + \beta_{31} u_{1i} u_{4i}.$$

We present details of only three of the possible hypotheses as follows:

$$M_0: \qquad \alpha = \beta_1 = \beta_2 = \beta_3 = \beta_{11} = \beta_{21} = \beta_{31} = 0,$$
$$M_1: \qquad \alpha = \beta_{11} = \beta_{21} = \beta_{31} = 0,$$
$$M_2: \qquad \beta_{11} = \beta_{21} = \beta_{31} = 0.$$

The details of the formal comparisons of the hypotheses M_0, M_1 and M_2 with the maximal model M_3 are given in Table 10.2. The simplest model which is not rejected is model M_1 and we adopt this as our working model, even though the slope parameter for cholesterol is not significantly different from zero, but it is borderline. Hence we use the measurements creatinine, cholesterol and log(triglyceride) to predict NEP dosage.

Table 10.2 *Tests of some hypotheses within the maximal model M_3 on the basis of standard F tests*

Model	Residual sum of squares	Residual d.f.	TS	P
M_3	120.9	50		
M_2	125.6	53	0.65	0.58
M_1	129.7	54	0.91	0.47
M_0	189.4	57	4.05	0.001

On the basis of model M_1 we then produce a 95% prediction interval for the stabilising dose in the referred patient. It is 4.91 ± 3.25 units. This is a wide interval, reflecting the substantial conditional variability in the NEP dosage in the data, and thus there is a large uncertainty attached to predictions of NEP dosage using the model.

10.4.2 Incidence of side effects

We consider logistic regression models, with incidence of side effects as the response variable and sex, log(triglyceride) concentration and dosage of NEP as explanatory variables. Let v_i denote the side effects indicator variable and u_{1i}, u_{2i} and u_{3i} denote, respectively, the sex, log(triglyceride) and NEP dosage for the ith patient. Then the maximal model is

$$v_i | u \sim Bi(1, \theta_i),$$

where

$$M_3: \qquad \text{logit}(\theta_i) = \mu + \alpha u_{i1} + \beta_1 u_{2i} + \beta_2 u_{3i} + \beta_{11} u_{1i} u_{2i} + \beta_{21} u_{1i} u_{3i}.$$

We present details of only three of the possible hypotheses as follows:

$$M_0: \qquad \alpha = \beta_1 = \beta_2 = \beta_{11} = \beta_{21} = 0,$$
$$M_1: \qquad \beta_{11} = \beta_{21} = 0,$$
$$M_2: \qquad \beta_{11} = 0.$$

The details of the formal tests of the hypotheses M_0, M_1 and M_2 within the maximal model M_3 are given in Table 10.3. The simplest model which is not rejected is model M_1, but it is borderline, and we adopt model M_2 as our working model. Therefore we use the variables sex, log(triglyceride), NEP dosage and an interaction between sex and NEP dosage to predict the incidence of side effects.

Table 10.3 *Tests of some hypotheses within the maximal model M_3 on the basis of asymptotic likelihood ratio tests*

Model	Residual deviance	Residual d.f.	TS(d.f.)	P
M_3	47.66	52		
M_2	47.99	53	0.33(1)	0.57
M_1	53.18	54	5.52(2)	0.06
M_0	80.13	57	32.47(5)	5×10^{-6}

Using model M_2, and taking the predicted value of 4.91 as the NEP dosage for this patient, we then conclude that for the referred patient the estimated chance of her experiencing a side effect is 55%, and a 95% confidence interval for the true chance is 21% to 85%.

10.5 Cutaneous malignant melanoma

Details of melanoma patients were drawn from the records of the West of Scotland section of the Scottish Melanoma Group, which records details of all patients presenting with primary cutaneous malignant melanoma (CMM) in Scotland, and are given in data set `malmel`. A total of 4332 patients, diagnosed as having invasive primary cutaneous malignant melanoma, were identified starting in 1979 and followed up until December 31st 1998. During this period there were 971 deaths due to CMM, 672 deaths due to other causes and 2775 patients were still alive. The survival times of patients in the last two categories were taken as censored. The effects of five factors – deprivation status, Breslow thickness, age group, histogenetic type and sex – are of interest and this information was recorded at the initial presentation. The method of Carstairs and Morris was used to determine a deprivation 'score' for each patient, giving seven categories from the most affluent (1) to the most deprived (7). There were five histogenetic types, type 1 to type 5, which are superficial spreading melanoma, nodular/polyploid, lentigo maligna melanoma, acral/mucosal and other/unspecified. Ages were grouped into six categories: <35, 35-44, 45-54, 55-64, 65-74 and >75 years. The Breslow factor had six categories: the first five were defined in terms of the thickness of the tumour, namely <1.5, 1.5-2.49, 2.5-3.49, 3.5-4.99 and >5.0, in millimetres, while the sixth category indicated the presence of stage 2 spreading of the tumour. In the statistical analysis these variables are treated as being of categorical type.

We will investigate two aspects of prognosis in this study: given an individual referred patient who presents with primary CMM and a given profile of the five factors, (a) what are his or her chances of surviving five years? and (b) what are his or her survival prospects in the future?

10.5.1 Five-year survival

In investigating the issue of five-year survival we consider only patients who presented before the end of 1993 in order that the five-year survival status of each patient is known. Thus, data from 2938 patients were utilised and are available in data set `mel5`. We consider a binary logistic regression model in which the five-year status u_i is the response variable and the five factors: deprivation, thickness, age, type and sex, denoted in order by v_1, v_2, v_3, v_4, v_5, are the explanatory factors. Therefore we assume that, conditional on the five-factor combination $pqrst$, the five-year status of the ith patient is u_i, with

$$u_i|v \sim Bi(1, \theta_{pqrst})$$

where θ_{pqrst} is the conditional probability that a patient is alive five years on from initial presentation. Given that there are many possible factor combinations we take the model containing all two-way factor interactions

$$M_4: \quad \text{logit}(\theta_{pqrst}) = \mu + \alpha_p + \beta_q + \gamma_r + \delta_s + \epsilon_t + (\alpha_p\beta_q) + (\alpha_p\gamma_r) + (\alpha_p\delta_s) + (\alpha_p\epsilon_t) + (\beta_q\gamma_r) + (\beta_q\delta_s) + (\beta_q\epsilon_t) + (\gamma_r\delta_s) + (\gamma_r\epsilon_t) + (\delta_s\epsilon_t),$$

subject to corner-point constraints, as a feasible maximal model. There is a large number of possible sub-models in the full lattice and we present results only for the following:

$$
\begin{aligned}
M_0 &: & \mathrm{logit}(\theta_{pqrst}) &= \mu, \\
M_1 &: & \mathrm{logit}(\theta_{pqrst}) &= \mu + \beta_q + \gamma_r + \delta_s + \epsilon_t, \\
M_2 &: & \mathrm{logit}(\theta_{pqrst}) &= \mu + \alpha_p + \beta_q + \gamma_r + \delta_s + \epsilon_t, \\
M_3 &: & \mathrm{logit}(\theta_{pqrst}) &= \mu + \beta_q + \gamma_r + \delta_s + \epsilon_t + (\beta_q\gamma_r).
\end{aligned}
$$

The details of the formal comparisons of the sub-models M_0, M_1, M_2 and M_3 within the maximal model M_4 are given in Table 10.4. The simplest model which is not rejected is model M_3 and we adopt this as our working model.

Table 10.4 *Comparison of some sub-models with the maximal model M_4 on the basis of asymptotic likelihood ratio tests*

Model	Residual deviance	Residual d.f.	TS(df)	P
M_4	2533	2747		
M_3	2704	2897	172(150)	0.11
M_2	2751	2916	218(169)	0.01
M_1	2759	2922	227(175)	0.01
M_0	3708	2937	1176(190)	$< 10^{-7}$

We will use the model as a basis of assessing the chances of five-year survival for some individual patients. Before proceeding it is useful to consider how good this model is likely to be if used to estimate five-year survival status. In order to investigate this matter the data were split randomly into training and test sets of size 1938 and 1000 respectively. The model M_3 was fitted to the training data and then used to estimate the five-year survival status of the 1000 patients in the test set. The status of each patient was computed using the Bayes classifier. Overall, the estimated classification accuracy was 76%, and 87% of patients who survived five years were correctly predicted to survive five years, but only 52% of those who died within five years were correctly classified. Thus, if used to predict the five-year survival status the procedure has fairly good specificity but disappointing sensitivity.

We now consider the prognosis of four referred patients whose case information is given in Table 10.5 together with the estimated odds of survival beyond five years. Thus in terms of five-year survival the prognosis for patient N1 looks good with strong odds in favour, but with odds in favour for patient N4 being less convincing. Unfortunately the prognosis for patient N2 does not look good, with clear odds against, and patient N3 has a 50-50 chance of surviving five years. We now turn our attention to the more general matter of the survival prospects of these patients in the future.

Table 10.5 *Odds of five-year survival for four referred patients with given combinations of factors*

Patient	Deprivation	Breslow thickness	Age group	Type	Sex	Odds
N1	most affluent	<1mm	<35 yrs	acral/ mucosal	female	19 to 1 for
N2	most affluent	stage 2	65-74 yrs	acral/ mucosal	male	6 to 1 against
N3	most affluent	stage 2	<35 yrs	acral/ mucosal	female	1.1 to 1 against
N4	most deprived	< 1mm	65-74 yrs	SSM	male	3 to 1 for

10.5.2 Survival prospects

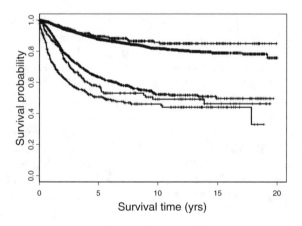

Figure 10.3 *Kaplan-Meier estimates of the survival function for the different histological types. The curves are ordered from highest to lowest as type 3, type 1, type 2, type 4 and type 5.*

We consider the survival of the patients with CMM over time and we use the data from all 4332 patients. Kaplan-Meier plots of survival probability

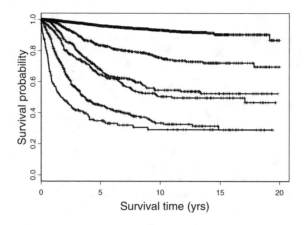

Figure 10.4 *Kaplan-Meier estimates of the survival function for the different cate-gories of Breslow thickness. The curves are generally ordered from highest to lowest according to increasing thickness of the tumour, with the stage 2 curve the lowest.*

against time are given in Figures 10.3 and 10.4 for the different histological types and different Breslow categories, respectively.

Patients of histological type 3 have good survival prospects, closely followed by those of type 1. The patients with the other three types have notably poorer prospects, with the survival probability falling more steeply initially and then flattening out at about 50%. Patients with tumours less than 1.5 mm thick have the best survival prospects, followed by those whose tumours are between 1.5 and 2.5 mm thick. The survival probability over time continues to be smaller as the thickness of the tumour increases. If the tumour is more than 5 mm thick or the patient is in stage 2 then the chance of survival falls markedly in the time period 0-5 years and then flattens out at about 30%.

The other factors also influence the survival function. Females have a higher chance of survival over time than males. The most affluent patients have a notably higher chance of survival over time than the other deprivation groups and the survival curves are lower as the deprivation level increases.

Cox proportional hazard models were fitted to the data. We take as a feasible maximal model

$$M_2: \quad \log \frac{h(t|v)}{h_0(t)} = \mu + \alpha_p + \beta_q + \gamma_r + \delta_s + \epsilon_t + (\beta_q \gamma_r).$$

Here $h(t|v)$ denotes the instantaneous hazard function at time t given that the factors in v have levels p, q, r, s and t and $h_0(t)$ is the baseline hazard function. As usual, the parameters are subject to corner-point constraints. The model contains main effects for all five factors as well as an interaction between the

Table 10.6 *Comparison of some sub-models with the maximal model M_2 on the basis of asymptotic partial likelihood ratio tests*

Model	Residual deviance	Residual d.f.	TS(df)	P
M_2	13454	4286		
M_1	13515	4311	61 (25)	$< 10^{-4}$
M_0	14691	4332	1237(46)	$< 10^{-7}$

factors Age group and Breslow thickness. More complicated models were also considered but this resulted in problems due to suspected over-fitting caused by the sparsity of data in some combinations of the factors.

There are many sub-models but we present results here for only the following:

$$M_0 : \quad \log \frac{h(t|v)}{h_0(t)} \;=\; \mu,$$

$$M_1 : \quad \log \frac{h(t|v)}{h_0(t)} \;=\; \mu + \alpha_p + \beta_q + \gamma_r + \delta_s + \epsilon_t.$$

The details of the formal comparisons of the sub-models M_0 and M_1 within the maximal model M_2 are given in Table 10.6. Both of the simpler models are rejected and so we adopt model M_2 as our working model.

We now consider the survival prognosis of the four referred patients considered in Table 10.4. Their estimated survival curves are given in Figure 10.5. Patient N1 is female, is less than 35, is in the most affluent category, has the smallest thickness category of tumour and is of histological type 4. Her prognosis is very good with a high chance of survival over a 20 year period. Patients N2 is male, is aged 65-74, is in the most affluent deprivation category but is of histological type 4 and has stage 2 secondary spreading of his tumour. His prognosis is therefore not too good, with rapidly decreasing survival probability in the first five years which remains less than 30% afterwards. Patient N3 is female, less than 35, is in the most affluent category, but like patient N2 she has histological type 4 and stage 2 spreading. Her prognosis is a little better than that of patient N2. Patient N4 is male, is aged 65-74, is in the most deprived category, has histological type 1 and has the smallest category of thickness of tumour. His prognosis is good with a probability of survival that is likely to be above 80% over a 20 year period.

10.6 Bibliographic notes

The statistical methods of this chapter depend largely on the theoretical ideas set out in Chapters 2, 3 and 4 and few additional references are necessary. Most

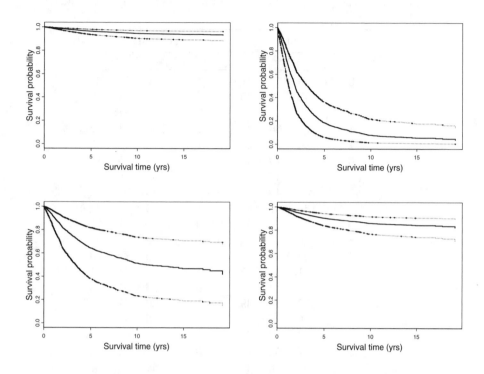

Figure 10.5 *Estimated survival curves, with 95% pointwise confidence intervals, for the referred patients N1 (top left), N2 (top right), N3 (bottom left)and N4 (bottom right).*

of the statistical analysis were performed as routine consultation within our universities and remained unreported in the literature. For further details of the techniques of survival analysis used in Section 10.3 and 10.5 see Collett (2003b).

For further discussion of the important current problem of cutaneous malignant melanoma, see

http://www.ehendrick.org/healthy/melanoma.

For further information on the method of Carstairs and Morris see

http://datalib.ed.ac.uk/EUDL/carstairs.html.

10.7 Problems

Problem 10.1 A clinic believes that three measurements may indicate which of two treatments 1 and 2 would best suit particular patients. To test this hypothesis the clinic has allocated 50 patients at random, 25 to each treatment. The success (1), failure (0) pattern and the indicants are set out below. You are asked to investigate the clinic's hypothesis and make recommendations about the use of the indicants.

Treatment 1				Treatment 2			
Outcome	Indicants			Outcome	Indicants		
0	40	42	21	1	36	70	21
0	52	63	30	1	26	74	19
1	39	52	14	0	65	61	35
1	44	66	34	1	50	51	42
1	26	73	20	1	20	46	26
0	35	79	50	1	39	75	17
1	37	46	37	0	58	56	36
1	51	45	23	1	45	51	42
1	35	67	48	1	44	71	34
0	41	44	30	0	45	67	37
1	40	51	24	1	39	53	41
1	34	61	21	1	30	72	23
0	51	51	35	1	48	61	31
1	54	65	34	0	63	51	35
1	43	49	39	1	26	37	25
0	46	65	33	1	43	45	30
0	47	49	33	1	46	50	32
1	27	52	14	0	50	71	44
0	53	78	26	1	41	61	18
1	20	67	20	1	47	60	25
1	30	62	43	1	61	41	31
0	34	54	11	0	41	42	27
1	44	53	21	1	26	74	18
1	43	73	27	1	23	76	11
1	34	53	26	1	32	54	26

Problem 10.2 A thyroid clinic is attempting to determine effective doses of a new drug for the treatment of under-active thyroid gland. There is a conjecture that the effective dose of the drug may depend on three indicant measurements of thyroid activity i1, i2, i3. In a study of 18 female and 20 male patients for whom these indicants have been measured the eventual effective dose has been recorded. The table below gives complete details of the study.

Females				Males			
Indicants			Effective	Indicants			Effective
i1	i2	i3	dose	i1	i2	i3	dose
51	208	150	178	73	177	168	347
42	210	331	410	51	239	356	566
33	235	589	619	77	150	241	401
61	180	193	266	72	197	114	333
65	190	262	351	82	119	49	170
52	169	249	257	71	171	205	381
39	203	457	503	72	194	384	519
74	163	138	209	64	210	487	788
46	217	326	409	60	259	350	683
59	146	184	308	67	189	137	242
49	170	280	344	85	128	221	276
63	188	339	397	88	106	210	329
53	231	309	364	57	211	323	488
45	266	338	350	74	192	274	409
51	215	221	205	70	144	101	310
49	206	179	243	71	168	132	273
64	210	280	322	78	79	277	312
57	210	317	395	60	237	307	561
60	232	185	387				
73	196	237	384				

You have been asked to investigate the extent, if any, that effect dose depends on the indicants and on gender.

The clinic has two new patients, a woman with indicants 35, 243, 347 and a man with indicants 74, 182, 422. What would your recommendation be for treatment of these two patients?

Problem 10.3 Refer to Problem 1.4 and provide a report to the clinic on the effectiveness of the two treatments.

Problem 10.4 Reconsider the melanoma study from Section 10.5. What are the survival prospects for a 70 year-old female who is most deprived, has a Breslow thickness of < 1 mm and is of histogenetic type acral/mucosal?

Problem 10.5 In a clinical trial comparing the success rates of two treatments for a particular ailment for which there is no existing treatment, treatment 1 has 65 successes and 87 failures, while treatment 2 has 90 successes and 63 failures. What conclusion would you reach about the value of these two treatments? You are subsequently given access to patient files and you discover that there are two possible indicants of treatment, each recorded as either high H or low L. On classifying the patients into categories HH, HL, LH, LL you can reset the data in the following format.

Treatment 1

	Patient category			
	HH	HL	LH	LL
Success	35	18	7	5
Failure	10	10	34	33

Treatment 2

	Patient category			
	HH	HL	LH	LL
Success	15	10	35	30
Failure	20	18	13	12

Would your report to the clinic now change in view of this additional information?

CHAPTER 11

Assessment

11.1 Introduction

In all the previous chapters we have been concerned with how statistical concepts, principles and analysis may be applied to a great variety of problems in clinical medicine, both in practice and research. It is, however, still true to say that in clinical practice the majority of the inferences and decisions made are not processed through any prescriptive statistical system but are in fact the intuitive or 'reasoned' judgements of clinicians, radiologists, steroid chemists, laboratory technicians, etc. In cases where there are prescriptive statistical methods such as in diagnosis, where there may be eventually a true assessment for a case, it is of interest to ask to what extent the clinician's judgement diverges from the normative assessment. This is an extension of the idea of observer error studied in Chapter 6. There we were concerned with the quality of the observation; here we are concerned with the much more complex problem of comparing inferences or decisions. Such studies are currently popular in clinical medicine, and we shall examine a number of studies of different types in diagnosis, prognosis, in calibration and assay and in treatment allocation. The general structure of such performance analysis is discussed in Section 11.2. We have found that such analyses have a considerable educational impact and comparisons of different groups of subjects can be very illuminating.

There are many areas in medicine where no inference made or action taken could be described as invalid since no absolute normative model can reasonably be postulated nor can we hope to elicit sufficient information from the decision-maker to formulate a personal normative model against which to make comparisons. Inference or action is then essentially a matter of opinion. At first sight it is not at all obvious that statistical analysis could possibly have a contribution to make in this area. The technique, however, of performance simulation analysis can often throw considerable light on how the clinician may be making inferences or decisions. Reporting back this information and comparing the simulation analysis of different clinicians can bring to light inconsistencies and discrepancies which hopefully may lead to more reasoned and better clinical practice.

Assessment of performance falls naturally into two possible categories.

(1) Assessment of performance on inferential tasks.
(2) Assessment of performance on decision tasks.

Inferential tasks involve assessing the relative probabilities of several outcomes, for example in differential diagnosis, while decision tasks relate to choice of a course of action from several possibilities, for example in treatment assessment the choice between medication and surgery.

When it is possible to formulate a rational model according to which a subject with the given information ought to be making inferences then we can compare the subject's actual conclusions with the corresponding normative inference. Radical differences between subjective and normative inferences have been recorded in a number of studies. Many of these studies have been conducted in artificial situations, subjects typically being presented with inferences about urns of different compositions with small monetary rewards for correct inferences. Despite all attempts at realism these must suffer from the criticism that the subjects are making their inferences or decisions outside the natural environment of their real-life problems. In the examples we shall study here we try to avoid this artificiality by taking as subjects clinicians making sequential inferences in a diagnostic situation with which they are familiar

There may not be sufficient understanding of the inferential process to allow the statistician to construct a normative model so that subjects may rightly claim that their inferences are as valid as any other. For example, classification of certain psychiatric conditions may be a matter of subjective opinion. In such circumstances it may still be possible to make useful analyses of a subject's performance. We shall consider this situation in terms of category 2 above, studies of decision-making performance, and show how the construction of performance simulation models can give insights into the consistency of the subject and provide possible explanations of inferential behaviour.

Theory will be developed to analyse within and between observer variability in performance for both (1) and (2). Practical examples will be presented along with simulated ones to demonstrate the usefulness and relevance of the latter method in this area. A special aspect that will also be investigated is the extent to which all the information available is utilized by each subject and how this varies between subjects.

11.2 Inferential tasks, statements and trials

11.2.1 Inferential tasks

In an inferential task (such as medical diagnosis or antibiotic assay) a subject (clinician, biochemist) is presented with a case (patient, blood sample) for which an inferential statement (diagnostic assessment, assessment of antibiotic concentration) concerning the true index (true disease type, true concentration of antibiotic) is required. The subject is aware that the case has associated with it a unique but unknown index belonging to a known index set U (set of feasible diseases, assumed or defined to be mutually exclusive; range of possible concentrations). To help the subject arrive at an inferential statement for a particular case the subject has available information concerning the case, data on a number of features (results of diagnostic tests, clearance circle diameters) which can thus be regarded as a feature vector in some defined feature space V.

Inferential statements may take many different forms but we shall confine attention to studies whereby the subject can be induced to make a probabilistic statement about the unknown true index.

11.2.2 Previous experience and training sets

The subject will normally have some training and experience in the kind of inferential task under study, and this is seldom quantifiable. Examples again are clinicians and biochemists with skills in diagnosis and assay. But inferential tasks can be selected so that the relevant experience and training is under the control of the experimenter, and hence quantifiable. Where diagnostic tests unfamiliar to the clinician have been evolved the subject can be presented with information on the complete training set of cases whose diagnoses and test results are known. In antibiotic assay a training set is an essential ingredient of the task: since clearance diameter is known to vary from batch to batch of infected medium, it is essential for the subject to know the concentrations and clearance diameters of a training set of cases, often referred to in assay work as 'the standards'.

We write D to denote the training set of n cases for each of which the true index and feature vector are known. In some cases this training set is effectively infinite, as for example in the Doctor's Trilemma example of Section 11.7.1, and then alternative simpler ways of presenting D can be used.

11.2.3 Inferential trials

In an inferential trial a subject S is presented with a test set of n unrelated or independent cases and on the basis of their feature vectors $v_1, \ldots, v_n$ is asked to make inferential statements about their unknown indices $u_1, \ldots, u_n$. As indicated earlier we concentrate on inferential statements that require the subject to provide density functions, say $s_1, \ldots, s_n$ on U, for the n test cases. The performance data thus consist of the set

$$\{(v_i, s_i) : i = 1, \ldots, n\}.$$

11.3 Measures of normative comparison

11.3.1 Normative model and system

In situations where a normative model can be specified standard statistical procedures can be applied to use the data D of the training set to obtain a fitted model or normative system which can be applied to the cases of a test set to produce inferential statements about these cases. The technical statistical details of the construction of the normative system need not concern us here until we consider specific areas of study. A normative system can thus be expressed in the form of a conditional density function $p(u|v, D)$ over U for a test case with feature vector v.

When the normative system is applied to the feature vectors $v_1, \ldots, v_n$ of the test set it produces normative statements, say $r_1, \ldots, r_n$, corresponding to the subject's inferential statements $s_1, \ldots, s_n$.

11.3.2 Nature of comparisons

Comparison of how a subject's performance departs from normative performance thus requires the construction of measures of the extent of the statements s_i from the normative statements r_i $(i = 1, \ldots, n)$. In the tasks so far defined we have considered the feature vector information being supplied in one piece and there being a single final inferential statement. Later we shall consider tasks where the feature vector information is supplied in sequence to the subject with the requirement that an inferential statement is supplied after each step in the sequence. In such circumstances when considering a typical step we shall have information about the probabilities assigned to the unknown index before as well as after the feature information is released. To deal with this at the present stage of our discussion we therefore suppose that for each case i the subject makes a composite inference statement q_i prior to receiving the feature vector v_i for the ith case $(i = 1, \ldots, n)$.

For a single test case therefore we have to suppose that there is a prior composite inferential statement $q(u)$ on U, that on the basis of knowledge of the feature vector v for the case we have to compare the subsequent inferential statement $s(u)$ on U with the corresponding normative inferential statement $r(u)$ on U.

11.3.3 Measures of performance

Degree of uncertainty

Associated with any composite inferential statement, say $q(u)$ on U, there is a degree of uncertainty $H\{q(u)\}$ or $H(q)$ remaining in the identification of the true index:

$$H(q) = -\sum_U q(u) \log q(u) \quad \text{or} \quad -\int_U q(u) \log q(u) du,$$

where $q(u) \log q(u) = 0$ if $q(u) = 0$.

Inference discrepancy

Since the subject records an inferential statement $s(u)$ on U which, according to the normative system, should be $r(u)$ on U we require, in order to assess the subject's ability in inference, a measure of the difference between $s(u)$ and the target $r(u)$. This is provided by an information theory measure, the Kullback-Liebler directed divergence measure:

$$I(r, s) = \sum_U r(u) \log \frac{r(u)}{s(u)} \quad \text{or} \quad \int_U r(u) \log \frac{r(u)}{s(u)} du,$$

with the property that $I(r, s)$ is always non-negative and equal to zero if, and only if, $s = r$.

Information gain index

We can quantify such notions as 'underusing the information available', 'reading too much into the data', 'going contrary to the data' in terms of an information gain index $G(q, r, s)$. Suppose that $H(q) > H(r)$ so that the normative system has removed $H(q) - H(r)$ of uncertainty or equivalently gained this amount of information about the index. The subject on the other hand has gained an amount $H(q) - H(s)$ of information in the move from q to s. Consider now the ratio

$$G(q, r, s) = \frac{H(q) - H(s)}{H(q) - H(r)}.$$

If $G(q, r, s) > 1$ then the subject has removed more uncertainty than the normative move and so can be said to be acting liberally or reading too much into the data. If $0 < G(q, r, s) < 1$ then the subject is acting conservatively or underusing the data. If $G(q, r, s) < 0$ then the subject is increasing the uncertainty when it ought to be being reduced and so the subject is running contrary to the evidence.

The same kind of argument applies to $G(q, r, s)$ when $H(q) - H(r) < 0$. Hence we can use the information gain index $G(q, r, s)$ to determine whether a subject's interpretation of the information is liberal $(G > 1)$, conservative $(0 < G < 1)$ or contrary $(G < 0)$.

Feature selection discrepancy

In a number of inferential problems the subject may be faced not only with problems of updating an inferential statement on the basis of the observed feature vector v, but also that of selecting which feature from a set of alternatives should be chosen. For example, in diagnosis the clinician would almost certainly have to choose which of a number of diagnostic tests should be carried out.

Suppose that from a starting density function $p(u)$ on U any one of a set F of features is available. Consider the choice $f \in F$. If outcome v is observed and leads to a normative posterior assessment $p(u|v)$ then the reduction in uncertainty or gain in information is $H\{p(u)\} - H\{p(u|v)\}$. In comparing the relative merits of different feature selections we do not know the outcome v and so we have to measure the merit of f in terms of the expected gain of information for f from the starting density $p(u)$:

$$K\{f, p(u)\} = \int_V [H\{p(u)\} - H\{p(u|v)\}] \, p(v).$$

The larger this is the more informative the feature is and so a normative choice $f^* \in F$ is obtained as

$$f^* = \arg \max_F K\{f, p(u)\}.$$

Note that f^* depends on $p(u)$: what is an optimum choice from one $p(u)$

may be poor from some other starting position. If a subject, at a declared assessment $p(u)$ and faced with a choice of feature, chooses f then the amount by which the expected gain of information falls short of the expected gain of information from the optimum f^* gives a measure

$$K\{f^*, p(u)\} - K\{f, p(u)\}$$

of the subject's inability to select the most informative feature. The subject, however, cannot do worse than choose f_* defined by

$$f_* = \arg \min_F K\{f, p(u)\}.$$

We can then measure the feature selection ability relative to the worst possible choice by recording the subject's feature selection discrepancy

$$S\{f, p(u)\} = \frac{K\{f^*, p(u)\} - K\{f, p(u)\}}{K\{f^*, p(u)\} - K\{f_*, p(u)\}}. \tag{11.1}$$

The measure S is confined to the range $0 \leq S \leq 1$, the value 1 corresponding to the worst possible selection and the value 0 to the normative selection.

11.3.4 Measures associated with normal assessments

For U a finite or discrete set, such as in the diagnostic inferential tasks already cited, the computations of the measures described are comparatively simple summations. When, as in prognostic, assay and calibration studies, U may be a real line or a higher dimensional space then evaluation of the measures for univariate or multivariate normal assessment and distributions can prove useful in their own right or as approximations. We have the following results:

$$H(q) = \begin{cases} \frac{1}{2}\{1 + \log(2\pi\sigma^2)\} & \text{when } q(u) \text{ is } N^1(\lambda, \sigma^2), \\ \frac{1}{2}\{1 + \log\det(2\pi\Sigma)\} & \text{when } q(u) \text{ is } N^d(\lambda, \Sigma). \end{cases}$$

When $r(u)$ is $N^d(\lambda, \Sigma)$ and $s(u)$ is $N^d(\mu, \Omega)$ then

$$I(r, s) = \frac{1}{2}\{\text{trace}(\Omega^{-1}\Sigma) - \log\det(\Omega^{-1}\Sigma)\} + \frac{1}{2}(\lambda - \mu)\Omega^{-1}(\lambda - \mu)^{\text{T}}.$$

The simplification for the univariate case when $r(u)$ is $N^1(\lambda, \sigma^2)$ and $s(u)$ is $N^1(\mu, \omega^2)$ is

$$I(r, s) = \frac{1}{2}\{(\sigma/\omega)^2 - \log(\sigma/\omega)\} + \frac{1}{2}((\lambda - \mu)/\omega)^2.$$

Note that the first bracketed part separates out a component of the inference discrepancy which measures departure of the subject's assessment of covariance structure from the normative covariance value. The second component does not, however, give an absolute measure of the disagreement of means because of its involvement with the subject's variance or covariance assessment ω or Ω; it gives instead a standardised measure akin to a signal-to-noise ratio.

Since $G(q, r, s)$ is a simple construction of H values there is no need to provide an explicit expression.

When $p(u)$ is $N^d(\lambda, \Sigma)$ the form of $K\{f, p(u)\}$ depends upon whether in the inferential task it is more appropriate to specify $p(v|u)$, say as $N^d(\alpha + uB, \Gamma)$, or to specify $p(u|v)$ as $N^d(\gamma + v\Delta, \Omega)$. In the first case,

$$K\{f, p(u)\} = \frac{1}{2} \log \left(I + \Gamma^{-1} B\Sigma B^T \right),$$

and in the second case

$$K\{f, p(u)\} = \frac{1}{2} \log \det \left(\Omega^{-1}\Sigma \right).$$

11.4 Sequential inferential tasks

The measures of performance of Section 11.3 have been defined on the basis of the feature vector being presented as a whole for a single inferential task. If it is meaningful to present the feature vector components one at a time or in successive blocks then the subject can be faced with a sequential inferential task, being required to update the initial assessment $q(u)$ immediately after each component $v_1, \ldots, v_n$ has been presented, resulting in successive subjective assessments, say $s_1(u), \ldots, s_n(u)$. We can then clearly analyse the subject's performance after each such subjective assessment.

Such a sequential performance analysis can take two forms. The first is a relative one in which at the jth stage we treat the subject's present view $s_{j-1}(u)$ attained after stage $j - 1$ as the starting $q_j(u)$ in the evaluation of the normative assessment $r_j(u)$ against which $s_j(u)$ is to be judged. Secondly there is an accumulating or absolute performance analysis which in the normative updating $r_j(u)$ after the jth stage uses as starting assessment the previous normative updating $r_{j-1}(u)$ rather than the subject's $s_{j-1}(u)$. Which is more appropriate will depend to some extent on the nature of the particular inferential task. On the whole we prefer the relative analysis because it builds successively on the subject's immediately held belief and so has a greater opportunity of identifying particular circumstances in which discrepancies from the normative occur.

The definition of feature selection discrepancy lends itself to sequential inference tasks. At each stage of a sequential inference task, instead of presenting the subject with the next component, we may ask which of the components not so far revealed the subject believes is likely to remove the most uncertainty. At the jth stage with the current subjective assessment at $s_{j-1}(u)$ if the subject chooses feature f_j from the set F_j of features available, then replacement of $f, F, p(u)$ by $f_j, F_j, s_{j-1}(u)$ in the definition of S at (11.1) produces the appropriate feature selection discrepancy for the jth stage.

11.4.1 Subject assessment profiles for a sequential inferential task: Doctor's trilemma

Subjects were given information about a series of independent diagnostic tests for differentiating three possible disease types A, B, C. Table 11.1 shows the

Table 11.1 *Conditional probabilities of a positive response on each test given each type*

Type	Test Number									
	1	2	3	4	5	6	7	8	9	10
A	0.4	0.8	0.7	0.4	0.6	0.5	0.3	0.2	0.4	0.1
B	0.4	0.7	0.4	0.8	0.5	0.9	0.5	0.3	0.8	0.5
C	0.6	0.6	0.6	0.5	0.2	0.4	0.8	0.7	0.2	0.9

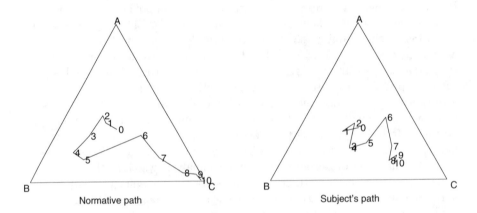

Figure 11.1 *A comparison of the normative sequential inferential path and one produced by a subject.*

conditional probabilities of a positive result on each of the ten tests for each type of disease. Each subject was asked to draw their diagnostic path showing their probability assessment within a ternary diagram ABC starting at the assumed incidence rate $(1/3, 1/3, 1/3)$. The results from tests 1-10 were given in sequence and the subject updated after each test. We illustrate the exercise with one of the test result sequences:

$$- + - + - - + + - + .$$

In Figure 11.1 we show the normative, Bayesian path based on these results and also a subject's path. We can then compute and show in the assessment of this subject's performance in terms of inference discrepancy and information gain index set out in Section 11.3. Figure 11.2 compares the progress of the normative removal of uncertainty with the much poorer performance by the subject. There is substantial inference discrepancy I, apparently increasing

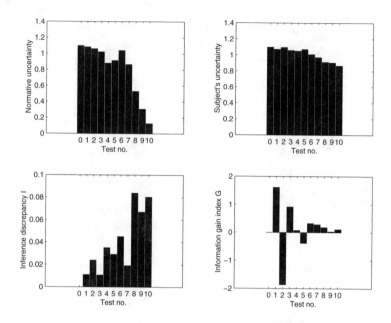

Figure 11.2 *Sequential measures of performance for the subject in Figure 11.1.*

towards the later tests, these being the tests which are on the whole more discriminating. Also the information gain index G shows examples of reading too much into the data, of conservative and contrary use of the information.

In another study at each stage the subject was asked to choose the test thought to be most informative and to move to the next point of a diagnostic path towards a possible earlier diagnosis. In the study reported the subject chose the tests in the order:

$$6 \ 8 \ 10 \ 4 \ 9 \ 3 \ 7 \ 1 \ 2 \ 5$$

with the following sequence of results:

$$+ \ - \ + \ + \ - \ + \ + \ + \ - \ -.$$

Figure 11.3 shows the normative and subject's paths. The profile of performance assessments is shown in Figure 11.4. Note that the test number refers to the sequence as carried out, so that test number 1 in Figure 11.4 refers to the original test number 6 and so on. This subject hardly reduces any of the initial uncertainty, has serious inference discrepancies, shows a whole range of reading too much into the data, being conservative and contrary, in much the same way as the previous subject. In choice of tests there is no great skill, with only three correct choices in the sequential process.

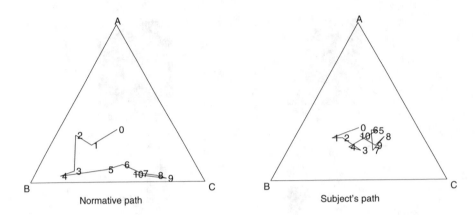

Figure 11.3 *A comparison of the normative sequential inferential path and one pro-duced by a subject.*

11.5 Some specific inferential tasks

In this section we define areas of clinical medicine where inferential tasks occur.

11.5.1 Diagnostic inferential tasks

First we emphasize that in these tasks diagnosis is presented as an inference rather than a decision problem, the subject being required, for a sequence of patients, to assign probabilities to the possible disease types on the basis of patient information released either sequentially or as a whole. For a valid performance analysis it is necessary to know exactly what information about a case is known to the subject. It is therefore not possible to allow the subject to see the patient lest visual or other information unknown to the analyst is being acquired. Thus information must be supplied verbally or on some visual display unit. To the extent that there is no contact with the patient it could be claimed that such studies do not put clinician subjects into their natural inference-making setting but most subjects seem to regard the tasks presented as fair tests of diagnostic skills. Moreover when interest is in comparing the inferential skills of clinicians with those of other professions direct access to patients is clearly not possible.

Performance analysis studies of diagnostic inference differ in a number of respects.

  (i) The extent to which the experience of the subject in the particular di-
      agnostic area has already been acquired and so is not determinable or

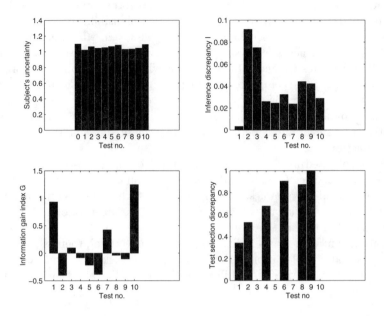

Figure 11.4 *Sequential measures of performance for the subject in Figure 11.3.*

cannot be completely supplied by the analyst (see the previous comments
in Section 11.2).

(ii) The extent to which the information on a new case can be supplied
sequentially.

(iii) In a sequential task the extent to which the choice of the next feature is
required of the subject.

(iv) The extent to which any assumptions of the normative assessments are
valid.

It is clear that any real or simulated task in this diagnostic area can be
easily presented, the only constraint being that for real diagnostic tasks we
have available an appropriate and sufficient training set on which to base
normative assessments. One aspect of normative assessments is that predictive
rather than estimative assessments are to be recommended.

11.5.2 Predictive and prognostic inferential tasks

Since we shall be describing below a calibrative inferential task which calls
for a density-function type assessment similar to those required here we shall
confine ourselves to the bare outline of such tasks.

Suppose that we give a subject who is aware of the concept of the normal
density function a set of observations from a normal distribution set out on a

horizontal scale and then pose the following task. Another observation is about to be recorded. Can the subject draw a pattern of plausibilities, essentially an unscaled density function, on the horizontal scale given, whose heights show the subject's assessments of the relative plausibilities of the various possible values? This requires a composite assessment which we can convert to proper density form $s(u)$ to be compared against the normative assessment $r(u)$. One point worth noting here is that the usually fitted normal curve with sample mean and standard deviation is, being an estimative form, not an appropriate normative assessment and is better replaced by the predictive form, a Student density function.

More complicated inferential tasks here involve regression-type situations. In such a task the set U will usually be the real line, the set of possible responses or dependent variables, while V is one- or higher-dimensional and consisting of possible explanatory, concomitant or covariate variables. A typical simple inferential task in this area is to provide the subject with a regression-type scattergram with v-axis horizontal and u-axis vertical, then ask the subject, after suitable explanation of the meaning of the task, to provide a density function $s(u)$ or 'pattern of plausibility' for the possible u values corresponding to a given v.

11.5.3 Calibrative inferential tasks

The type of task here is best described in terms of a specific simple example that we have given to a variety of subjects with some very interesting results. For this task each subject receives a copy of Figure 11.5 which is the training set, data for the 'standard curve' for an assay or calibration and the background to the problem is explained to the subjects. The problem concerns the assay of the concentration u of an antibiotic in a patient's blood. Droplets of standard preparations of known concentrations u_i of the antibiotic are placed on a prepared infected medium on Petri dishes and, after cooking for 24 hours, the diameters v_i(mm) of the circles cleared, which are of course related to the concentrations in a statistical rather than a deterministic way, are recorded.

In Figure 11.5 these (u_i, v_i) points are plotted. The subject is then made aware that the problem is to try and infer something about the unknown concentration of antibiotic in a patient's blood from knowledge only of the diameter of the clearance circle from a single droplet. He is invited to make use of numbered patterns of variability, similar to those shown in Figure 11.6, and supplied to him on a transparent sheet and to place what he regards as an appropriate pattern on the horizontal u axis. The meaning of such patterns is explained to him in some detail, for example,

(i) that the mode of the pattern selected should naturally be placed above the concentration regarded as the most plausible;

(ii) that with such patterns the relative heights of the curve above any two concentrations should reflect the subject's view of the relative plausibilities of these concentrations;

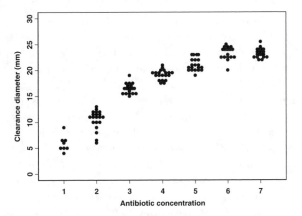

Figure 11.5 *Training data for the calibrative task of estimating the concentration of antibiotic given value(s) of the clearance diameter.*

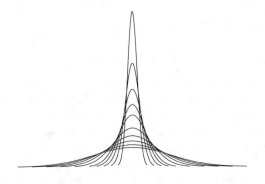

Figure 11.6 *Possible normal curves given to the subjects who undertake the calibrative task.*

(iii) that the 'narrower' the pattern chosen the more precise the subject is regarding the method of assay;

(iv) that, since only a finite number of patterns can be provided, he is free to choose an in-between pattern by 'interpolation' recording his choice to one decimal place; for example, a pattern 4.3 is intermediate between pattern 4 and pattern 5 but nearer to pattern 4 than 5.

At the outset the subject is told that all concentrations are equally likely. In our studies two tasks are given. First the subject is told that the diameter from a single droplet of the patient's blood was 19 mm and is asked to to identify his pattern by writing down the most plausible value and the pattern curve number. In the second he is told three diameters of 18.5, 18.5 and 20 mm. Again he is asked to select, on the basis of this information, his pattern by again noting his selected most plausible value and pattern curve number. The assessments of performance can, of course, be easily quantified by comparison of the selected curve $s(u)$ with the normative curve $r(u)$, such as the calibrative density or a normal approximation to it. The measures of Section 11.3 are then appropriate.

One interesting and surprising feature of the results is that in each of a number of different groups – statistical students in various years, clinicians, physicists – approximately one-half choose a wider pattern in the second task than in the first, contrary to the common sense view that more experimentation should provide a more precise inferential statement. This is clearly a phenomenon that is worth further investigation. One possible explanation is that with the single diameter some subjects have a tendency to forget about or underestimate the variability in diameter for a given dose, whereas when they are presented with three diameters showing variability they then take account of this variability.

11.6 Distributions of inferential statements

When studying a single subject performing different inferential tasks or a number of different subjects performing the same task we are faced with a set of inferential statements $s_1, \ldots, s_n$, each a probability distribution over a set U. For statistical analysis of such data it is clearly an advantage to consider probability distributions over U. Consider first the situation where U is a finite set with D categories. Then $s_1, \ldots, s_n$ are probabilistic data in the sense that they can be represented in the d-dimensional simplex S^d as defined in Section 4.2, where $d = D - 1$. In other words we are dealing here with compositional data.

The logistic-normal distributions, as defined in Section 4.2, then provide a rich class of distributions for the analysis of such inferential statements. There are, indeed, some grounds for expecting that the pattern of variability of inferential statements may follow such logistic-normal distributions. If, for given u, the distribution of the components $v_1, \ldots, v_n$ of the feature vector are independently distributed with density functions $p(v_j|u)$ then from prior probabilities $p(u)(u \in U)$ we have, by Bayes's formula,

$$o_i = \log \frac{p(u_i|v)}{p(u_D|v)} = \log \frac{p(u_i)}{p(u_D)} + \sum_{j=1}^{n} \log \frac{p_j(v_j|u_i)}{p_j(v_j|u_D)}.$$

Provided that the distributions $p_j(v_j|u)$ satisfy sufficient regularity conditions for the central limit theorem to be valid and that n is a reasonable size, then the o_i, being sums, will tend to be normally distributed, and so the true inferential statement will follow logistic-normal variability. Of course in practice the independence assumption will not be valid, so that logistic-normality of true inferential statements would have to rely on a central limit property for dependent sums. But we suspect that subjects have considerable difficulty in taking account of dependence in their assessments so that if their subjective process does correspond to some rough and ready form of Bayes's formula it is likely to be in approximately independent form. All this is speculative and it seems doubtful whether the subjective process can ever be investigated in this amount of detail. But at least there is a prima facie case for investigating logistic-normality of distributions of inferential statements associated with a finite set U.

For U non-finite, such as the real line in the calibration problem, the description of the variability of inferential statements, now probability distributions over the real line, is much more difficult. If the task takes the form of the selection of a normal curve then an inferential statement is equivalent to (m, s), where m and s are the mean and standard deviation of the selected normal curve. For this task we then have to select some suitable joint distribution for (m, s) and it is possible that some normal-Wishart form may be appropriate.

11.7 Two studies involving inferential tasks

We now illustrate the application of logistic-normal analysis to the inferential statements of groups of subjects in performing diagnostic tests.

11.7.1 Doctor's trilemma

The subjects were 48 first-course statistics students and each was presented with four tasks, the four cases requiring a diagnosis between three types with information from the ten independent binary tests presented sequentially. Each test could have a positive or a negative result. The test results for the tasks of classifying four new patients are shown in Table 11.2 and the information on the conditional probabilities of a positive result on each test given each of the three types is given in Table 11.1.

Each of the 24 possible orders of presentation of the cases was allocated to two students, the allocating being at random. The trial was conducted in two sessions. In each task the subjects were told that the types are equally likely. At the first session, early in the course and before students had met the appropriate technical tool of Bayes's formula, each student tackled his first two cases. The remaining two cases were presented at the second session, some six weeks later, and after meeting Bayes's formula in lectures. Subjects were not informed that Bayes's formula was the appropriate tool and were not allowed to write anything on paper except their inferential statements. No feedback

Table 11.2 *Ten binary test results for four new patients*

Patient	Test Number									
	1	2	3	4	5	6	7	8	9	10
N1	−	−	−	−	−	−	+	+	−	−
N2	−	+	+	+	−	−	−	+	−	+
N3	+	+	−	−	+	−	−	+	−	+
N4	+	+	+	+	+	+	−	−	+	+

was given to the subjects as to their diagnostic performance after the first session.

If s_{ij} denotes the inferential statement of the ith subject on the jth presented task then a model Ω for the analysis of the various effects is as follows:

$$s_{ij} \sim L^2(\mu + \alpha_i + \beta_j + \gamma_{k(i,j)}, \Sigma),$$

where $k(i,j)$ is 1 or 2 according as the case comes before or after knowledge of Bayes's formula. The usual form of identifiability restrictions apply:

$$\sum_{i=1}^{48} \alpha_i = 0, \qquad \sum_{j=1}^{4} \beta_j = 0, \qquad \gamma_1 + \gamma_2 = 0.$$

Here the α_i and β_j denote subject and task effects and non-zero values of γ_1 and γ_2 will indicate some effect associated with knowledge of Bayes's formula.

For testing any hypothesis ω within the model Ω the usual chi-squared approximation at significance level α for the generalised likelihood ratio test can be expressed in the form

$$192 \log \frac{\det \hat{\Sigma}_\omega}{\det \hat{\Sigma}_\Omega} > \chi^2(r, 1 - \alpha),$$

where $\hat{\Sigma}_\omega$ and $\hat{\Sigma}_\Omega$ are the maximum likelihood estimates of Σ under ω and Ω, r is the number of independent constraints on the parameters required to specialise Ω to ω and $\chi^2(r, 1 - \alpha)$ is the $(1 - \alpha)$th quantile of the chi-squared distribution with r degrees of freedom. Figure 11.7 gives the complete lattice of hypotheses with the test quantities and their degrees of freedom in parentheses. Moving up the lattice we can reject all hypotheses except $\gamma_k = 0$. Thus we must conclude from this that there are significant subject and task effects but that there is no significant evidence of a 'Bayes effect' on subjective performance, though the shortfall of the test quantity 5.12 from the critical value 5.99 is perhaps small enough to encourage the undertaking of more and larger studies.

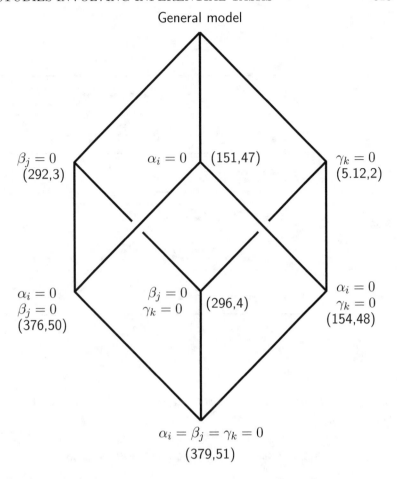

Figure 11.7 *Lattice of hypotheses associated with the Doctor's Trilemma study. At each node the appropriate value of the chi-squared test statistic is shown with the associated number of degrees of freedom.*

11.7.2 Statistician's syndrome

In this analysis three groups of subjects, 56 professional statisticians, 11 second-year statistics students and 9 clinical consultants, were each presented with five tasks involving the differential diagnosis of three types based on six quantitative features. The complete training set of 36 cases, 12 of each type, was given together with the information that for each of these equally-prevalent types the distributions of the features were normally distributed, the three mean vectors and covariance matrices also being given to the subjects. Of the presented information the task information is displayed in Table 11.3, the summary statistics are shown in Table 11.4 and the raw data are shown in Figure 11.8, and are available in data set statsyn.

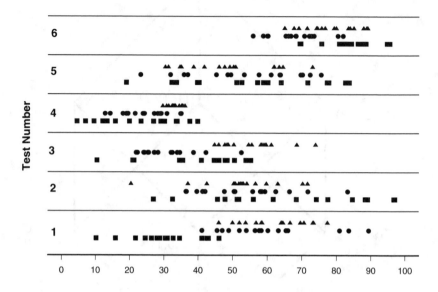

Figure 11.8 *Plot of the raw data used in the Statisticians' Syndrome diagnostic challenge.*

Table 11.3 *Test results for five new patients with Statistician's syndrome*

Patient	Test Number					
	1	2	3	4	5	6
N1	47.1	46.1	59.3	35.2	61.4	84.6
N2	64.3	71.2	63.2	34.0	19.6	64.5
N3	38.3	62.0	25.0	19.2	49.2	69.3
N4	42.7	38.0	25.1	10.8	31.4	80.5
N5	45.5	55.3	48.0	26.1	59.8	60.2

For each group there are highly significant subject and task effects. The extensive between-subject variability can be easily seen in Figure 11.9 which shows in terms of triangular coordinates the inferential statements of the 56 statisticians for cases N1, N2, N4 and N5, the true types of these cases being A, C, A and B respectively. If, for a given task, group g has inferen-

Table 11.4 *Summary information for Statistician's Syndrome in the forms of sample means(standard deviations) and correlation matrices*

Type	Test Number					
	1	2	3	4	5	6
A	30.4(9.8)	65.6(22.2)	39.7(12.8)	21.8(11.4)	56.3(19.5)	83.6(7.8)
B	60.6(13.9)	53.7(13.3)	30.8(8.2)	24.5(6.6)	53.6(15.8)	68.2(7.3)
C	62.4(9.2)	52.3(12.2)	55.9(8.1)	33.3(2.0)	48.7(13.2)	78.1(7.7)

$$
A \quad
\begin{bmatrix}
1 & 0.24 & -0.14 & 0.19 & -0.53 & 0.30 \\
  & 1 & -0.25 & 0.57 & -0.82 & 0.40 \\
  &   & 1 & 0.11 & 0.42 & -0.72 \\
  &   &   & 1 & -0.40 & -0.17 \\
  &   &   &   & 1 & -0.53 \\
  &   &   &   &   & 1
\end{bmatrix}
$$

$$
B \quad
\begin{bmatrix}
1 & 0.24 & -0.14 & 0.19 & -0.53 & 0.30 \\
  & 1 & -0.25 & 0.57 & -0.82 & 0.40 \\
  &   & 1 & 0.11 & 0.42 & -0.72 \\
  &   &   & 1 & -0.40 & -0.17 \\
  &   &   &   & 1 & -0.53 \\
  &   &   &   &   & 1
\end{bmatrix}
$$

$$
C \quad
\begin{bmatrix}
1 & 0.24 & 0.52 & 0.16 & 0.21 & -0.31 \\
  & 1 & 0.47 & 038 & -0.49 & -0.32 \\
  &   & 1 & -0.11 & -0.46 & -0.16 \\
  &   &   & 1 & 0.16 & -0.20 \\
  &   &   &   & 1 & 0.39 \\
  &   &   &   &   & 1
\end{bmatrix}
$$

tial statements which distributed according to the logistic-normal distribution $L^2(\mu_g, \Sigma_g)$ then interest is in testing $\mu_1 = \mu_2 = \mu_3$ and $\Sigma_1 = \Sigma_2 = \Sigma_3$. We have made such comparisons among our three groups for each task with the following results. For only one of the tasks is there no significant differences among the groups. For all of the remaining four tasks there are significant differences between the mean vectors, highly significant at the 0.1 per cent level for three of these tasks, though for only one task is there a significant difference, at the 5 per cent level, between the covariance matrices.

Thus there is evidence not only that subjects within a group vary but that there can be significant between-group differences in the performance of subjects. Since a normative statistical system can for each task supply a normative

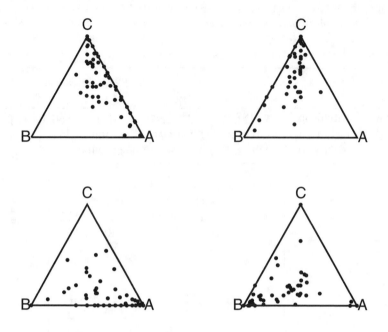

Figure 11.9 *Patterns of variability in the responses of 56 professional statisticians when faced with cases N1 (top-left), N2 (top-right), N4 (bottom-left) and N5 (bottom-right) of the Statisticians' Syndrome diagnostic study.*

inferential statement translatable into a logratio value μ we can test whether a group's μ_g is significantly different from μ. For all three groups and all five tasks there are significant differences of groups means from the normative value.

11.8 Bibliographic notes

The concept of assessment of performance in clinical practice is probably the least familiar of the contents of this monograph and so we give a reasonably full set of references of the subject. In the 1960's the resurgence of Bayesian inference led to an interest in how subjects behave in relation to simple inference and decision tasks, where well established conditional probability theory provides normative or optimal inferences and decisions. The problems presented to the subjects in such early studies were usually simple and highly artificial, seldom related to real situations. A typical study at this time is Phillips and Edwards (1966). With extensive work in consultation on diagnostic problems in clinical medicine came the opportunity to compare the diagnostic performance of clinicians with the application of statistical analysis. An early study in this area, to differential diagnosis in non-toxic goitre, is described in Taylor, Aitchison and McGirr (1971). The measures of performance in such a study are based largely on the information ideas contained in Kullback and Liebler (1951) and Lindley (1956). The original definitions of measures of subjective performance contained in Taylor, Aitchison and McGirr (1971) were simplified for easier interpretation in Aitchison (1981). For other studies in this general area, see Aitchison (1974, 1978) and Aitchison and Kay (1973, 1975).

The possibility of comparing performance of various groups of individuals was made possible by developments in compositional data analysis as in Aitchison (1986).

For other related studies in performance, as for example in treatment selection, see Aitchison et al. (1973), Aitchison and Moore (1976), Moore et al. (1974) and Taylor et al. (1975).

11.9 Problems

Problem 11.1 In the process of diagnosing a patient a doctor has reached a stage where she is placing probabilities 0.5, 0.1, 0.4 on the three possible diseases A, B, C. As a next step she has to choose between two tests, 1 and 2, which yield positive or negative results according to the following probability pattern.

Probability of + and − results for the different disease types.

Disease type	Test 1		Test 2	
	+	−	+	−
A	0.2	0.8	0.7	0.3
B	0.3	0.7	0.5	0.5
C	0.6	0.4	0.1	0.9

For each test illustrate the moves in her diagnostic path for each of the possible outcomes.

Which test should she choose if she wishes to maximise the expected gain of information about the patient's disease?

Problem 11.2 Review Section 11.3.4. with the various distribution of lognormal instead of normal form. In what way are the measures of performance altered?

Problem 11.3 The test results for a new case in the Doctor's Trilemma exercise of Section 11.7.1 were

$$- + - + - - + + - +$$

Compute and plot the diagnostic path for this case within an ABC ternary diagram.

Problem 11.4 One subject presented with the case in Problem 11.3 drew a diagnostic path based on steps leading from the starting probabilities (1/3, 1/3, 1/3) to the following assessments

After test	Diagnostic assessment		
	A	B	C
1	0.16	0.58	0.26
2	0.25	0.45	0.30
3	0.17	0.50	0.33
4	0.18	0.48	0.34
5	0.23	0.36	0.41
6	0.40	0.15	0.45
7	0.21	0.21	0.58
8	0.12	0.27	0.61
9	0.16	0.21	0.63
10	0.11	0.25	0.64

Construct a performance profile of this subject showing the uncertainty H, the inference discrepancy I, the information gain index G after each stage.

Problem 11.5 Either use the Doctor's Trilemma framework of Section 11.5.1 or construct a similar situation of your own. Encourage some of your friends to act as subjects, allowing them to attempt to choose optimum tests at each stage. For each subject construct a H, I, G, S profile and attempt to explain the nature of performance to each of your subjects.

Problem 11.6 A clinic is currently using an expensive, time-consuming, but accurate method of determining the (a, b, c) composition of a certain type of tissue in patients, and has been investigating the possibility of using the tissue specimens to create a response in a certain medium to produce what is believed to be a related (A, B, C) composition. In a trial with 25 standard (a, b, c) tissues the corresponding (A, B, C) responses were recorded as below.

Standard proportions			Response proportions		
a	b	c	A	B	C
0.66	0.15	0.19	0.71	0.14	0.15
0.33	0.61	0.06	0.40	0.55	0.05
0.50	0.44	0.06	0.48	0.43	0.09
0.40	0.39	0.21	0.42	0.36	0.22
0.68	0.23	0.09	0.68	0.24	0.08
0.50	0.27	0.23	0.54	0.18	0.28
0.51	0.18	0.31	0.57	0.15	0.28
0.61	0.20	0.19	0.67	0.14	0.19
0.54	0.22	0.24	0.45	0.24	0.31
0.52	0.36	0.12	0.53	0.35	0.12
0.39	0.49	0.12	0.31	0.58	0.11
0.31	0.39	0.30	0.32	0.35	0.32
0.26	0.17	0.57	0.23	0.15	0.62
0.65	0.14	0.21	0.70	0.13	0.17
0.41	0.30	0.29	0.33	0.36	0.31
0.60	0.24	0.16	0.64	0.22	0.14
0.71	0.16	0.13	0.68	0.19	0.13
0.40	0.32	0.28	0.36	0.39	0.25
0.51	0.36	0.13	0.51	0.37	0.12
0.44	0.38	0.18	0.52	0.28	0.20
0.47	0.26	0.27	0.40	0.37	0.23
0.62	0.27	0.11	0.67	0.24	0.09
0.47	0.27	0.26	0.48	0.27	0.25
0.58	0.29	0.13	0.69	0.21	0.10
0.57	0.32	0.11	0.62	0.28	0.10

The clinicians believe that from the (A, B, C) compositional response to a new patient's tissue of unknown (a, b, c) composition they can reconstruct the (a, b, c) composition. Design an assessment trial to investigate this claim.

Regardless of the outcome of such an investigation what would your recommendation be to the clinic on this assay problem?

Data and Software

The data sets which have been analysed, together with the data sets in the end of chapter problems, are available from the book web-site at the following address.

www.crcpress.com/e_products/downloads

Almost all of the work was performed in MATLAB or S-Plus or R. The packages nlme and WinBUGS were also used, as were the Venables and Ripley (2002) libraries MASS, nnet and class. S/R scripts and WinBUGS programmes are also available from the book web-site.

A.1 Aldosterone

This problem involves the calibration of two methods of determining the concentration of aldosterone in blood samples. The methods are a radioimmunoassay method (RIA) and a double isotope method (DI) and data are available from 72 blood samples. The data set aldo has 72 rows and 2 columns named RIA and DI; see Section 7.2.

A.2 Angiotensin II

This problem concerns the determination of the concentration of angiotensin II in samples of blood plasma using radioimmunoassay. Data are available for 16 samples of blood plasma. The data set angio has two columns named CONC and PERBD and 16 rows; see Section 7.5.

A.3 Auditory dysfunction

This is a problem of differential diagnosis of auditory dysfunction on the basis of electrocochleography in which only a composite diagnosis is available for the four types of hearing state: normal hearing, conduction hearing loss, Menière's disease and hair-cell damage. Data are available on 93 subjects consisting of four derived measures from action potentials together with a type composition. The data set hearing has 93 rows and 9 columns, with the first containing case numbers, the next four containing the derived measures and the latter four containing the composite type information; see Section 9.6.

A.4   Bacteria

This problem concerns the reproducibility of observers in counting bacterial colonies on petri plates. Data, in the form of numbers of colonies, are available for 20 plates with each of three observers providing a count for each plate. The data set bact has 3 columns named PLATE, OBSERVER and COUNT and 60 rows; see Section 6.7.

A.5   Bilateral hyperplasia

It is required to describe the experience of measurements of cortisol and cortisone in 27 patients who have bilateral hyperplasia. The data set bilhyp has two columns named CSOL (cortisol) and CSONE (cortisone) and 27 rows; see Section 5.3.1.

A.6   Calcium contents

This problem concerns the description of the variability of the calcium contents CH and CF of the heel and forearm in relation to Gender (G), Age (A), Weight (W), Height (H), Surface area (SA), Strength of forearm (MF), Strength of leg (ML), Diameter of os calcis (OS), Area of os calcis (AC) and Diameter of radius and ulna (DR). Data are available for 127 patients and the data set bones has 12 columns, named G, A, W, H, SA, MF, ML, OS, AC, DR, CH and CF, and 127 rows; see Section 5.4.2. Data in the same format as bones are available for four new patients in data set newbones.

A.7   Cells

This problem involves an observer error study of cell counts in areas of tissue. Data are available for 10 cases and three observers and the numbers of labelled and unlabelled cells that are counted are given for each combination. The data set cells has four columns, named CASE, OBS, LABCNT and UNLABCNT, and 30 rows; see Section 6.5.

A.8   Cervical cancer

This problem is a randomised survival study of patients with cervical cancer conducted to compare the usefulness of two treatments A and B. Data are available on 105 patients and contained in the data set cancer which has three columns and 105 rows. The columns contain for each patient the censoring status (STATUS), the survival time (TIME) and their treatment (TREAT); see Section 10.3.

A.9 Conn's syndrome

This problem is one of differential diagnosis of patients with Conn's syndrome. Data are available on concentrations of sodium (Na), potassium (K), carbon dioxide (CO2), renin (Ren) and aldosterone (Aldo) in blood plasma, together with systolic (SysBP) and diastolic (DiasBP) blood pressures, for 31 cases with Conn's syndrome from clinic 1 (20 with an adenoma (a) and 11 with bilateral hyperplasia (b)). The data set conn has nine columns, named Case, Na, K, CO2, Ren, Aldo, SysBP, DiasBP and Type, with 31 rows; see Table 1.1.

Data are also available on 21 patients from clinic 2, 17 of whom have an adenoma and 4 have bilateral hyperplasia, and also for 22 undiagnosed cases. These data are available in the data set newconn in the same format as data set conn, but with Type being coded as c, d and e for the adenoma, bilateral hyperplasia and undiagnosed patients, respectively; see Sections 1.2, 8.2 and 9.2-3.

A.10 Crohn's disease

The problem here is one of differential diagnosis between patients with ulcerative colitis and those with Crohn's disease. Specimens were collected from the guts of 33 patients – 11 with ulcerative colitis, 11 with Crohn's disease and 11 normal subjects – and the cells from these specimens were classified as into three types: I, A and M. The data set crohn has four columns, named I, A, M and Type, and 33 rows; see Section 5.5.1.

A.11 Crown rump length

This is a problem of determining the age of a foetus by means of its crown rump length as determined by sonar techniques. Data are available from 194 mothers, some of whom were assessed on more than one occasion. Data set foetal has three columns, named Patient, Maturity and CRL, and 339 rows; see Section 7.4.

A.12 Cushing's syndrome

This is a problem of differential diagnosis involving patients with Cushing's syndrome. Data are available for 87 patients on the 14 steroid metabolites defined in Table 1.3. Data set cush has sixteen columns containing the case identifiers in column 1, values of the 14 steroid metabolites in the next 14 columns and the Type of disease in column 16. Type is labelled as a (adenoma), b (bilateral hyperplasia), c (adrenal carcinoma), d (ectopic carcinoma) and n (normal). See Sections 1.10, 8.5 and 9.7 for more details. Data on the 14 steroid metabolites for 30 normal children are available in data set cushkids; see Section 5.5.2.

A.13   Cutaneous malignant melanoma

This is a problem involving the survival prognosis of patients with cutaneous malignant melanoma. Complete data are available on 4332 patients in the data set `malmel` which has 4332 rows and 8 columns, named DEP7 (deprivation status), SEX, BRSLW5 (Breslow thickness), HIST4 (histogenetic type), AGEGRP (age group), SURVYRS (survival time), STATUS (observed (1) or censored (0)). Data on four new patients are available in data set `newmel`. Data set `mel5` contains data on a subset of 2938 of the patients for whom five-year survival could be determined. This has the same format as data set `malmel` except that there is a column named FIVE recording five-year survival (1= yes, 0 = no) in place of the column containing censoring status; see Section 10.5.

A.14   Diagnostic ratio

This problem concerns observer error studies of heart X-rays. The are 65 X-rays and the six measurements defined in Section 6.3 are made on each X-ray by five observers. Data set `dratio` has 325 rows and 9 columns. The first column indicates the X-ray. Columns 2–7 contain the six heart measurements. Column 8 contains the observer code and the ninth column gives the diagnostic ratio. These data are discussed in Sections 6.3–4. The data set `dratio2` contains replicated assessment on 15 of the heart X-rays by two of the observers; there are 60 rows and 4 columns containing information on the X-ray, radiologist, replicate and diagnostic ratio; see Section 6.3.

A.15   Glucose

This problem concerns the calibration of two methods of determining glucose concentration. Data are available from 52 individuals in the form of glucose concentration as determined by the oxidase method and two or three corresponding measurements made using the reflectance meter method. Data set `gluc` has three columns, named as Subject, OXI (oxidase method) and RM (reflectance meter), and 162 rows; see Section 7.3.

A.16   Goitre

This is a problem of the differential diagnosis of patients with non-toxic goitre in the presence of missing data. There are three types of disease: Hashimoto's disease (1), simple goitre (2) and thyroid carcinoma (3). Data are available from 143 patients in the form of four tests together with the known type (1, 2 or 3). The data set `goitre` has 143 rows and five columns, the first four of which contain the results of the four tests and the fifth contains the type of goitre; see Section 9.5.

A.17 Haemophilia

This is a problem of differential diagnosis of women as carriers or non-carriers of haemophilia. Data in the form of results of two coagulation tests are available for 43 women, 20 of whom are known to be carriers (c) while the other 23 are non-carriers (n) of haemophilia. Data set haemo has four columns, named Case, FactorI, FactorIV and Type, and 43 rows; see Sections 5.3.2 and 8.4. Data on 15 new patients are available in data set newhaem.

A.18 Hormone

This problem concerns the variability of the measurements of an anti-diuretic hormone in relation to gender and urine osmolarity. Data are available on 75 patients in data set adhorm which contains 75 rows and three columns: ADH, UO and Sex. Data are available for 6 new patients in data set newadh; see Section 5..4.1.

A.19 Keratoconjunctivitis sicca

This is a problem of diagnosing whether or not rheumatoid arthritis patients have Keratoconjunctivitis sicca (kcs). Data on ten binary symptoms are available on 77 patients, 40 of whom have kcs while the remainder do not have kcs. The data set kcs has 77 rows and 12 columns. The first column contains the case identifiers, the next 10 columns contain presence/absence (1/0) of the symptoms and the twelfth column contains the true type (y for kcs and n for non-kcs). Data are available on forty further patients, 23 of whom have kcs and 17 of whom do not, in data set newkcs; see Section 8.3.

A.20 Nephrology

This problem involves the prediction of dosage of the drug NEP and also the occurrence of side-effects. Data set kidney contains data from 58 patients on concentrations of creatine (CREAT), cholesterol (CHOL) and triglyceride (TRIG) along with NEP dose (NEP), sex (SEX) and presence of side-effects (SIDE); it has 58 rows and 6 columns; see Section 10.4.

A.21 Potassium

This problem concerns describing the experience of concentrations of potassium in blood plasma. Data set potass has a single column containing measurements of potassium concentration from 200 healthy patients; see Section 5.2.1.

A.22 Pregnenetriol

This problem concerns describing the experience of urinary excretion rates of pregnenetriol in 37 healthy patients. Data set `preg` has a single column containing measurements of the urinary excretion rates for 37 healthy individuals; see section 5.2.2.

A.23 Statistician's syndrome

Data set `statsyn` contain the training data and data for the five new patients on the six tests in Statistician's syndrome. Rows 1–16, 17–32 and 33–48 contain the data for types A, B and C, respectively, and rows 49–53 contain the test results for 5 new patients; see section 11.7.2. In a study of statisticians at a conference each of 56 volunteers were given data on 5 new cases and asked to plot their assessment of the types in ternary diagrams. The resulting data are available in data set `ssresults` which has 275 rows and 5 columns. The first two columns contain the subject and case numbers and the last three columns contain the assessed probabilities for types A, B and C; see Section 11.7.2.

A.24 Tobramycin

This is a problem of determining concentration of tobramycin from the clearance diameter. Each of 20 patients contributed blood samples which were tested at six known concentrations of tobramycin and the clearance diameter recorded. Data set `tobra` has 120 rows and 3 columns named PATIENT, CONC (concentration) and CLEAR (clearance diameter); see Section 9.6.

A.25 X-rays

This problem concerns observer error in two studies involving diagnoses made on the basis of large and small X-rays by three observers. Data set `xrays` contains data for 90 patients. For each patient there is a large X-ray and a corresponding small X-ray, and three observers have reached correct or wrong diagnoses on both sizes of X-ray. Data set `xrays` has 90 rows and six columns, named AL, AS, BL, BS, CL and CS respectively. These columns contain binary data (1 for a correct and 0 for a wrong diagnosis) for each of the observers A, B and C on large and small X-rays; see Section 6.6.

References

Abrahamowitz, M. and Stegun, I.A. (1972). *Handbook of Mathematical Functions: with formulas, graphs and mathematical tables.* Dover Publications. New York.

Agresti, A. (2002). *Categorical data analysis (2nd edition).* Wiley. New Jersey.

Aitchison, J. (1974). Hippocratic Inference. *IMA Bulletin* **10**, 48-53.

Aitchison, J. (1977). A calibration problem in statistical diagnosis: the system transfer problem. *Biometrika* **64**, 461-472.

Aitchison, J. (1978). *The Truth, the Whole Truth and Statistical Inference.* An inaugural lecture from the Chair of Statistics. Libra Press. Hong Kong.

Aitchison, J. (1979). A calibration problem in statistical diagnosis: the clinic amalgamation problem. *Biometrika* **66**, 357-366.

Aitchison, J. (1981). Some distribution theory related to the analysis of subjective performance in inferential tasks. In *Statistical Distributions in Scientific Work.* Eds. C. Taillie, G.P. Patil and B. Baldessari. **5**, 363-385. D. Reidel Publishing Company, Dordrecht, Holland.

Aitchison, J. (1986). *The Statistical Analysis of Compositional Data.* Chapman and Hall. London. Reprinted, with a new foreword and a postscript with post-1986 developments and publications, in 2003 by The Blackburn Press, New Jersey.

Aitchison, J. (1990). Relative variation diagrams for describing patterns of variability of compositional data. *J. Math. Geol.* **22**, 487-512.

Aitchison, J. (1997). The one-hour course in compositional data analysis or compositional data analysis is easy. In *Proceedings of the Third Annual Conference of the International Association for Mathematical Geology.* Ed. Vera Pawlowsky Glahn. 3-35. CIMNE. Bercelona.

Aitchison, J. (2001) Simplicial inference. In *Algebraic Structures in Statistics.* Eds. M. Viana and D. Richards. Contemporary Mathematics Series of the American Mathematical Society.

Aitchison, J. and Aitken, C.G.G. (1976). Multivariate binary discrimination by the kernel method. *Biometrika* **63**, 413-420.

Aitchison, J. and Begg, C.B. (1976). Statistical diagnosis when basic cases are not classified with certainty. *Biometrika* **63**, 1-12.

Aitchison, J. and Dunsmore, I.R. (1975). *Statistical Prediction Analysis.* Cambridge University Press. Cambridge. UK.

Aitchison, J. and Greenacre, M. (2002). Biplots for compositional data. *Appl. Statist.* **51**, 375-382.

Aitchison, J., Habbema, J.D.F. and Kay, J.W. (1977). A critical comparison of two methods of statistical discrimination. *Appl. Statist.* **26**, 15-25.

Aitchison, J. and Kay, J.W. (1973). A diagnostic competition. *IMA Bulletin* **9**, 382-383.

Aitchison, J. and Kay, J.W. (1975). Principles, practice and performance in decision-making in clinical medicine. In *Proceedings of the 1973 NATO conference on The*

Role and Effectiveness of Decision Theories in Practice. Eds. K.C. Bowen and D.J. White. 252-272. English Universities Press. London.

Aitchison, J. and Lauder, I.J. (1979). Statistical diagnosis from imprecise data. *Biometrika* **66**, 475-483.

Aitchison, J. and Lauder, I.J. (1985). Kernel density estimation for compositional data. *Appl. Statist.* **34**, 129-137.

Aitchison, J. and Moore, M.F. (1976). The analysis of decision-making performance. *J. Math. Statist. Psych.* **29**, 53-65.

Aitchison, J., Moore, M.F., West, S. and Taylor, T.R. (1973). Consistency of treatment allocation in thyrotoxicosis. *Quart. J. Medicine* **42**, 575-583.

Aitchison, J. and Shen, S.M. (1980). Logistic-normal distributions: some properties and uses. *Biometrika* **67**, 261-272.

Aitkin, M.A., Anderson, D., Francis, B. and Hinde, J. (1989). *Statistical Modelling in GLIM.* Clarendon Press. Oxford. UK.

Anderson, J.A. (1972). Separate sample logistic discrimination. *Biometrika* **59**, 19-35.

Anderson, J.A., Whaley, K., Williamson, J. and Buchanan, W.W. (1972), A statistical aid to the diagnosis of Keratoconjunctivitis sicca. *Quart. J. Med.* **41**, 175-189.

Anderson, T.W. (1984). *An Introduction to Multivariate Statistical Analysis (2nd edition).* Wiley. New York.

Barnett, V. (1982). *Comparative Statistical Inference.* Wiley. New York.

Baxter, R.H. (1974). The use of a reflectance meter for the diagnosis of neonatal hypoglycaemia. *Ann. Clin. Biochem.* **2**, 8-10.

Bayes, T. (1763). Essay towards solving a problem in the doctrine of chances. *Phil. Trans Roy. Soc. Lond.* **53**, 370-418.

Berkson, J. (1944). Application of the logistic function to bioassay. *J. Amer. Statist. Assoc.* **39**, 357-365.

Bliss, C.I. (1934). The method of probits. *Science.* **79**, 38-39

Bowman, A.W. and Azzalini, A. (1997). *Applied Smoothing Techniques for Data Analysis.* Oxford University Press. Oxford. UK.

Box, G.E.P. and Cox, D.R. (1964). An analysis of transformations (with discussion). *J. R. Statist. Soc. B* **26**, 531-550.

Boyle, J.A., Greig, W.R., Franklin, D.A., Marden, R. McG., Buchanan, W.W. and McGirr, E.M. (1965). Construction of a model for computer-aided diagnosis: application to the problem of non-toxic goitre. *Quart. J. Med.* **35**, 565-588.

Brown, J.J., Chinn, R.H., Dasterdeck, G.O., Fraser, R., Lever, A.F., Robertson, J.I.S. and Tree, M. (1969). Hypertension with hyperaldosteronism and low plasma renin concentration. Analysis of a series of eighty-two patients. *Proc. R. Soc. Med.* **62**, 1258

Brown, J.J., Chinn, R.H., Davies, D.L., Dasterdeck, G.O., Fraser, R., Lever, A.F., Robertson, J.I.S., Tree, M., and Wiseman, A. (1968). Plasma electrolytes, renin and aldosterone in the diagnosis of primary hyperaldosteronism with a note on plasma-corticosterone concentration. *The Lancet* **2**, 55-59.

Brown, P.J. (1982). Multivariate calibration. *J. R. Statist. Soc. B* **44**, 287-321.

Brown, P.J. (1993). *Measurement, regression and calibration.* Oxford University Press. Oxford. UK.

Campbell, N.A. (1985). Updating formulae for allocation of individuals. *Appl. Statist.* **34**, 235-236.

Clarke, M.R.B. (1971). Algorithm AS 41: Updating the sample mean and dispersion matrix. *Appl. Statist.* **20**, 206-209.

Collett, D. (2003a). *Modelling Binary Data (2nd edition)*. Chapman and Hall/CRC. London.

Collett, D. (2003b). *Modelling Survival Data in Medical Research (2nd edition)*. Chapman and Hall/CRC. London.

Conn, J.W. (1955). Primary aldosteronism, a new clinical syndrome. *J. Lab. Clin. Med.* **45**, 3-17.

Cook, R.D. and Weisberg, S. (1982). *Residuals and Influence in Regression*. Chapman and Hall. London.

Cox, D.R. and Hinkley, D.V. (1974). *Theoretical Statistics*. Chapman and Hall. London.

Cox, D.R. (1975). Partial likelihood. *Biometrika* **62**, 269-276.

Damkjaer-Neilsen, M., Binder, C. and Starup, J. (1969). Urinary excretion of different corticosteroid-metabolites in oral contraception and pregnancy. *Acta Endocrinologia* **69**, 473-485.

Damkjaer-Neilsen, M., Lund, J.O. and Munch, O. (1972). Urinary excretion of tetrahydrocortisone in normal subjects and in patients with adrenal insufficiency and Conn's syndrone. *Acta Endocrinologia* **71**, 498-511.

Dawid, A.P. (1976). Properties of diagnostic data distributions. *Biometrics* **32**, 647-658.

Day, N.E. and Kerridge, D. F. (1967). A general maximum likelihood discriminant. *Biometrics* **23**, 313-323.

Dempster, A.P., Laird, N.M. and Rubin, D.B. (1977). Maximum likelihood from incomplete data via the EM algorithm (with discussion). *J. R. Statist. Soc. B* **28**, 1-38.

Dunn, G. (1989). *Design and Analysis of Reliability Studies: The Statistical Evaluation of Measurement Errors*. Oxford University Press. Oxford. UK.

Dunsmore, I.R. (1966). A Bayesian approach to classification. *J. R. Statist. Soc. B* **28**, 568-577.

Filliben, J.J. (1975). The probability plot correlation coefficient test for normality. *Technometrics* **17**, 111-117.

Finney, D.J. (1971). *Probit Analysis (3rd edition)*. Cambridge University Press. Cambridge. UK.

Finney, D.J. (1976). Radiological assay. *Biometrics* **32**, 721-740.

Fisher, R.A. (1936). The use of multiple measurements in taxonomic problems. *Ann. Eugen.* **7**, 179-188.

Gabriel, K.R. (1971) The biplot-graphic display of matrices with application to principal component analysis. *Biometrika* **58**, 453-467.

Gabriel, K.R. (1981) Biplot display of multivariate matrices for inspection of data and diagnosis. In *Interpreting Multivariate Data*. Ed. V. Barnett. 147-173. Wiley. New York.

Gaddum, J.H. (1933). *Reports on biological standards. III. Methods of biological assay depending on quantal response*. Spec. Rep. Ser. Med. Res. Com. Lond. **183**.

Geisser, S. (1964). Posterior odds for multivariate normal classification. *J. R. Statist. Soc. B.* **26**, 69-76.

Gelman, A., Carlin, J.C., Stern H. and Rubin D.B. (1995). *Bayesian Data Analysis*. Chapman and Hall. New York.

Gilks, W.R., Richardson, S. and Spiegelhalter, D.J.(eds.) (1996). *Markov Chain Monte Carlo in Practice*. Chapman and Hall. London.

Hamilton, M. (1956). *Clinicians and Decisions*. Leeds University Press. Leeds. UK.

Healey, M.J.R. (1972). Statistical analysis of radioimmunoassay data. *Biochem. J.* **130**, 207-210.

Hermans, J., Eggermont, J.J., Hagedooren, J. and Odenthal, D.W. (1975). Probabilistic differential diagnosis of auditory dysfunction on the basis of electrococheography. *Meth. Inform. Med.* **14**, 87-95.

Hoel, P.G. (1971). *Introduction to Mathematical Statistics*. Wiley. New York.

Hollingsworth, T.H. (1959). Using an electronic computer in a problem of medical diagnosis. *J. R. Statist. Soc. A.* **122**, 221-231.

Jeffreys, H. (1961). *Theory of Probability (3rd edition)*. Oxford University Press. Oxford. UK.

Johnson, R.A. and Wichern, D.W. (1998). *Applied Multivariate Statistical Analysis*. Prentice-Hall. Upper Saddle River, New Jersey.

Krzanowski, W.J. (1975). Discrimination and classification using both binary and continuous variables. *J. Amer. Statist. Assoc.* **70**, 782-790.

Kullback, S. and Liebler, R.A. (1951). On information and sufficiency. *Ann. Math. Statist.* **22**, 525-540.

Lauder, I.J. (1981). Latent variable models for statistical diagnosis. *Biometrika* **68**, 365-372.

Lauder, I.J. (1983). Direct kernel assessment of diagnostic probabilities. *Biometrika* **70**, 251-256.

Lindley, D.V. (1956). On a measure of the information provided by an experiment. *Ann. Math. Statist.* **27**, 986-1005.

MacKie, R.M., Bray, C.A., Hole, D.J., Morris, A., Nicolson, M., Evans, A. and Doherty, V. (2002). Incidence of and survival from malignant melanoma in Scotland: an epidemiological study. *The Lancet* **360**, 587-591.

McCullagh, P. and Nelder, J.A. (1989). *Generalized linear models (2nd edition)*. Chapman and Hall. London.

Mardia, K.V., Kent, J.T. and Bibby, J.M. (1979). *Multivariate Analysis*. Academic Press. New York.

Moore, M.F., Aitchison, J., Parker, L.S. and Taylor, T.R. (1974). Use of information in thyrotoxicosis treatment allocation. *Meth. Inf. Med.* **13**, 88-92.

Morrison, D.F.(1976). *Multivariate Statistical Methods (2nd edition)*. McGraw-Hill. New York.

Patterson H.D. and Thompson, R. (1971) Recovery of inter-block information when block sizes are unequal. *Biometrika* **58**, 545-554.

Phillips, L.D. and Edwards, W. (1966). Conservatism in a simple probabilistic inference tasks. *J. Exp.Psych.* **72**, 346-354.

Pickering, G. (1968). *High Blood Pressure*. Churchill. London.

Pinheiro, J.C. and Bates, D.M. (2000). *Mixed-Effects Models in S and S-PLUS*. Springer. New York.

Pregibon, D. (1981). Logistic regression diagnostics. *Ann. Statist.* **9**, 705-724.

Prentice, R.L. (1976). A generalisation of probit and logit methods for dose-response curves. *Biometrics* **32**, 761-768.

Racine-Poon, A. (1988). A Bayesian approach to nonlinear calibration problems. *J. Amer. Statist. Assoc.* **83**, 650-656

Rao, C.R. (1965). *Linear Statistical Inference and its Applications*. Wiley. New York.

Robinson, H.P. and Fleming, J.E.C. (1975). A critical evaluation of sonar crown-rump length measurements. *Brit. J. Obstetrics. and Gynaecology* **82**, 702-710.

Schollnik, D.P.M. (2002). Actuarial modelling with MCMC and BUGS. *North American Actuarial Journal* **5**, 96-125.

Searle, S.R., Casella, G. and McCulloch, C.E. (1992) *Variance Components*. Wiley. New York.

Seber, G.A.F. and Wild, C.J. (1989). *Nonlinear Regression*. Wiley. New York.

Silverman, B.W. (1986). *Density Estimation for Statistics and Data Analysis*. Chapman and Hall. London.

Silvey, S.D. (1975). *Statistical Inference*. Chapman and Hall. London.

Simonoff, J.S. (1996). *Smoothing Methods in Statistics*. Springer. New York.

Spiegelhalter, D.J., Thomas, A., Best, N. and Lunn, D. (2003). *WinBUGS User Manual: Version 1.4*. Medical Research Council. Cambridge. UK.

Stephens, M.A. (1982). EDF statistics for goodness of fit and some comparisons. *J. Amer. Statist. Assoc.* **69**, 730-737.

Taylor, T.R., Aitchison, J. and McGirr, E.M. (1971). Doctors as decision-makers: a computer-assisted study of diagnosis as a cognitive skill. *Brit. Med. J.* **3**, 35-40.

Taylor, T.R., Aitchison, J., Parker, L.S. and Moore, M.F.(1975). Individual differences in selecting patients for regular haemodialysis. *Brit. Med. J.* **2**, 380-381.

Titterington, D.M. (1976). Updating a diagnostic system using unconfirmed cases. *Appl. Statist.* **25**, 238-247.

Titterington, D.M. (1980). A comparative study of kernel-based density estimates for categorical data. *Technometrics* **22**, 259-268.

Venables W.N. and Ripley B.D. (2002). *Modern Applied Statistics with S*. Springer. New York.

Wand, M.P. and Jones M.C. (1995). *Kernel Smoothing*. Chapman and Hall. London.

Author index

Subject index